To My Dad——

    And also my friend, who taught me independence but was always there when I needed him.

G.F.F.

To Bradley——

    And those who have touched my life through his affliction.

To Kelly——

    Who proves that little girls really are made of sugar 'n' spice.

To Ryan——

    Who carries the family banner into the next generation. Steel true, blade straight—and slide headfirst on close plays at second base.

J.D.C.

EXERCISE AND CORONARY
HEART DISEASE

EXERCISE AND CORONARY HEART DISEASE

ROLE IN PREVENTION, DIAGNOSIS, TREATMENT

Second Edition

By

GERALD F. FLETCHER, M.D.

Director of Internal Medicine
Georgia Baptist Medical Center
Atlanta, Georgia
Professor of Medicine (Cardiology)
Emory University School of Medicine

and

82 9595

JOHN D. CANTWELL, M.D.

Associate Director of Cardiac Rehabilitation
Georgia Baptist Medical Center
Atlanta, Georgia
Clinical Assistant Professor in Medicine (Cardiology)
Emory University School of Medicine

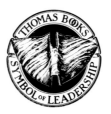

CHARLES C THOMAS • PUBLISHER
Springfield • Illinois • U.S.A.

Published and Distributed Throughout the World by

CHARLES C THOMAS • PUBLISHER
Bannerstone House
301-327 East Lawrence Avenue, Springfield, Illinois, U.S.A.

First Edition, 1974
Second Edition, 1979

*With THOMAS BOOKS careful attention is given to all details of
manufacturing and design. It is the Publisher's desire to present books that are
satisfactory as to their physical qualities and artistic possibilities and
appropriate for their particular use. THOMAS BOOKS will be true to those
laws of quality that assure a good name and good will.*

Library of Congress Cataloging in Publication Data
Fletcher, Gerald F.   1935-
    Exercise and coronary heart disease.
    Includes index.
    1. Coronary heart disease. 2. Exercise tests. 3. Exercise therapy. I. Cantwell,
John D., joint author. II. Title.
RC685.C6F55 1978   616.1′23′0624   78-494
ISBN 0-398-03775-2

Printed in the United States of America
M-3

PREFACE

CORONARY ATHEROSCLEROTIC HEART DISEASE continues to be pandemic in much of the world, especially in the United States where it claims the lives of over 700,000 persons annually; 40 to 50 percent of these persons never reach a hospital. This disease alone is the cause of 40 percent of all deaths. It is largely due to the frequent occurrence of coronary heart disease that American men rank eighteenth on a worldwide list of life expectancy. Coronary atherosclerotic disease frequently develops early in life as evidenced by autopsy studies of American men killed in the Korean War,[1] British pilots killed in air crashes,[2] and Chilean men and women who died in automobile accidents.[3]

Current statistical data verifies that changes in life-style of Americans is coincident with a "declining vascular mortality."[4] This seemingly began in January of 1964, when the Surgeon General of the United States Public Health Service warned of the health hazards of tobacco consumption, particularly cigarette smoking,[5] and when, a few months later, the American Heart Association recommended limited dietary intake of saturated fats and cholesterol. A decline in mortality from coronary heart disease, the leading cause of death, started the same year the warnings were issued and has continued through 1975. As Walker has so well stated, "the fact that two events tend to occur together certainly does not establish a causal relation between them; neither does it exclude one."[4]

This recent decline in coronary mortality is the first recorded in American history. There are certainly many other factors likely implied with this, such as coronary care units, rescue units, improved cardiac surgical techniques, and exercise programs. However, it is apparent that reduced smoking and change in diet paralleled the reverse trend in coronary mortality.[6, 7]

vii

The purpose of this book is to define and elaborate on the role of exercise in the prevention, diagnosis, treatment, and rehabilitation of patients with "coronary" disease. In recent years, there has been a surge of interest in exercise. There also is supportive evidence (to be discussed) that exercise is beneficial and instrumental in altering coronary heart disease mortality and morbidity. It is our intention to discuss the role of exercise in its proper perspective in all the areas of "coronary" management. We make emphasis of the fact that "proper perspective" means safely prescribed exercise along with control of cigarette smoking, high blood pressure, dietary fat intake, body weight, and other coronary risk factors. We feel that exercise used in this perspective will serve as a catalyst in this multirisk factor modification approach.

It is our sincere hope that this book will be of particular use to the primary care physician, for it is s/he to whom the patient usually turns for medical advice regarding exercise, who frequently advises the type and degree of exercise, and who will share in the ultimate consequences.

REFERENCES

1. Enos, W.F., Holmes, R.H., and Beyer, J.: Coronary disease among United States soldiers killed in action in Korea. *JAMA, 152:*090-1093, 1953.
2. Mason, J.K.: Asymptomatic disease of coronary arteries in young men. *Br Med J, 2:*1234-1237, 1963.
3. Viel, B., Donoso, S., and Salcedo, D.: Coronary atherosclerosis in persons dying violently. *Arch Intern Med, 122:*97-103, 1968.
4. Walker, W.J.: Changing United States life-style and declining vascular mortality: Cause or coincidence? *N Engl J Med, 297, 3:*163-165, July, 1977.
5. *Smoking and Health: Report of the Advisory Committee to the Surgeon General of the Public Health Service.* Washington, D.C., United States Department of Health, Education and Welfare, 1964.
6. United States Department of Agriculture: *Agricultural Statistics 1976.* Washington, D.C., United States Government Printing Office, 1976, pp. 106, 142, 384, 414, 561.
7. Bureau of Health Education: *1975 Adult Use of Tobacco.* Atlanta, DHEW Center for Disease Control, 1976, p. 20.

ACKNOWLEDGMENTS

WE WOULD LIKE to express our appreciation to Barbara Johnston, M.N. and to Edward Watt, Ph.D., for their contributions in research and acquisition of background material, to Mary Lewis and JoAnn Bryant for editorial assistance and typing, to Bob Beveridge for photography, to members of the Georgia Baptist Cardiac Rehabilitation team for their personal efforts in patient care, and to the members of the outpatient gym exercise program for their enthusiasm and perseverance in properly prescribed physical training.

G.F.F.
J.D.C.

CONTENTS

Page

Preface..*VII*

Acknowledgments..*IX*

Chapter

1. Historical Aspects of Exercise and Coronary Heart Disease. 3
2. Exercise Physiology in Normals and in Patients With
     Coronary Heart Disease... 11
3. Sedentary Living—A Coronary Risk Factor?......................... 27
4. Effect of Exercise on Coronary Risk Factors......................... 47
5. Exercise Stress Testing—A Review................................. 72
6. Guidelines to Exercise Training.................................... 122
7. Coronary Risk Factor Detection and Exercise Prescription
     in a Preventive Cardiology Clinic................................... 127
8. Postinfarction Rehabilitation—Hospital Phase..................... 143
9. Outpatient Exercise Therapy for Coronary Disease—A
     Prescription... 168
10. Dangers of Exercise.. 215
11. An Outpatient Gym Exercise Program for Patients with
     Recent Myocardial Infarction—An Update....................... 225
12. Survey of Current "Cardiac" Exercise Programs in the
     United States.. 250
13. Cardiac Rehabilitation in Other Countries......................... 289
14. Summary... 319
     Subject Index... 322
     Author Index... 333

EXERCISE AND CORONARY
HEART DISEASE

Chapter 1

HISTORICAL ASPECTS OF EXERCISE AND CORONARY HEART DISEASE

T HE ARCHIVES OF ancient history have referred to the effects of exercise on many occasions. Cicero (106-43 B.C.) stated, "exercise and temperance can preserve something of our early strength even in old age." [1] Timaeus said of the body, "by moderate exercise reduces to order according to their affinities the particles and affections which are wandering about." [2] Richard Steele (1672-1729) stated, "reading is to the mind what exercise is to the body," [3] and Addison (1672-1719) said, "exercise ferments the humours, casts them into their proper channels, throws off redundancies, and helps nature in those secret distributions, without which the body cannot subsist in its vigour, nor the soul act with cheerfulness." [4]

Using exercise to improve the cardiovascular system and to promote longevity has been debated for many centuries. Chauncey Depew, who lived for ninety-four years, once stated, "I get my exercise acting as a pallbearer to my friends who exercised." [5] Easton, however, in 1799, reported 1,712 instances of longevity over one hundred years of age and remarked, "It is not the rich and the great, not those who depend on medicine, who become old: but such as use much exercise. For an idler never attains a remarkable great age." [6]

Exercise as an adjunct to good physical health attained popularity early in American history. In 1785, Thomas Jefferson, while minister to France, wrote to his nephew, "Walking is the best possible exercise. Habituate yourself to walk fast without fatigue." [7] In 1854, concerning treatment of fatty degeneration of the heart, Stokes said that a person must adapt to early hours and graduated exercise. [2]

3

Since his death in 1974, Doctor Paul Dudley White has become part of history, and his influence will continue in both professional and lay circles. He was a strong advocate of exercise and believed that exercise was beneficial, both physiologically and psychologically. He felt that walking was beneficial, especially because of its "venous squeezing" effect; that the lower extremity veins have valves and that walking helped move the blood in the veins and provoked better circulatory dynamics. He advocated that people who walk a great deal have less early arteriosclerosis and that people today have a life that is much too easy—using elevators instead of stairs and having lunch brought in rather than going out. He felt that "work alone never killed a man unless he is already sick."

Doctor White advised walking as probably the best exercise and was averse to activities with weight lifting. His own personal exercise included climbing stairs, walking to lunch, gardening, cutting trees and splitting logs, shoveling snow, and "working in the soil."

He believed that "one feels so much better with exercise" and his formula for long life was to "work hard mentally, physically, and spiritually." He referred to our easy way of living as a "real pity." He felt that our ancestors were in better physical health because of their active lives spent in clearing the forests and plowing the land. He felt that exercise was the "best tranquilizer there is." In farewell comments to his many friends and acquaintances, he was never known to say "take it easy" but rather to say "take it hard." [8] Doctor White is shown in Figure 1-1 performing one of his many active exercise habits.

Over the years it has become generally accepted that those persons who have physically active occupations enjoy better physical health; such an assumption, however, is not totally supported by sound evidence. Isolated case histories such as that of Clarence DeMar,[9] the marathon runner of the early 1900s, provide striking examples of the benefits of long-term physical conditioning. DeMar participated in marathon races (such as seen in Figure 1-2) for forty-nine years, and at his death (of metastatic rectal cancer) at age seventy, his coronary arteries at autopsy were two to three times the normal diameter.

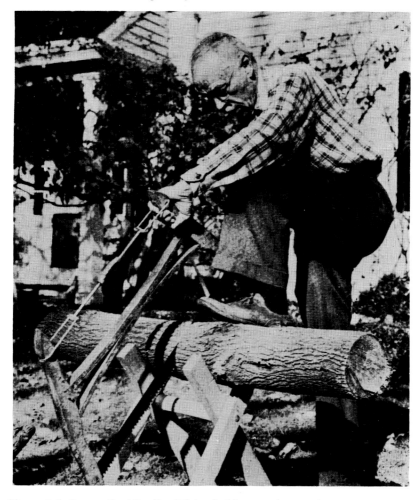

Figure 1-1. Doctor Paul Dudley White, in his seventies, performing one of his favorite pastimes—"sawing logs." Courtesy of *Cardiovascular and Metabolic Diseases,* December 3, 1973.

One of the most important aspects of exercise activities has been that of "testing" the individual. Utilization of walk tests, step tests, and treadmill tests are means by which normal and cardiac patients are evaluated for their safe exercise limits.

Historically, the Chinese, Romans, and Greeks first used the

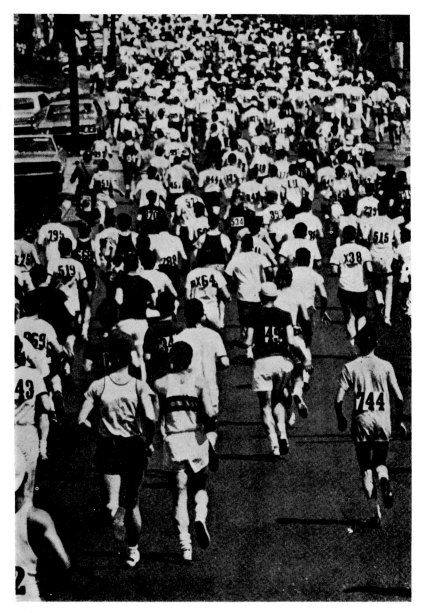

Figure 1-2. A group of runners in the Boston Marathon, an event in which Clarence DeMar participated on numerous occasions.

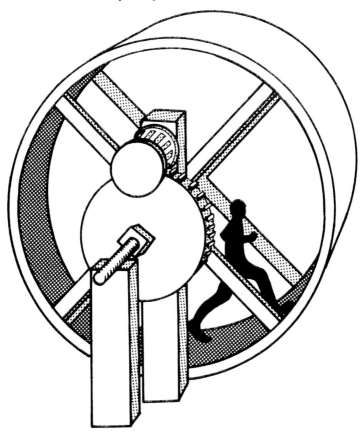

Figure 1-3. Artist's sketch of a squirrel cage treadmill used for pumping. Courtesy of the British Museum, London.

treadmill for irrigation and construction projects over 2,000 years ago.[5] In 1818, William Cubitt, a British civil engineer designed an elongated "stepping wheel" on which dozens of prisoners could work side by side. In accord with this, "treading the wheel" for punishment became prevalent throughout English prisons. (Figures 1-3 and 1-4 show examples of "treading" used for punishment.) In 1846, however, because reformers considered treading the wheel a cruel, inhumane, and unhealthy practice, Edward Smith began to investigate

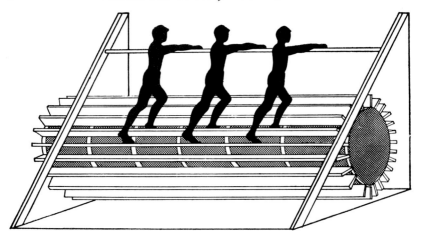

Figure 1-4. Artist's sketch of the treadmill at Brexton Prison. From C.B. Chapman, Edward Smith (1818-1874) Physiologist, human ecologist, reformer, *Journal of the History of Medicine and the Allied Sciences, 22:*1-26, 1967.

physical performance by utilizing new physiologic techniques during treadmill exercise.[10] These studies were the first systematic inquiry into the respiratory and metabolic response of the human to muscular exercise, and they laid the groundwork for the extensive studies that have followed in the evaluation of exercise performance in patients with coronary heart disease. Smith's early studies include measurements of inspired air, respiratory rate, respiratory stroke volume, pulse rate, and oxygen production. By 1857, measurements were made for other types of exercise including swimming, rowing, and horseback riding.[11]

With the acquisition of exercise habits early in history and the insight into methods of evaluation of exercise performance, observations[12] began to reveal in some instances a higher mortality rate in people with sedentary occupations compared to those who were physically active. These observations were to be the forerunners of more studies relating physical inactivity to mortality and morbidity from coronary heart disease.

As history has been influential in other fields of medicine, it appears that such trends have also developed in the relation of exercise to coronary heart disease. Although little or no specific mention is made of coronary heart disease in the preceding paragraphs, it can be assumed that historically, as is certainly true today, a considerable percentage of human mortality was secondary to diseases of the heart and blood vessels—especially coronary disease. Sudden death has been a subject of recent interest; this most likely was prevalent in early history and, as is thought to be true today, was likely related in many instances to undiagnosed coronary atherosclerotic disease.

As the following chapters relate various aspects of exercise in the management of coronary heart disease, the reader should keep in mind the many historical aspects of exercise and good health. The scientific approach to prescribing the proper quantity and quality of exercise for the patient with coronary heart disease should be considered as a progressive extension of basic historical concepts.

REFERENCES

1. Cicero, An Old Age, X34, trans. James Logan. In Strauss, M. (Ed.): *Familiar Medical Quotations.* Boston, Little, 1968, p. 169.
2. Fox, S.M. III, and Skinner, J.S.: Physical activity and cardiovascular health. *Am J Cardiol, 14:*731-746, 1964.
3. Parmley, L.F.: Proceedings of the National Conference on Exercise in the prevention, in the evaluation, in the treatment of heart disease. *J SC Med Assoc, 65:*i, 1969.
4. In *The Spectator,* Vol II, No. 115 (July 12, 1911), ref. 4, p. 165.
5. Adams, C.W.: Symposium on exercise and the heart (Introduction). *Am J Cardiol, 30:*713-715, 1972.
6. Easton, J.: *Human Longevity,* London, Salisburg, 1799, pp. xi, xxvi.
7. Alexander, J.K.: Exercise and coronary heart disease, *Cardiovasc Res Cent Bull, 8:*2-7, 1969.
8. White, Paul Dudley: Personal communication, 1969.
9. Currens, J.H., and White, P.D.: Half a century of running: Clinical, physiological and autopsy findings in the case of Clarence DeMar ("Mr. Marathon"). *N Engl J Med, 265:*988-993, 1961.
10. Chapman, C.B.: Edward Smith (1818-1874) Physiologist, human ecologist, reformer. *J Hist Med, 22:*1-26, 1967.
11. Smith, E.: Inquiries into the quantity of air inspired throughout the day

and night, and under the influence of exercise, food, medicine and temperature. *Proc Roy Soc Med, 8*:451-456, 1857.

12. Smith, E.: Report on the sanitary circumstances of tailors in London. In *6th Ed. Rep Med Officer Primary Council with Appendix, 1862*. London, H.M. Stationery Office, 1864, pp. 416-430.

Chapter 2

EXERCISE PHYSIOLOGY IN NORMALS AND IN PATIENTS WITH CORONARY HEART DISEASE

I N DEALING WITH patients, we as physicians are obligated to consider what goals we are trying to attain through exercise and what parameters we are trying to achieve in the cardiovascular system.[1] These goals should be made clear when we discuss exercise with our patients, and the patients should be provided with a basic understanding as to how the normal and abnormal cardiovascular systems respond to exercise.

The external stress that may be imposed on the human body through some types of exercise may not actually alter the work of the heart itself or enhance "conditioning" of the cardiovascular system. For example, gardening, raking leaves, mowing grass, and household domestic chores are types of exercise that individuals cannot refer to as "good exercise." These types of activity may impose fatigue and musculoskeletal strain on a subject, but they do not necessarily cause high caloric expenditure. There is also a possible harmful isometric effect that will be later elaborated upon in this chapter. To the contrary, jogging, swimming, brisk walking, and sprinting cause higher levels of caloric expenditure and are considered dynamic and more efficient types of exercise. The calories expended per hour for various types of physical activity are listed in Figure 2-1, in which data is taken in part from Falls.[2] Similar information is seen in Figure 2-2, which is the work classification scheme of Wells et al.[3]

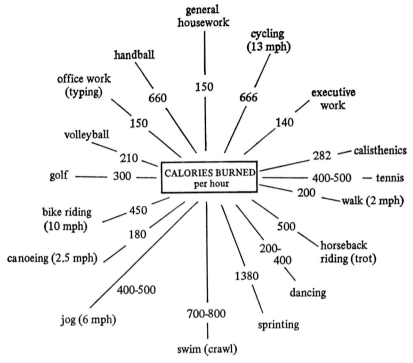

Figure 2-1. Chart showing the calories utilized per hour for various types of physical activity. From H.B. Falls, Proceedings of the national conference on exercise in the prevention, in the evaluation and in the treatment of heart disease. The relative energy requirements of various physical activities in relation to physiological strain, *Journal of the South Carolina Medical Association,* *65*:8, 1969.

NORMALS

Regarding the cardiovascular system in recommending exercise and evaluating exercise, one should consider those factors that determine the work done by the heart, that is the *myocardial oxygen consumption.* Sarnoff et al.[4] and Monroe et al.[5] have clearly shown through precise physiological measures that heart work or myocardial oxygen consumption is directly related to the heart rate, systemic systolic blood pressure or intraventricular pressure, and the inotropic or contractile state

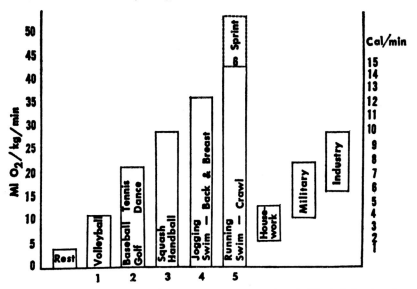

Figure 2-2. Bar graph showing oxygen consumption (ml/kg/min) related to calories expended per minute for various levels of physical activity. From Wells et al., Lactic acid accumulation during work; a suggested standardization of work classification, *Journal of Applied Physiology, 10:*51-55, 1957.

of the myocardium. These principles were transposed to the clinical setting quite vividly some years ago through the work of Robinson.[6] He found, in his group of 15 patients with angina pectoris exposed to various types of progressive exercise training followed with periodic exercise testing, that the threshold at which pain developed was always related to a fixed level of systolic blood pressure and heart rate. Regardless of the increased duration of the exercise or the work load reached on the treadmill, the work level that precipitated angina pectoris in his patients was always at the same heart rate and systolic blood pressure.

The *circulatory dynamics* of exercise have been of interest for many years. In 1957, Mitchell et al.[7] related evidence that maximal oxygen intake is a measure of cardiac capacity and the ability to increase the arteriovenous oxygen difference, not of the ability of the vascular bed to accommodate left ventricular output. Because of this, they felt that maximal oxygen consumption had clinical usefulness in evaluating patients with cardiovascular disease. In 1963, Frick et al.[8] studied 14 young men with sedentary habits. At the end of a two-month period of intensive physical training, they found that 11 of the 14 subjects had an increase in heart volume, higher cardiac output at rest, and reduced heart rate at rest. After a period of physical training, 3 subjects had a larger stroke volume and significantly lower heart rate during exercise. In 1968, Saltin et al.[9] studied 5 young normals extensively in a longitudinal study lasting three months. During the bed rest period of twenty days there was a pronounced decrease in maximal oxygen uptake, stroke volume, and cardiac output. At the end of a following fifty-five-day training period, 2 previously trained subjects were able to attain the same level of maximal oxygen uptake as they had reached in the initial control studies. Three previously sedentary subjects reached levels after training that were higher than their control values. In these latter 3 subjects, the increase in maximal oxygen uptake after training was attributable to an increase in stroke volume and to widening of the arteriovenous oxygen difference. In addition to these aforementioned apparent hemodynamic benefits of training in normal young people, similar studies from the same laboratory by Siegel et al.[10] have shown a maximal oxygen uptake increase of 19 percent in 9 healthy, blind, sedentary men who participated in a fifteen-week quantitative physical training program.

Studies on older physically well-trained individuals have shown, in contrast to younger normals, that aerobic work capacity decreases with increasing age.[11] This is a basic principle to be aware of when testing individuals in the older age group, especially because of their statistical predilection to coronary disease.

In recent years, physiological studies in normals, both in animals and in humans, have continued; they repeatedly give us more data supportive of the beneficial effects of exercise.

In 1972, Wollenberger et al.[12] reported studies in dog mitochondria. They concluded that one was justified in predicting that the return from an exhausted, hypoxiclike cellular state to the normal resting condition (a process in which mitochondrial repair presumably involving macromolecular synthesis appears to be a notable feature) should occur more rapidly and easily in trained than in untrained muscle. Korge et al.,[13] in studies using rat hearts, reported data on water, sodium and potassium transmembrane distribution, magnesium, calcium, zinc and copper content, and sodium, potassium, and ATPase activity in the myocardium, along with adrenocortical and blood gas activity. They found that the effect of physical exertion on these factors depended upon the duration of work. Moderate work was characterized by potassium accumulation in myocardial cells without significant elevation in water and sodium activity. They also found an increase in sodium and potassium ATPase and adrenocortical activity, along with a metabolic acidosis. In acute heart overload, they found intracellular edema with increased sodium, with a decrease in sodium, potassium, and ATPase activity. These changes in myocardial metabolism were accompanied by a decrease in adrenocortical activity and development of metabolic alkalosis.

Scheuer et al.[14] has reported data in rats comparing a group trained in moderate swimming to a sedentary group. The trained hearts displayed a greater mechanical response to tachycardia and to increases in pre– and afterload, probably secondary to an increase in coronary blood flow and oxygen delivery. They found that conditioned rat hearts had increased ATPase activity and increased rates of superprecipitation of actomyosin, probably by alteration of availability of sulfhydryl at the active site of myosin. The results reflected that conditioned hearts were resistant to hypoxemia and converted chemical energy to external work with greater efficiency.

Korge et al.,[15] in 1974, studied the effect of physical conditioning on the cardiac response to acute exertion in rats. He found that training increased the potassium content in heart cells and was dependent on the duration of exercise. The change was not associated with hypertrophy. The study also revealed that chronic physical overload decreased the hearts' ability to accumulate potassium with exercise. They concluded that potassium accumulation in heart cells is an essential adaptive reaction to physical exertion, and the extent of potassium uptake depends on the functional state of the heart. Horwitz et al.[16] studied the left ventricular dynamics during recovery from exercise in dogs. They found an increase in left ventricular end diastolic diameter with exercise recovery and concluded that with strenuous exercise there was a sympathetically mediated increase in contractility which decreased promptly during recovery. The Frank-Starling mechanism, however, continued to be a factor.

Segel, Mason et al., in 1975,[17] studied cardiac glycogen metabolism in rats and reported that glycogen super-recompensation in the heart with exercise is related to the severity of the exercise. Later, in 1976, McRitchie et al.[18] studied the role of arterial baroreceptors with exercise in dogs. They found that the arterial baroreceptor reflex is "turned off" with exercise and does not significantly modify exercise response.

In studies of normal humans, similarly revealing and encouraging data in exercise physiology and metabolism continue to be reported.

In 1972, Simpson, Hames et al.[19] studied platelet aggregation in physically active and inactive groups in Evans County, Georgia. Each group was studied on a treadmill to compare the effects of such exercise on adrenalin-induced platelet aggregation. Though the sample of subjects was small (7 and 8 in each group), the data showed the more physically active group to have significantly less platelet aggregation at peak exercise than the less physically active group. They concluded that eleven to twelve metabolic equivalents of exercise may decrease the tendency to thromboembolic vascular disease.

Rose et al.[20] studied 127 trained subjects versus 157 nontrained to evaluate postexercise potassium levels. Their data suggested that cardiovascular fitness reduces the magnitude of electrolyte shift with acute anaerobic exercise, supporting the thesis of the objective effect of physical training.

Barnard et al.,[21] in 1973, studied 10 healthy Los Angeles area firemen. Sudden vigorous exercise (by jumping on a treadmill without warm-up) resulted in "ischemic" electrocardiographic changes. With warm-up, the same group had no ischemic changes. It was concluded that the increase in systolic blood pressure in the group without warm-up (with the associated heart rate increase) is secondary to a massive sympathetic discharge. This was not seen in the testing after warm-up and supports the value of the "warm-up period" in exercise programming for normal subjects.

Hurych et al.,[22] in the same year, studied 16 normal subjects and found that with graded exercise there was 100 percent increase in pulmonary blood flow and 40 percent increase in pulmonary blood volume. These studies support the associated pulmonary dynamic changes in exercise and the need to always consider both the cardiac and pulmonary status of individuals who are exercising.

Davies et al.,[23] in 1975, studied the cardiopulmonary response to exercise in 17 obese young women. The results showed that oxygen consumption for a given work load was increased but that ventilation was normal. However, the maximal oxygen consumption was decreased, and it was felt that obesity causes a reduction in physiological performance at a near-maximal effect. Therefore, the potential changes of excessive exercise in obese individuals are emphasized.

Keul and Doll, in 1975,[24] did a significant study in 19 normal humans (aged twenty to thirty years) to delineate myocardial substrate uptake in men during exercise under hypoxic conditions. They found that the limiting factor in performance was the skeletal muscle oxygen deficiency. The heart, to the contrary, tolerated hypoxic air (12.7% O_2) as it used other substrate. This was chiefly through carbohydrate being converted to energy, manifest by an increased ratio of lactate and glucose and probably by beta-hydroxybutyrate being extracted by the heart. Therefore, it was felt that the substrate and oxygen supply of the heart is not endangered for healthy persons at altitudes of 4,250 meters, as the limiting factors will be skeletal muscle rather than cardiac muscle.

It is therefore obvious that in recent years, research in normal exercise physiology in animals and humans has been revealing and has dealt more with the intimate details of cellular and metabolic function. Investigation of mitochondria, electrolytes, enzymes, platelets, cardiac substrates, baroreceptors, and ventricular and pulmonary dynamics in normals are all supportive of the beneficial effects of exercise and, hopefully, will be transposed in part to the abnormals.

HEART DISEASE

Regarding studies in cardiovascular hemodynamics in patients with heart disease, a number of authors have related their experiences. Naughton et al.,[25] in 1966, studied 24 men with well-documented myocardial infarctions; 12 participated in a physical conditioning program, and the remainder remained sedentary. After eight months, the trained cardiac patients showed significant training effects as reflected by the systolic and diastolic blood pressure and heart rate during rest, standing, and comparable levels of energy expenditures. The response of the cardiac patient compared to that of a group of healthy normals indicated that the presence of disease did not necessarily affect the physiologic response of the subject.

In 1966, Varnauskas et al.[26] investigated the hemodynamic and metabolic effects of physical training in 9 patients with coronary disease. In addition to clinical improvement after training, they reported a hemodynamic adjustment toward a hypokinetic state and reduction in work of the left ventricle. Later, in 1968, Frick et al.[27] assessed the hemodynamic effects of physical training in 7 patients after myocardial infarction. The training was followed by a reduction in exercise heart rate and tension time index, enhanced stroke volume, and improved left ventricular function. Concomitant with these hemodynamic changes, exercise tolerance was improved.

More recently, Clausen et al.[28] studied the effect of physical training on the distribution of cardiac output in patients with coronary artery disease. This was done by measurement of cardiac output and regional blood flow parameters in liver and skeletal muscle at rest and during exercise. In 7 of these patients, reported values were taken during a physical training program of four to ten weeks duration. After training, cardiac output was reduced at moderate work loads (13.1%) but increased during heavy exercise (5.5%). Similar changes were seen in muscle blood flow, which was decreased at submaximal loads (14.9%) and increased at maximal (8.6%). Hepatic blood flow showed, in contrast, a less pronounced reduction at both work loads after training (difference 7.2%). They felt that these noted effects of training could be explained as peripheral regulatory alterations without implying primary improvement in cardiac performance. They suggest that local changes in trained muscles are important for the reduction in myocardial pressure work caused by physical conditioning.

Detry et al.,[29] in 1971, reported the results of training in 12 patients with coronary heart disease. The rate-pressure product and the left ventricular work decreased after training, whereas stroke volume was unchanged and arteriovenous oxygen (A-VO$_2$) difference increased. The classic posttraining brady-cardia was compensated by an increased A-VO$_2$ difference which resulted from both a higher arterial oxygen content and an increased peripheral oxygen extraction. They concluded that benefits with physical training in coronary patients at submaxi-mal exercise levels result from enhanced arterial oxygen content and peripheral extraction, and, secondarily, from lower hemodynamic stress on the ischemic myocardium.

More recently, in 1973, Thompson and Lown[30] reported a significant study in dogs regarding exercise during experimen-tal acute myocardial infarction. They experimentally occluded the proximal left anterior descending coronary artery in 39 dogs. Twenty of the dogs were run to exhaustion, one to six hours after occlusion and twice daily for a three-week duration. The other 19 dogs had no exercise. In each group, 1 dog developed a ventricular aneurysm, and 1 in the control group suffered rupture of the left ventricle. There was no difference in the size of infarction when comparing the exercised group to the control group. This study, therefore, affords excellent con-trolled data regarding the lack of harmful effects of extreme exercise in dogs subjected to experimental coronary arterial occlusion. Though the coronary circulation in dogs likely is different when compared to humans, such data may be supportive of the lack of harmful effects of exercise in the recent postinfarction state in humans. Wyatt et al.[31] have recently reported the effects of conditioning and deconditioning in dogs. Coronary angiogram studies showed an increase in coronary artery cross-sectional diameters ($p<0.05$) in the 8 conditioned dogs as well as trends for increases in myocardial capillary density and perimeter. The results, therefore, suggest that physical conditioning may improve myocardial blood supply and that regular physical exercise may be required to maintain these effects.

In 1974, Auchincloss[32] studied oxygen consumption in patients with coronary artery disease by graded treadmill testing and compared this to hemodynamic studies. He found a low oxygen consumption in 21 of 40 patients and in 12 of 16 such patients with an elevated left ventricular and diastolic pressure ($p<0.05$). He found no correlation with number of coronary vessels with disease. His data suggest that a decreased left ventricular performance is associated with a diminished rise in oxygen consumption with exercise testing. Such data is helpful in evaluating patients in exercise programming, for if oxygen consumption does not increase with training, then it is likely that left ventricular performance is impaired.

Adams et al.[33] commented recently on the long-term physiological adaptation to exercise, with special reference to performance and cardiorespiratory function in health and disease. These authors concluded that after myocardial infarction, most trained patients can achieve the performance levels of sedentary normals. Their response to training, however, is often restricted, presumably because residual disease causes myocardial dysfunction. They also concluded that successful coronary artery bypass surgery seldom normalizes work performance and cardiorespiratory function, although it may alleviate symptoms. Physical training in conjunction with bypass surgery, they feel, effects a further improvement in work performance.

More data of late is available on pressure and volume changes before and after physical training in the studies of Bergstrom et al.[34] They studied 34 trained and 34 nontrained post-myocardial-infarction patients. Their results showed no difference with regard to work capacity; however, the blood volume and total hemoglobin increased in the trained group.

Therefore, considerable data continues to appear in the literature regarding the effects of exercise in coronary artery disease, both in animals and in humans. The study of Thompson and Lown,[30] reporting the lack of harmful effects of exhaustive exercise in dogs after left anterior descending coronary artery ligations, is one of the most contributory in recent years. In addition, the hemodynamic study of Auchincloss,[32] confirming the diminished rise in oxygen consumption with training in patients with poor left ventricular performance, is most helpful in exercise programming. Lastly, data supporting increased blood volume and increased total hemoglobin in trained patients in the postinfarction state is of note.[34]

ISOMETRICS

Investigations into the physiological aspects of exercise have involved studies of isometrics. Siegel et al.[35] studied 6 normal subjects, 27 patients with coronary atherosclerotic heart disease, and 6 patients with idiopathic congestive cardiomyopathy. The method of study involved maximal isometric handgrip exercise. Results showed that isometric handgrip caused rapid and significant increases in systolic (22 to 39 mm Hg) and diastolic (27 to 36 mm Hg) blood pressure and heart rate (fifteen to twenty beats per minute). It was concluded that isometric handgrip exercise is a simple cardiovascular stress test which is applicable at the bedside, exerting its effect by increased blood pressure or afterload. Other observations[36] have concluded that such increases in pressure may be undesirable in patients with coronary artery disease or with borderline hemodynamic function.

Other investigation into types of exercises for coronary patients have included those studies involving the onset of angina pectoris in relation to circulatory adaption during arm and leg exercise. Wahren and Bygdeman[37] studied this in 10 patients with signs of coronary artery disease. Both arm and leg exercise elicited angina pectoris in all patients. Anginal pain

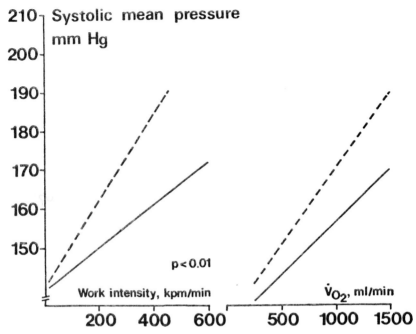

Figure 2-3. Graph showing regression of the systolic mean pressure for leg exercise and arm exercise on internal work performed and on pulmonary oxygen uptake. The broken lines represent arm exercise, and the solid lines represent leg exercise. From J. Wahren and S. Bygdeman, Onset of angina pectoris in relation to circulatory adaptation during arm and leg exercise, *Circulation, 44*:432-441, 1971.

appeared at a smaller work load and a lower pulmonary oxygen uptake during arm exercise than during leg exercise, and heart rate, peak systolic, diastolic mean, diastolic, and mean arterial pressures all increased more steeply in relation to work load during arm exercise than during leg exercise. An example of this data is shown in Figure 2-3. This was attributed in part to the lower mechanical efficiency and higher sympathetic outflow during arm exercise. It was felt that these factors may reflect a larger component of static work with trunk muscles during arm exercise.

Therefore, it appears that different types of exercise elicit different responses from the heart and peripheral circulation.

Evidence is suggestive of the fact that dynamic exercise, as opposed to isometric, is more efficient in conditioning the cardiovascular system and imposes less harmful stress on the myocardium, especially with regard to the increase in systemic blood pressure or afterload.

PRACTICAL APPLICATION

In accord with such clinical and hemodynamic observations, leaders in exercise programming are being urged to design their training activities to deal with the simple factors of blood pressure and heart rate, that is to design training with the end point being to increase heart rate to a certain level in order to condition the heart. Dynamic exercises are preferred to those which involve isometric maneuvers. Figure 2-4 shows examples of various heart rates for given ages based on the data of Sheffield et al.[38] that are currently in use in training programs.

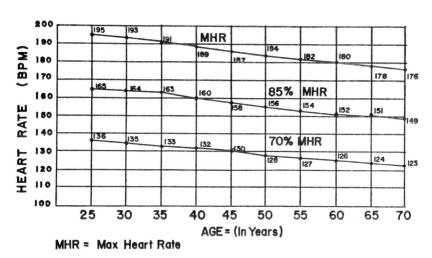

MHR = Max Heart Rate

Figure 2-4. Graph showing various levels of heart rate in beats per minute (BPM) expressed as maximum heart rate, 85 percent of maximum, and 75 percent of maximum. The heart rate is plotted with age in years. Based on data from Sheffield et al., Hemodynamic consequences of physical training after myocardial infarction, *Circulation, 37:*192-202, 1968.

These rates are depicted for the 70 and 85 percent of maximal heart rate (MHR) levels; it is felt that the 70 percent MHR level is best used as an end point for exercise, and the 80 percent MHR levels are best reserved for an exercise testing end points in the presence of a physician. Using these parameters through selected exercise over a long period of training (such as jogging), it has been shown that a person can achieve a progressively greater level of exercise with less acceleration of the heart rate, thus reducing the work of the heart for a given level of exercise. Likewise, through such physical training, maximal blood pressure elevation can be decreased for the same level of exercise, again decreasing the work of the heart. Therefore, with the more scientific approach to exercise, more benefits can be achieved with fewer complications—complications that are frequently associated with inefficient efforts.

REFERENCES

1. Fletcher, G.F.: Exercise and the heart. *ACCESS, 2, 5:* 1970.
2. Falls, H.B.: Proceedings of the national conference on exercise in the prevention, in the evaluation and in the treatment of heart disease. The relative energy requirements of various physical activities in relation to physiological strain. *J SC Med Assoc, 65:*8, 1969.
3. Wells, J.G., Balke, B., and Van Fossan, D.D.: Lactic acid accumulation during work; a suggested standardization of work classification. *J Appl Physiol, 10:*51-55, 1957.
4. Sarnoff, S.J., Braunwald, E., Welch, G.F., Jr., et al.: Hemodynamic determinants of oxygen consumption of the heart with special reference to the tension time index. *Am J Physiol, 192:*148-156, 1958.
5. Monroe, R.G., and Frence, G.N.: Left ventricular pressure-volume relationships and myocardial oxygen consumption in the isolated heart. *Circ Res, 9:*362-374, 1961.
6. Robinson, B.F.: Relation of heart rate and systolic blood pressure to the onset of pain in angina pectoris. *Circulation, 35:*1073-1083, 1967.
7. Mitchell, H.J., Sproule, B.J., and Chapman, C.B.: The physiological meaning of the maximal oxygen intake test. *J Clin Invest, 37:*538-547, 1958.
8. Frick, M.H., Konttinen, A., and Sarajas, H.S.: Effects of physical training on circulation at rest and during exercise. *Am J Cardiol, 12:*142-147, 1963.

9. Saltin, B., Blomqvist, G., Mitchell, J.H., et al.: Response to exercise after bed rest and after training. *Circulation, 38: Suppl 12:*1-55, 1968.
10. Siegel, W., Blomqvist, G., and Mitchell, J.H.: Effects of a quantitated physical training program on middle-aged sedentary men. *Circulation, 41:*19-29, 1970.
11. Grimby, G., and Saltin, B.: Physiological analysis of physically well trained middle-aged and old athletes. *Acta Med Scand, 179:*513-526, 1966.
12. Wollenberger, A.: Responses of the heart mitochondria to chronic cardiac overload and physical exercise. *Recent Adv Stud Card Struct Met, 1:*213-222, 1972.
13. Korge, P., Roosson, S., and Oks, M.: Heart adaptation to physical exertion in relation to work duration. *Acta Cardiologica XXIX:*303-320, 1974.
14. Scheuer, J., Penpargkul, S., and Bhan, A.: Experimental observations on the effects of physical training upon intrinsic cardiac physiology and biochemistry. *Am J Cardiol, 33:*744-750, 1974.
15. Korge, P., Masso, R., and Rooson, S.: The effect of physical conditioning on cardiac response to acute exertion. *Can J Physiol Pharmacol, 53:*745-752, 1973.
16. Horwitz, L.D., Atkins, J.M., and Dunbar, S.A.: Left ventricular dynamics during recovery from exercise. *J Appl Physiol, 39, 3:*449-452, 1975.
17. Segel, L.D., Chung, A., et al.: Cardiac glycogen in Long-Evans rats: diurnal pattern and response to exercise. *Am J Physiol, 229, 2:*398-401, 1975.
18. McRitchie, R.J., Vatner, S.F., et al.: Role of arterial baroreceptors in mediating cardiovascular response to exercise. *Am J Physiol, 230, 1:*85-89, 1976.
19. Simpson, M.T., Hames, C.G., et al.: Physical activity, catecholamines, and platelet stickiness. *Recent Adv Stud Card Struct Met, 1:*742-752, 1972.
20. Rose, K.D., Ursick, J.A., and Maca, R.D.: Exercise and serum potassium flux: myocardial metabolic implications. *Recent Adv Stud Card Struct Met, 1:*673-683, 1972.
21. Barnard, R.J., MacAlpin, R., et al.: Ischemic response to sudden strenuous exercise in healthy men. *Circulation, 48:*936-949, 1973.
22. Hurych, J., Stanek, J., et al.: Changes in cardiopulmonary blood volume during graded exercise. *Eur J Cardiol, 1, 1:*71-77, 1973.
23. Davies, C.T.M., Godfrey, S., et al.: Cardiopulmonary responses to exercise in obese girls and young women. *J Appl Physiol, 38:*373-376, 1975.
24. Keul, J., and Doll, E.: Myocardial substrate in men during exercise under hypoxic conditions. *Recent Adv Stud Card Struct Met, 7:*261-266, 1975.
25. Naughton, J., Shanbour, K., Armstrong, R., et al.: Cardiovascular responses to exercise following myocardial infarction. *Arch Intern Med, 117:*541-545, 1966.
26. Varnauskas, E., Bergman, H., Houk, P., et al.: Hemodynamic effects of physical training in coronary patients. *Lancet, 2:*8-12, 1966.
27. Frick, M.H., and Katila, M.: Hemodynamic consequences of physical

training after myocardial infarction. *Circulation, 37:*192-202, 1968.

28. Clausen, J.P., and Trap-Jensen, J.: Effects of training on the distribution of cardiac output in patients with coronary artery disease. *Circulation, 42.*611-624, 1970.

29. Detry, J.M.R., Rousseau, M., Vandenbrouche, G., et al.: Increased arteriovenous oxygen difference after physical training in coronary heart disease. *Circulation, 44:*109-118, 1971.

30. Thompson, P.L., Jenzer, H.R., Lown, B., and Lohrbauer, L.A.: Exercise during acute myocardial infarction: an experimental study. *Cardiovasc Res 7.*642-648, 1973.

31. Wyatt, H.L., and Mitchell, J.: Influences of physical conditioning and deconditioning upon the coronary vasculature of dogs. *Am J Cardiol, 39:*262, 1977.

32. Auchincloss, J.H., Gilbert, R., and Bowman, J.L.: Response of oxygen uptake to exercise in coronary artery disease. *Chest, 65:*5, May, 1974.

33. Adams, W.C., McHenry, M.M., and Bernauer, E.M.: Long-term physiologic adaptations to exercise with special reference to performance and cardio-respiratory function in health and disease. *Am J Cardiol, 33:*765-775, 1974.

34. Bergstrom, K., Bjernulf, A. and Erikson, U.: Work capacity and heart and blood volumes before and after physical training in male patients after myocardial infarction. *Scand J Rehabil Med, 6:*51-64, 1974.

35. Siegel, W., Gilbert, C.A. and Nutter, P.O., et al: Use of isometric handgrip for the indirect assessment of left ventricular function in patients with coronary atherosclerotic heart disease. *Am J. Cardiol 30:*48-54, 1972.

36. Lind, A.R.: Cardiovascular response to static exercise (editorial). *Circulation 41:*173-176, 1970.

37. Wahren, J. and Bygdemon, S.: Onset of angina pectoris in relation to circulatory adaptation during arm and leg exercise. *Circulation 44:*432-441, 1971.

38. Sheffield, L.T., Ratman, D., and Reeves, T.J.: Hemodynamic consequences of physical training after myocardial infarction. Circulation *37:*192-202, 1968.

Chapter 3

SEDENTARY LIVING:
A CORONARY RISK FACTOR?

INTEREST IN PHYSICAL activities and fitness in this country is not a recent phenomenon, for as noted in Chapter 1, early leaders such as John Quincy Adams and Thomas Jefferson expressed strong opinions in favor of habitual exercise.

The past decade has witnessed the jogging craze, the bicycle boom, and the resurgence of tennis. Mass-participation sports continue to be popular the world over. In Sweden, 9,000 persons participate in the Vasa cross-country ski race every March for little reward other than self-satisfaction and a cup of blueberry soup. Not to be outdone, in 1972, the Danes started an eight-mile footrace around Eremitage Castle, the hunting ground of the Royal Family; the entry roll has increased manyfold, matching that of the Vasa. The Boston Marathon, originating in 1897, has attracted over 2500 runners in recent years on Patriots' Day; 10 percent of these runners are physicians.

In spite of the fads and the exercise extravaganzas, most citizens in the United States remain either apathetic, skeptical, or confused. Perhaps the latter is related to medical warnings, prevalent early in the century, against the development of the "athlete's" heart. Neil Armstrong, whose very survival on the moon was so dependent on scientific precisions, once was quoted to the effect that he rarely exercised because man has only so many heartbeats in a lifetime and he (Armstrong) didn't want to waste his. (When questioned by Doctor Cantwell, Armstrong indicated that he was merely repeating what someone had said to him and that he did not concur with this statement.) Satchel

Paige, the legendary baseball pitcher, advised us to "keep the juices jangling" but to "avoid running at all times."

Amid the juxtaposition of exercise enthusiasm and indifference, wherein lie the facts relating to exercise and the heart? Perhaps the best approach is to first take a look at the animal experimental data pertaining to physical activity and training which has recently been summarized so admirably by Froelicher.[1] In brief, the data can be analyzed under several categories.

ANIMAL EXPERIMENTAL DATA

Effect of Exercise on the Size of Heart Muscle Fibers

Multiple studies[1-4] confirm the fact that the animal heart responds to chronic exercise by enlarging. Wild animals, for instance, have larger heart/body ratios than do less active domestic animals.[5] An age factor seems to be important, however, in that while exercise induces cardiac hypertrophy in younger animals, there is actually a loss in cardiac size and weight in older animals.[6] While most feel that exercise-induced cardiac enlargement reflects hypertrophy of myocardial cells and fibers, several studies suggest that hyperplasia (an increased number of fibers) may also occur.[7]

Effect of Exercise on the Coronary Arterial System

At least three types of investigations have dealt with enhancement of the coronary microcirculation following exercise training. Leon and Bloor[6] looked at the age factor in some detail and evaluated the exercise frequency factor in several groups of rats. The rats were divided into three age groups which corresponded to the human brackets of teens, twenties to forties, and fifties to seventies. Each age bracket contained a control group, a group that swam for one hour per day, and a group that swam for one hour two days per week. The results indicated increased capillary numbers, capillary/fiber ratios and coronary lumen areas in young adult rats but not in their older counterparts.

Tomanek[7] ran a group of rats on a treadmill for forty minutes per day over a three-month period. He demonstrated an increased ratio of coronary microvessels to myocardial fibers, implying an enhanced blood supply to the heart muscle. He also noted that the greatest increase in capillary development occurred in the younger rats. Poupa[8] compared tame and wild rats and rabbits, finding a greater capillary network in the wild, more active animals. The capillary development was more impressive in younger animals, suggesting that these small vessels were more responsive to growth stimuli at an early age.

The above studies suggest that the microcirculation of cardiac muscle in animals will be significantly enhanced only if exercise is started in youth. The luminal area of the larger coronary arteries will enlarge in the teen group and in the young adults who exercise on a daily rather than a twice-weekly basis.

The effect of exercise on the coronary *collateral circulation* of animals has likewise been evaluated by multiple research groups. The most widely quoted study of this type was performed by Doctor Richard Eckstein in 1957.[9] Using a surgical technique, Eckstein narrowed the large coronary arteries in one hundred dogs. Those who developed signs of a myocardial infarction on subsequent electrocardiograms were divided into two groups. The dogs in group A were exercised on a treadmill for five hours per week over a one-and-one-half– to two-month period. Dogs in group B were kept in small cages over a similar time period. The collateral circulation around the narrowed vessels was markedly enhanced in the exercise group as compared to the rest group. Cobb et al.[10] attempted to duplicate Eckstein's work by studying the collateral vessel development radiographically in 50 dogs, half of whom were in an exercise group and half in a control group. The former ran on a treadmill for forty minutes daily over a three-month period. When the coronary arteries in both groups were then injected with radiographic dye, there was no enhancement of collateral growth in the exercise group. One drawback to such a study, however, is that small collateral vessels cannot be demonstrated by angiographic technique. Burt and Jackson[11] were interested in seeing if an animal could develop the collateral vessels through exercise without first having had a large coronary artery partially occluded. Using a technique which was otherwise similar to Eckstein's, they were unable to demonstrate any exercise-induced collateralization, implying that one needed the ischemia of a narrowed vessel to stimulate the growth of the collateral vasculature. Kaplinsky et al.[12] studied the effects of total occlusion of a major coronary artery in 40 dogs. Twenty-six of the dogs survived the insult and were subsequently equally divided into exercise and control groups. Coronary arteriograms were performed at the end of the study, the animals were sacrificed, and pathologic studies were then made of the coronary arteries. Both groups developed extensive networks of collateral vessels, but the exercise group had no better development than the control group. Perhaps if a vessel is suddenly totally occluded, as opposed to the partial occlusions induced by Eckstein, exercise does not enhance collateral formation.

The effect of exercise on the size of the *large coronary arteries* was studied by Tepperman et al.[13] and by Stevenson et al.[14] The former conducted a sophisticated experiment in which they compared two exercise groups of rats with two control groups. One exercise group ran a mile per day for thirty-six days, while the other group swam for thirty minutes on a daily basis for ten weeks. The animals were sacrificed at the end of the study, and vinyl acetate was injected into the coronary arteries. Potassium hydroxide was used to digest all of the heart tissue except for the coronary arteries, which were then weighed. Both exercise groups had significantly greater weights of the coronary arteries as compared to the control groups. Stevenson et al.[14] studied rats in a similar fashion, analyzing different frequencies and intensities of treadmill and swimming activities. They were able to show increases in coronary arterial tree sizes in all exercise groups as compared to nonexercise groups. However, in the strenuous swimming group, rats who swam for eight hours per week actually developed larger coronary artery diameters than those who swam sixteen hours per week. This study provides food for thought as the possibilities of a maximum exercise tolerance, beyond which no significant increases in the size of large coronary arteries accrue.

Effect of Exercise on Myocardial Performance, Efficiency, and Mitochondrial Morphology

Exercised rats, when compared to controls, are able to perform greater amounts of cardiac work and have an enhanced stroke volume.[15] When heart rates in both groups were artificially increased by cardiac pacing, the hearts of physically trained rats were able to utilize more oxygen and produced less lactic acid than did the control hearts.

Holloszy[16] has described an increase in both size and number of skeletal muscle mitochondria after exercise training. In addition, there is a quantitative increase in the respiratory enzymes per gram of muscle tissue. The mitochondria of rat heart muscle were studied after various intensities of exercise.[17] While most of the exercised rats increased both size and number of myocardial mitochondria (similar to skeletal muscle), some mitochondrial degeneration occurred in the intensively exercised rats, suggesting that overexercise might have harmful effects. In another study, digitalis seemed to prevent such degenerative changes.[18] Banister et al.[4] showed that the degeneration of mitochondria is more noticeable shortly after exhaustive exercise is begun and is much less once a training effect is achieved.

Summary and Practical Application of Animal Studies

In taking an overview of the animal experimental data, several concepts are apparent. First, the evidence is overwhelming that exercise has a beneficial effect on the animal heart, be it an increase in the coronary macro– or microcirculation, in the mitochondria, or in cardiac performance. Comparing young and old animals, it appears that exercise produces more impressive changes in the former. If we can extrapolate this to the human, one could build a case for developing exercise habits at an early age. The animal data also raises the question as to whether overexercise can actually be harmful. Again putting this into human perspective, is the man who jogs twenty miles per week doing less for his heart than the man who jogs ten miles per week? From the available report on Clarence DeMar, who customarily ran over ten miles per day for many years, he did not show any cardiac deterioration (although electron microscopy was not performed). Furthermore, treadmill studies in our laboratory on marathon runners, some of whom put in up to 150 miles of road work per week, show them to be in a much higher level of physical conditioning than the average jogger.

Researchers at the University of California in San Diego feel that too many animal studies have been done on dogs and that actually the pig's heart more closely resembles that of man. There are other similarities. The eating habits of pigs more closely emulate those of man than do those of dogs. If one takes a dog to the beach, the animal will frolic and romp about. Humans and pigs are more likely to root about. One group of pigs will be exercised on treadmills, while the control group will remain relatively sedentary. Results at the end of this five-year study should be of great interest.

Let us turn now to the epidemiology studies in humans pertaining to physical activity levels and the incidence and prevalence of coronary heart disease. Excellent review articles have been written by Fox et al.[19] and by Froelicher et al.[20] The latter categorized the research into retrospective studies, prospective studies, autopsy evaluation, and rehabilitation studies. This classification will be used below in a brief review.

EPIDEMIOLOGY STUDIES IN MAN

Retrospective Studies

This type of study evaluates a group of persons after the development of coronary disease, seeking out factors in their past which might have predisposed them to the disease. One of the most often quoted studies of this nature is that of the London transport employees. Doctor Jerry Morris[21] conducted a review of the records of 31,000 men, ages thirty-five to sixty-four, and noted that the more sedentary busdrivers had an incidence of coronary disease 1.5 times that of the more active conductors who spent most of their day going up and down the steps of double-decked busses. Moreover, the sudden death rates and the death rates during the first two months after a myocardial infarction were twice as high in drivers. This study, though often the basis for the "hard sell" of exercise benefits, had certain significant weaknesses. For instance, there was no attempt to actually substantiate the activity differences between the two groups, nor was consideration given to off-the-job activities. Subsequent reviews of the data showed that the drivers had higher blood pressure and cholesterol levels than did the conductors, even when they first applied for the job.[22] Such differences could have made the drivers a higher risk for coronary disease for reasons other than the proposed difference in physical activity levels.

Doctor Henry Taylor from the University of Minnesota led a study on the mortality rates of white men employed by the United States Railroad Industry.[23] Death certificates for the years 1955 and 1956 were analyzed, and they showed that the more active sectionmen had less than half the death rates from coronary disease that the sedentary clerks had. Thus, it could be surmised that men in sedentary occupations have more coronary disease than do those engaged in moderate to heavy physical activity. Further analysis of the data was rather interesting, however. Additional questioning of relatives and associates and detailed quantitations of on-the-job energy expenditure revealed that certain clerks actually expended as much caloric energy per day as did the presumably more active sectionmen. More significant was the discovery that men with coronary disease symptoms either retired or withdrew from the position of sectionman and entered into that of a sedentary clerk. The death rates could, therefore, be explained by a bias in job transfers and retirement tendencies rather than by any protective influence of exercise.[24]

Another interesting retrospective study was that of Frank et al.[25] who studied 55,000 men, ages twenty-five to sixty-four, who were enrolled in the Health Insurance Plan of New York. Over a sixteen-month period, 301 had experienced myocardial infarctions. Questionnaires and personal interviews with either the patient or his widow as to on-the-job and leisure time activity allowed classification into categories of light, moderate, and heavy. The death rate following the infarction was 49 percent in the light activity group as opposed to only 13 percent in the heavy activity group. Thus, it would appear that even if physical activity did not prevent a coronary event, it might greatly enhance one's chances of survival. In a critique of the report, Keys indicated certain problems in its validity.[26] It seems that many of the men were ill prior to the infarction. It would be expected that the 22 percent with symptoms of coronary disease, the 19 percent with hypertension, and the 10 percent with diabetes mellitus would be less active than the others, providing not only a statistical bias for inactivity but also one for the severity of the infarction. Keys went on to reemphasize prior observations that widows tend to underestimate the degree of physical activity of their deceased husbands.

Doctor Curtis Hames, a private practitioner from Claxton, Georgia, had the foresight to arrange a coronary epidemiology study [27, 28] in Evans County, Georgia, after observing that his black patients appeared to have much less coronary disease than his white patients, despite a greater tendency toward hypertension and high saturated fat dietary intake in the former. Analysis of the data confirmed the clinical suspicion that indeed the black males had a much lower prevalence of coronary artery disease than the white males. After assessing the various risk factors through the use of the multiple logistics equation, Hames concluded that low social standards and relatively high physical activity habits appeared to account for at least some of the protective effect among the blacks.

A favorite subject for retrospective study has been the college athlete. Pomeroy and White[29] studied former Harvard football players and found no harmful cardiovascular effects from their prior strenuous activity. Indeed, those who continued to exercise in later life had fewer myocardial infarctions than the nonactive or formerly active groups. Prout[30] studied the records of 172 graduates of Harvard and Yale, each of whom had been members of the crew squad between the years 1882 and 1902. For each crew member, a classmate was picked at random to serve as a control. The average life span of the combined crew members was 67.85 years, significantly greater ($p<.02$) than the average life span of the combined controls (61.55 years). When the cause of death prior to age sixty was known, however, there was not a significant difference as to the incidence of cerebrovascular and cardiac disease between the controls (7 instances) and the oarsmen (6 instances). This study was somewhat limited by the inadequate listing of the cause of death in many instances. Schnohr[31] obtained information on 297 male athletic champions who were born in Denmark between 1880 and 1910 and compared their mortality with that of the general Danish male population. Although the causes of death were essentially the same among the athletes as among the general population, the mortality of the athletes was significantly lower under the age of fifty years. A recent study by Polednak[32] compared longevity and cardiovascular mortality among 681 former Harvard lettermen. Subdivision of the athletes by the type of sport revealed no significant differences in longevity. A unique finding was that men who earned three or more varsity letters had significantly higher coronary mortality rates than did the one– to two-letter athletes. This data is again somewhat restricted in view of the inaccuracy of death certificate data and by the lack of follow-up knowledge as to exercise habits after graduation.

A retrospective study of coronary deaths in New Mexico[33] showed a serial decline in deaths from the lowest to the highest altitude. One of their speculations was that "adaptation to reduced oxygen tension at higher altitudes is never complete, and, therefore, that exertions associated with the activities of daily living represent increased physical exercise." If this is so, why did women not show a similar decline in mortality, and why did studies in Colorado[34] not show an inverse relationship between altitude of residence and coronary death rates? The matter clearly needs additional study before firm conclusions can be drawn.

Those who feel that exercise alone is not a deterrent to coronary disease are quick to quote statistics from the "heart attack capital" of the world, North Kyrelia (Finland). The men residing in this region tend to be lean and muscular, engaging in outdoor work such as dairy farming and lumberjack activities. Their environment is "a natural setting so relaxing that a doctor in the United States might prescribe it for a vacation for a cardiac patient." According to Doctor Heikki Siltanen, a twenty-nine-year-old physician new to the area, coronary disease casts a huge shadow in this region: "No one feels safe. One of the great shocks you get in coming here from outside the area, as I did, is making school check-ups. You are shattered to find out how many very young children are without fathers."[36]

As has been shown in the Seven Countries study, these people are prone to high cholesterol levels. Their diet is high in saturated fat, as milk, butter, fatty sausage *(lenkkimakkara)*, and pastries are plentiful.

The World Health Organization has set up a study in this high-risk area to see if coronary events can be reduced by an active intervention program. The latter consists of the following:

1. A hypertension registry, with early detection through mass screening.
2. Dietary education programs, urging wives to use foods lower in saturated fats, bakers to reduce the sugar and butter content of their products, and sausage makers to develop low fat substitutes.
3. A ban on cigarette advertising, along with prohibition of smoking in public places.

The five-year results on coronary events in North Kyrelia will be compared to events in Kuopio, the "control" county.

Prospective Studies

In a prospective study, a population group is carefully evaluated and then closely followed for a period of time. Those persons developing coronary disease in the follow-up period are compared with those who are free of clinical disease, utilizing the initial screening data. The most widely publicized prospective study in the medical literature is certainly the Framingham study headed by Doctor William Kannel.[37] Over 5,000 men and women, initially free of coronary disease, have been followed since 1949. While those with sedentary life habits had significantly more coronary disease than their more active counterparts, there are certain limitations to the analysis. The level of physical activity was not precisely ascertained, and the physiological measurements (as level of obesity, vital capacity, handgrip strength, etc.) used to assess the degree of physical activity are somewhat arbitrary.

Paffenbarger[38] reported a sixteen-year follow-up study on San Francisco longshoremen. The study initially encompassed over 300 men, ages thirty-five to sixty-four years. It was possible to separate the workers into two levels of work activity, differing by over 900 calories in energy expenditure per day. During the follow-up period there were 291 deaths attributed to coronary disease. The less active group had a 33 percent higher coronary death rate than their more active colleagues. The differences due to activity were sustained even when blood pressure levels and smoking habits were taken into consideration. Unfortunately, serum cholesterol levels were not ascertained, leaving a big question as to whether or not this important risk factor could have accounted for the group differences.

The Seven Countries Study is an ongoing prospective study[39] involving a population of over 12,000 men, ages forty to fifty-nine, from the following countries: Japan, Greece, Yugoslavia, Italy, the Netherlands, Finland, and the United States. When the data was tabulated at the five-year point, Japan had the lowest rate of coronary decrease, while the United States and Finland had the highest rates. Physical activity levels could perhaps explain the low rate in the Japanese (who tend to be very active) and the high rates in the United States (noted for escalators and motor-driven bicycles) but certainly not the high rates in the Finns (the ultimate in physical fitness orientation). By using the multiple logistics equation, wherein all other measured factors were held constant while a single risk factor was being assessed, physical inactivity was considered a much less significant coronary risk factor than was hypertension and hypercholesterolemia.

The Goteborg, Sweden, study[40] is a fascinating project involving 834 men who were all born in the year 1913. In 1963, when the men were fifty-years-old, there were no clinical signs of coronary heart disease. Four years later, myocardial infarctions were diagnosed in 23 of the men, angina pectoris in 18 men, and new electrocardiographic abnormalities were present in 9 others. The incidence of myocardial infarction was significantly less in those whose occupations involved "heavy" physical activity than those in "medium" and "sedentary" job classifications. Unfortunately, leisure time activities were not considered in this study.

In an update of the Goteborg study, Tibblin et al.[41] described 19 deaths from ischemic heart disease and 31 survivors. Cigarette smoking and alcohol abuse were more common in the coronary patients than in the remaining subjects; similarly, systolic blood pressure, serum cholesterol, and triglycerides tended to be higher in the coronary group. There was no relationship between physical inactivity during work and coronary disease. The authors state that "in part this may be an expression of a limited variation in physical strain during ordinary work in an industrialized city" and go on to say that there was a "trend toward reduced effort during leisure time activities . . . among those who later had ischemic heart disease."

Exercise habits during leisure hours were, however, carefully reviewed in a recent publication by Morris et al.[42] Between 1968 and 1970, these investigators obtained weekend activity questionnaires on 16,882 men, ages forty to sixty-four. In the follow-up period to date, 232 of the men have developed clinical evidence of coronary disease. Each of the latter was matched with two colleagues who were not afflicted in terms of relative activity levels. Only 11 percent of the men who later developed coronary disease performed any vigorous weekend activity, versus 26 percent of the control group. In other words, men who reported vigorous activity during the single two-day weekend assessed had about one-third the risk of developing coronary disease than the less active group. The shortcomings of this study were apparent to the authors, who correctly surmised that misclassifications could easily occur when assessing the activity of only a single weekend. For example, the active sportsman who was inactive that weekend because of an upper respiratory infection would be underscored, whereas the sedentary chap whose wife finally goaded him into a weekend project would be falsely classified in an upward fashion. Another deficit was that some of the forms of arduous exercise such as "vigorously getting about" are extremely difficult to determine and more so to quantitate.

Pathology Studies

Of the pathology studies, that of Morris and Crawford [43] has been widely cited. In the mid-1950s, these investigators performed autopsies on 3,800 men, ages forty-five to seventy, who died of noncoronary causes. The last occupation of the deceased was estimated as involving light, moderate, or heavy physical exertion. An independent assessment as to the degree of coronary atherosclerosis was made, and the results indicated that so-called "silent" complete occlusions of a major coronary vessel, that is a complete occlusion without clinical awareness, were more common in those of the light activity group. However, all occupational groups had an equally high prevalence of less extensive coronary atherosclerosis, somewhat clouding the issue.

Another interesting autopsy study, previously alluded to, was that of Clarence DeMar. [44] DeMar was a remarkable man who competed in over 1,000 distance races over a sixty-year period. He competed in over one hundred marathon races, including thirty-four at Boston. His record of seven wins in the Boston marathon has never been equalled. When he died of metastatic bowel cancer at age seventy, his coronary arteries were found to be two to three times the diameter of the average man in his age category. Although he had some atherosclerosis, the overall

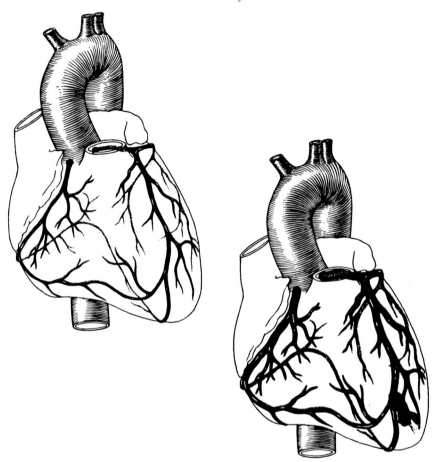

Figure 3-1. Artist's sketch of an autopsy study on Clarence DeMar, comparing his coronary vasculature (lower right) with that of a sedentary man of similar age (upper left).

vessel diameter was such that this was of little consequence (Fig. 3-1). While it is possible that DeMar inherited larger-than-average coronary vessels, there is nothing in his family history to suggest unusual physical development.

Recent studies by Hutchins et al.[45] suggest a direct linear relationship between heart weight and the cube of the normal coronary artery diameter. Hence, it seems likely that DeMar's large arteries were indeed related to his myocardial hypertrophy, produced by lifelong exercise habits.

Rehabilitation Studies

There are several rehabilitation studies[46-48] suggesting that exercise has a favorable influence on coronary disease. These will be reviewed in Chapter 9. Suffice it to say that such studies often have built-in selection bias in that those without previous interest or experience in exercise will tend to drop out, as will those whose symptoms make them unable to tolerate the exercise program. The future looks promising regarding the acquisition of hard data in the field of postcoronary rehabilitation studies. The World Health Organization is conducting a randomized controlled study in European cities such as Geneva, Switzerland, and Bordeaux, France. In the United States, the Department of Health, Education and Welfare is funding similar studies in at least four major medical centers. The project is directed by Doctor John Naughton. Georgia Baptist Hospital, via affiliation with Emory School of Medicine, has been actively engaged in this long-range (five– to ten-year) study.

The multiple studies regarding exercise in the prevention of coronary disease in man are summarized in Table 3-I. The trend of most studies is that physical inactivity may be a contributing factor toward the development of premature coronary disease. However, hard data is lacking to say unequivocally that physical inactivity is a major coronary risk factor. Hopefully, future studies will be devoid of the many weaknesses of previous reports. The "Seven Countries" study and the "Men Born in 1913" project (Goteborg) are in the final phases, and the end results are awaited with great interest.

The current shortcomings of our understanding as to the effects of exercise on coronary heart disease and upon longevity can be seen in the intriguing study by Doctor Alexander Leaf.[49] Doctor Leaf, while on sabbatical leave from Massachusetts General Hospital, traveled to Vilcabamba in the Ecuadorean Andes, Hunza, located in the Karakoren range of Kashmir, and

TABLE 3-I

EPIDEMIOLOGY STUDIES: PHYSICAL ACTIVITY AND CORONARY HEART DISEASE (CHD)

Type of Study	Major Author	Population Size	Occupation	Correlations of Physical Inactivity to CHD
Retrospective				
London Transport	Morris	31,000	Drivers vs. conductors	Yes
North Dakota	Zukel	20,000	Farmers vs. others	Yes
U.S. Railroad	Taylor	100,000	Switchmen vs. clerks	Yes
Evans Co.	Hames	5,000	Laborers vs. white collar	Yes
HIP of New York	Frank	301	Less active, intermediate, more active	Yes
Peoples Gas Co.	Stamler	1,500	Blue collar vs. white collar	Yes
College Oarsmen	Prout	172	Athletes vs. nonathletes	No (but athletes lived longer)
Danish athletes	Schnohr	307	Athletes vs. nonathletes	No (but athletes lived longer)
Harvard football	Pomeroy		Athletes vs. nonathletes	No CHD in athletes who kept active after graduation
Harvard athletes	Polednak	681	Athletes (1 or 2 letter) vs. Athletes (3 letters or more)	More CHD in lettermen with three letters or more
Prospective				
San Francisco	Paffenbarger	3,300	Cargo workers vs. clerks	Yes
Framingham	Kannel	5,000	Active vs. sedentary	Yes
Seven Countries	Keys	12,000	Active vs. sedentary	No
Goteborg	Werko	834	Active vs. sedentary	Yes
British Civil Servants	Morris	16,882	Active vs. inactive (leisure time)	Yes
Pathology				
England	Morris	3,800	Light, moderate, heavy	Yes
DeMar	White	1	Marathon runner	Enlarged diameter of coronary arteries
Rehabilitation				
Israel	Gottheiner	1,103	Coronary patients	Positive trend
Case Western Reserve	Hellerstein	100	Coronary patients	Positive trend
Canada	Rechnitzer	68	Coronary patients	Positive trend

Abkhazia in the Caucasus Mountains of Russia. These isolated areas were selected for study in view of their high incidence of centenarians per 100,000 population. While in the United States the incidence of centenarians is 3 per 100,000 people, the figure is 63 per 100,000 in Abkhazia. Some have questioned these figures, stating that records in these less developed countries are inaccurate and often exaggerated. Doctor Leaf surmised that a low calorie and low fat diet, psychosocial factors, and physical conditioning were among the possible secrets for such unusual longevity. Most of the centenarians continued to work and to exercise regularly at elevations of up to 6,000 feet, indicative of highly efficient cardiopulmonary function. Although once again "hard" clinical data is lacking in this study, it is of note that Doctor Leaf was so impressed by the effects of vigorous exercise in these people that he became a regular jogger upon returning to the United States. Doctor Leaf observed that these people "don't worry about anything they can't change," and he goes on to offer the following advice to those who strive for a long, healthy life: "Lose excess weight, get regular exercise that creates endurance, cut down on the meat and animal fat portion of the diet, and develop a consuming interest in something other than your work." [35]

REFERENCES

1. Froelicher, V.F.: Animal studies of effect of chronic exercise on the heart and atherosclerosis: A review. *Am Heart J, 84:*496-506, 1972.
2. Bloor, C.M., Pasyk, S., and Leon, A.S.: Interaction of age and exercise on organ and cellular development. *Am J Pathol, 58:*185-199, 1970.
3. Hakkila, J.: Studies of the myocardial capillary concentration in cardiac hypertrophy due to training. *Ann Med Exp Biol Fenn, 33: Suppl 10:*1, 1955.
4. Banister, E.W., Tomanek, R.J., and Cvorkov, N.: Ultrastructural modifications in rat heart: Responses to exercise and training. *Am J Physiol, 220:*1935-1940, 1971.
5. Poupa, O., Rakusan, K., and Ostadal, B.: The effect of physical activity upon the heart of vertebrates. In Brunner, E. (Ed.): Physical activity and aging. *Med Sports, 4:*202, 1970.

6. Leon, A.S., and Bloor, C.M.: Exercise effects on the heart at different ages (Abstr). *Circulation, 41* and *42: Suppl III:* 50, 1970.
7. Tomanek, R.J.: Effects of age and exercise on the extent of the myocardial capillary bed. *Anat Rec, 167:*55-62, 1970.
8. Poupa, O., Rakusan, K., and Ostadal, B.: The effect of physical activity upon the heart of vertebrates. In Brunner, E. (Ed.): Physical activity and aging. *Med Sports, 4:*202, 1970.
9. Eckstein, R.W.: Effect of exercise and coronary artery narrowing on coronary collateral circulation. *Circ Res, 5:*230-235, 1957.
10. Cobb, F.R., Ruby, R.L., and Fariss, B.L.: Effects of exercise on acute coronary occlusion in dogs with prior partial occlusion (Abstr). *Circulation, 37* and *38:*104, 1968.
11. Burt, J.J., and Jackson, R.: The effects of physical exercise on the coronary collateral circulation of dogs. *J Sports Med, 5:*203-206, 1965.
12. Kaplinsky, E., Hood, W.B., Jr., McCarthy, B., et al.: Effects of physical training in dogs with coronary artery ligation. *Circulation, 37:*556-565, 1968.
13. Tepperman, J., and Pearlman, D.: Effects of exercise and anemia on coronary arteries of small animals as revealed by the corrosion-case technique: *Circ Res, 9:*576-584, 1961.
14. Stevenson, J.A.F., Feleki, V., Rechnitzer, R., et al.: Effect of exercise on coronary tree size in the rat. *Circ Res, 5:*265, 1964.
15. Penpargkul, S., and Scheuer, J.: The effect of physical training upon the mechanical and metabolic performance of the rat heart. *J Clin Invest, 49:*1859-1868, 1970.
16. Holloszy, J.O.: Morphological and enzymatic adaptations to training: A review. In Larsen, O.A., and Malmborg, R.O. (Eds.): *Coronary Heart Disease and Physical Fitness.* Baltimore, University Park Press, 1971, pp. 147-151.
17. Arcos, J.C., Sohal, R.S., Sun, S.C., et al.: Changes in ultra-constructure and respiratory control in mitochondria of rat heart hypertrophied by exercise. *Exp Mol Pathol, 8:*49-65, 1968.
18. Aldinger, E.E., and Sohol, R.S.: Effects of digitoxin on the ultrastructural myocardial changes in the rat subjected to chronic exercise. *Am J Cardiol, 26:*369-374, 1970.
19. Fox, S.M. III, and Skinner, J.S.: Physical activity and cardiovascular health. *Am J Cardiol, 14:*731-746, 1964.
20. Froelicher, V.F., and Oberman, A.: Analysis of epidemiologic studies of physical inactivity as risk factor for coronary artery disease. *Prog Cardiovasc Dis, 15:*41-65, 1972.
21. Morris, J.N., Heady, J.A., Raffle, P.A., et al.: Coronary heart disease and physical activity of work. *Lancet, 2:*1053-1057, 1953.
22. Morris, J.N., Kagan, A., Pattison, D.C., et al.: Incidence and prediction of ischemic heart disease in London busmen. *Lancet, 2:*553-559, 1966.
23. Taylor, H.L., Klepetar, E., Keys, A., et al.: Death rate among physically

active and sedentary employees of the railroad industry. *Am J Public Health, 52:*1697, 1962.

24. Taylor, H.L., Blackburn, H., Brozek, J., et al.: Occupational factors in the study of coronary heart disease and physical activity. *Can Med Assoc J, 96:*825, 1967.

25. Frank, C.W., Weinblatt, E., Shapiro, S., et al.: Physical inactivity as a lethal factor in myocardial infarction among men. *Circulation, 34:*1022-1033, 1966.

26. Keys, A.: Physical activity and the epidemiology of coronary heart disease. In Brunner, D. (Ed.): Physical activity and aging. *Medicine and Sport,* Vol. 4. Baltimore, University Park Press, 1970, p. 250.

27. McDonough, J.R., Hames, C.G., Stubb, S.C., et al.: Coronary heart disease among Negroes and Whites in Evans County, Georgia. *J Chronic Dis 18:*443, 1965.

28. Hames, C.G.: Evans County cardiovascular and cerebrovascular epidemiology study: Introduction. *Arch Intern Med, 128:*883-886, 1971.

29. Pomeroy, W.C., and White, P.D.: Coronary heart disease in former football players. *JAMA, 167:*711-714, 1958.

30. Prout, C.: Life expectancy of college oarsmen. *JAMA, 220:*1709-1711, 1972.

31. Schnohr, P.: Longevity and causes of death in male athletic champions. *Lancet, 2:*1364-1366, 1971.

32. Polednak, A.P.: Longevity and cardiovascular mortality among former college athletes. *Circulation, 46:*649-654, 1972.

33. Mortimer, E.A., Jr., Monson, R.R., and MacMahon, B.: Reduction in mortality from coronary heart disease in men residing at high altitude. *N Engl J Med, 296:*581-585, 1977.

34. Morton, W.E., Davids, D.J., and Lichty, J.A.: Mortality from heart disease at high altitude: the effect of high altitude on mortality from arteriosclerotic and hypertensive heart disease. *Arch Environ Health, 9:*21-24, 1964.

35. *The Mayo Alumnus,* July, 1974, pp. 32-35.

36. *The Atlanta Journal and Constitution,* February 23, 1975.

37. Kannel, W.B.: Habitual level of physical activity and risk of coronary heart disease: The Framingham study. *Can Med Assoc J, 96:*811-812, 1967.

38. Paffenbarger, R.S., Laughlin, M.E., Gima, A.S., et al.: Work activity of longshoremen as related to death from coronary heart disease and stroke. *N Engl J Med, 282:*1109, 1970.

39. Blackburn, H., Taylor, H.L., and Keys, A.: Coronary heart disease in seven countries. XVI. The electrocardiogram in prediction of five-year coronary heart disease incidence among men aged 40-59. *Circulation, 41: Suppl 1:*154, 1970.

40. Werko, L.: Can we prevent heart disease. *Ann Intern Med, 74:*278-288, 1971.

41. Tibblin, G., Wilhelmsen, L., and Werko, L.: Risk factors for myocardial

infarction and death due to ischemic heart disease and other causes. *Am J Cardiol, 35:*514-522, 1975.

42. Morris, J.N., Adam, C., Chave, S.P.W., et al.: Vigorous exercise in leisuretime and the incidence of coronary heart disease. *Lancet, 1:*333-339, 1973.

43. Morris, J.N., Heady, J.A., Raffle, P.A.B., et al.: Coronary heart disease and physical activity of work. *Lancet, 2:*1053-1057, 1953.

44. Currens, J.H., and White, P.D.: Half a century of running: Clinical, physiological and autopsy findings in the case of Clarence DeMar ("Mr. Marathon"). *N Engl J Med, 265:*988-993, 1961.

45. Hutchins, G.M., Bulkley, B.H., Miner, M.M., et al.: Correlation of age and heart weight with tortuosity and caliber of normal coronary arteries. *Am Heart J, 94:*196-202, 1977.

46. Gottheiner, V.: Long range strenuous sports training for cardiac reconditioning and rehabilitation. *Am J Cardiol, 22:*426-435, 1968.

47. Hellerstein, H.K.: The effects of physical activity: Patients and normal coronary-prone subjects. *Minn Med, 52:*1335-1341, 1969.

48. Rechnitzer, P.A., Pickard, H.A., Paivio, A.U., et al.: Long-term follow-up study of survival and recurrence rates following myocardial infarction in exercising and control subjects. *Circulation, 45:*853-857, 1972.

49. Leaf, A.: Every day is a gift when you are over 100. *National Geographic, 143:*93-119, 1973.

Chapter 4

EFFECT OF EXERCISE ON CORONARY RISK FACTORS

N UMEROUS STUDIES[1-5] have led to the identification of multiple factors which seem to predispose one to premature coronary heart disease. A cross sampling of several such studies produces the following list of the more frequently implicated coronary risk factors:

1. Blood lipid abnormalities
2. Hypertension
3. Cigarette smoking
4. Carbohydrate intolerance
5. Physical inactivity
6. Overweight
7. Diet
8. Heredity
9. Personality and behavior patterns
10. Electrocardiographic abnormalities
11. Disorders in blood coagulation
12. Elevation in blood uric acid
13. Pulmonary function abnormalities

It has been difficult to assess the relative importance of a single factor in comparison to the others. Many of the factors are interrelated, such as blood lipid abnormalities, diabetes, heredity, and obesity. Individual studies taken alone can contribute to this confusion. For example, compare the relative importance of diet and physical inactivity: Irish men residing in their native country consumed more calories and saturated fat than did their blood brothers residing in the United States,[6] yet they had a significantly lower incidence of coronary heart disease. The latter was attributed by some to reflect their increased physical activity, which was mainly in the form of bicycle riding and manual labor. Exercise might also be the reason why the Masai tribesmen of East Africa have such a low incidence of atherosclerosis despite eating foods extremely high in saturated fats.[7] It may also be the reason why farm laborers in Evans County, Georgia, have less coronary disease than their more affluent constituents, in spite of the fact that they consume more saturated fat.[8] On the other hand, certain studies have indicated that regular exercise is no panacea against premature coronary disease. The Rendille tribesmen of Africa exercise vigorously each day, walking upwards of twenty-five miles. However, they consume a diet high in saturated fat and have a high incidence of atherosclerosis, suggesting that diet is perhaps a more significant risk factor than physical activity.[9] An evaluation of risk factors in young persons with premature myocardial infarctions (prior to age thirty-nine) revealed that four men had exercised vigorously on a daily basis for up to three years prior to the attack.[10] One individual jogged from two to five miles per day. Another point against the importance of physical activity was a report comparing 100 male military personnel who survived a myocardial infarction at age forty or less with a control group.[11] There was no significant difference in physical activity levels between the two groups. It should be pointed out that such reports can be misleading in that the accustomed degree of physical activity was determined by questionnaires rather than by direct interrogation.

Despite the deficiencies in the analysis of risk factors, they remain the most reliable simple screening device that we have available at present. Furthermore, the use of a multiple logistics equation has recently made it possible to assess the importance of a single risk factor while keeping the other factors constant. This sophisticated formula was used in the Seven Countries study,[12] and when the five-year data on over 12,000 men was tabulated, hypertension, serum cholesterol, and dietary levels of saturated fat seemed to be the most important factors.

In a recent study[13] of coronary risk factors in 240 young (under age forty) coronary patients from nine countries, 89 percent had at least one of the three major risk factors (hypertension, cigarette smoking, hypercholesterolemia). Eighty percent of the patients were smokers, while 25 percent had cholesterol levels in excess of 280 mg/dl.

Coronary heart disease is no doubt multifactorial in etiology. Likewise, the effect of exercise is also multifactorial, not only inducing beneficial hemodynamic changes but also interacting with the previously mentioned risk factors. It is therefore worthwhile to review the effect of exercise on the respective factors, for this might serve as an objective means of explaining the subjective improvements most physically fit persons profess. To do this, let us take the thirteen risk factors listed at the beginning of the chapter on an individual basis.

BLOOD LIPID ABNORMALITIES

Cholesterol

Lipoprotein electrophoresis techniques have enhanced our knowledge of the different types of hyperlipidemias.[14] Despite such techniques, the serum cholesterol and triglyceride levels remain the most practical screening tests.

Considerable data from numerous animal studies suggest that exercise has a beneficial effect in reducing serum and tissue cholesterol levels. Myasnikov[15] and Kobernick et al.[16] found that exercising rabbits had lower serum cholesterol levels and lesser degrees of coronary atherosclerosis than did the sedentary groups. In the latter study, 36 rabbits were placed on a cholesterol-rich diet for two months. Half were kept sedentary, while the others exercised for ten minutes per day on a rotating drum device, a level of exercise which was sufficient to produce the cholesterol lowering effect. Several investigators have used chickens as their study model.[17] In general, the exercised birds (some of which walked four miles per week) had reduced serum cholesterol levels and lesser degrees of large vessel atherosclerosis than did the matched controls. Gollnick[18] found that vigorous exercise could decrease the concentration of cholesterol in rat livers. Watt et al.[19] also studied rats and came up with several interesting observations. The rats were exercised on a motor-driven wheel over an eight-week period, and then underwent detraining over a similar time period. Training had a significant lowering effect on serum cholesterol, serum trigly-ceride and adipose triglyceride levels in the rats, but did not significantly affect the adipose levels in the heart or in skeletal muscle. The lowered lipid levels persisted during the eight-week detraining period, despite the fact that the body weight loss during training was regained.

In humans, decreases in serum cholesterol following an active physical conditioning program have been noted by many investigators. These include studies on prisoners,[20] air force officers,[21] postcoronary patients,[22, 23] and the general popula-tion.[24] The latter study indicated that the amount of decrease was related to the percentage of exercise sessions attended over a six-month period. The duration of individual exercise sessions and of the total physical conditioning period was quite variable. Siegel et al.[25] reported a mean decrease in serum cholesterol from 247 to 210 mg in 9 blind men who were exercised for only twelve minutes, three times per week, over a fifteen-week period. This was independent of any weight change. The latter is an important piece of information that too often is not referred to in reports of this nature. Campbell,[26] Berkson,[27] Mann,[28] and Golding[29] reported similar weight-independent changes in other studies. The study of Golding was a longitudinal study and encompassed more than nine years of observations.

Numerous other studies have shown an exercise-related lowering of serum cholesterol levels and deserve mention. Johnson[30] found that 11 swimmers had significantly lower cholesterol levels during training than at other times. Karvon-en[31] found that Finnish skiers had lower cholesterol levels than did nonathletes. Chailly-Bert[32] studied middle-aged men and found lower cholesterol levels in those who were more physically active. Three members of his sedentary group with hypercho-lesterolemia were exercised and experienced a significant lowering of serum cholesterol. Unlike the rat study of Watt et al.,[19] Rochelle[33] found that the decrease in human cholesterol levels during intensive physical training returned to pretraining levels within four weeks after the exercise regimen. Phillips[34] had a similar experience with 6 study patients. The serum cholesterol levels fell from an average of 298 mg% to 195 mg% during the eight weeks of running and handball activities but rose to baseline levels during the detraining period (also eight weeks). When retrained, the levels fell as before.

The effect of exercise frequency, duration, and intensity upon serum cholesterol levels has been studied in several centers. Daniel[35] divided male faculty members into control, mild, and moderate to heavy exercise groups. The exercise consisted of varying-speed treadmill work, five days per week, for seven weeks. While all three exercise groups had significantly lower cholesterol levels than the controls, there were no significant differences among the exercise groups themselves. Pollock[36] likewise found that there was no greater cholesterol-lowering effect in four exercise sessions per week than in two sessions. Konttinen[37] divided 187 Finnish military recruits into light and heavy exercise groups. Both showed significant decreases of serum cholesterol. Although the heavy exercise group did not have a greater decrease in serum cholesterol, they consumed more calories, which added a confusing factor to the interpretation.

Few studies have dealt with exercise and serum cholesterol levels in women. Pohndorf[38] followed a married couple (both of whom were physicians) for a ten-week period during which both swam 1,000 yards daily. The husband then underwent periods of detraining and retraining, while the wife kept active, though at a decreased frequency of exercise activity. Cholesterol levels decreased in both during training. The reduced level persisted in the woman despite less activity but returned to the baseline level in the man during detraining. Metivier[39] compared the effects of stationary bicycle, vibrating table, and free exercises in college women. Significant decreases in cholesterol levels occurred only with the latter type of exercise.

There have been many negative studies, including our own, regarding exercise and cholesterol levels. Despite sixteen hours of vigorous daily physical activity over a twenty-two week period, there was no significant decrease in the serum cholesterol of 101 marine trainees.[40] Holloszy et al.[41] studied 27 subjects over a six-month period of vigorous training and found no change in serum cholesterol nor in serum phospholipids. Studies comparing cross-country skiers[42] and college athletes[41] with age-matched nonathletes detected no difference in cholesterol levels. Skinner[43] reported no significant decrease in the serum cholesterol levels of 14 middle-aged men who exercised thirty minutes per session, five times weekly, for six months. Olson[44] randomly assigned 31 faculty members to sedentary and exercise groups. After a three-month period, there was no significant difference in serum cholesterol levels between the two groups. The active group participated in "recreational" swimming, however, and one can question the intensity of such activity. Brumbach[45] divided college men into two groups of 20 each. The groups were matched for initial cholesterol levels, relative physical fitness, weight, and age. The exercise group met three times weekly for ten weeks, participating in calisthenics, weight lifting, and running sessions. No significant cholesterol-lowering effect could be demonstrated in the latter group. Zauner and Swenson[46] trained 10 middle-aged men over an eight-week period, using activities similar to Brumbach's. After fourteen days of training, significant reductions of serum cholesterol were demonstrated. As training continued, however, the cholesterol level drifted upward toward the initial values.

It appears then that there is no uniform agreement as to whether exercise per se has a significant effect on the serum cholesterol level. Many of the preceding studies are difficult to interpret because true control groups were not mentioned, seasonal variations in lipid levels were not considered, and details of concomitant weight and dietary alterations are lacking.[47, 48] Furthermore, Mirkin[49] pointed out a marked fluctuation in serum cholesterol levels on a day-to-day basis during a long-distance running program.

Wood et al.[50] may have provided at least part of the answer to the exercise-cholesterol relationship by showing that vigorous exercise may actually increase high density lipoprotein (HDL) levels. Recent studies[51, 52] have shown an inverse relationship between high density lipoprotein levels and coronary risk. It is postulated that high density lipoprotein stimulates intracellular lecithin cholestryl acyl transferase (LCAT), thereby facilitating cholesterol removal from the cell. Perhaps the HDL molecule interferes with low density lipoprotein entry into the cell, or perhaps HDL is preferentially transported to the liver for excretion and less likely to be incorporated into atherosclerotic plaques. Such observations are speculative and need to be supported by further studies.

Triglycerides

In the well-controlled study of Holloszy et al.,[41] six months of physical training resulted in a significant decrease in serum triglycerides (from a mean of 208 mg% to a mean of 125 mg%) in fourteen men. This change was found to persist for only approximately two days following each exercise session, however. Oscai et al.[53] placed 7 middle-aged hyperlipidemic men on a fixed diet and studied the effects of interrupted exercise sessions on serum triglyceride, serum cholesterol, and lipoprotein electrophoretic measurements. The men covered three to four miles in forty minutes each day for four consecutive days and then rested from three to seven days. On the four exercise days, the mean serum triglyceride level fell progressively from 235 mg% to 104 mg%. During the rest period the triglyceride levels gradually returned to the baseline level, taking up to seven days in some instances. The serum cholesterol levels were unaffected by exercise. The abnormal lipoprotein patterns of type IV and type V were normalized by exercise but became abnormal again during the sedentary period.

Nikkila and Konttinen[54] studied two groups of Finnish army recruits. Both groups consumed high fat meals. One group marched for two hours, while the other group was inactive. The serum triglyceride levels were significantly reduced in the marchers. Daniel and Pollock[35, 36] compared the frequency and intensity of exercise with the triglyceride-lowering effect. The former divided 24 male faculty members into four groups. One group remained inactive, while the degree of activity was varied in the three exercise groups. All of the latter groups showed significant reductions in serum triglyceride levels as compared to the controls. The decreases were greater in the moderate and heavy work groups than in the mild work group. Pollock randomly assigned middle-aged persons into control and exercise groups. The latter were subdivided into two days/week and four days/week exercise sessions. Both exercise groups had significant triglyceride-lowering effects from exercise as compared to the controls. However, those who exercised four days/week had no greater reductions than did the twice-week exercise group. The usual postprandial increase in triglycerides was appreciably reduced by exercise in the group studied by Cohen et al.[55] Hoffman et al.[21] reported a triglyceride-lowering response to exercise but furnished no information concerning weight change and comparison with a control group.

In a study of forty-six men with type IV hyperlipoproteine-mia, Lampman et al.[56] compared the effects of physical training, diet, and combinations thereof, with the following results:

| | TRIGLYCERIDE | |
	Baseline	*After 6 weeks*
Physical training	163	136
Diet	229	145
Both	196	116

These changes seemed independent of alterations in total body weight or in body composition.

Several reports suggest either no change[57, 41, 58] or an increase in serum triglyceride levels following physical training.[24, 40] This probably can be explained by an accompanying increase in food intake. Although Siegel et al.[25] found a mean decrease in serum triglyceride of 137 to 82 mg%, they did not feel this to be of significance. They made no mention as to how long postexercise the samples were collected.

The trend of most current studies suggests a transient lowering effect on postexercise and postprandial triglyceride levels. This might serve as an indicator for the frequency of exercise sessions (every forty-eight hours at least). The elevations in serum triglycerides during exercise training are most likely related to dietary alterations.

HYPERTENSION

Comparisons of resting blood pressures in active and inactive population groups have yielded varying results. Taylor[59] found lower systolic blood pressures in 416 active railroad switchmen as compared to 298 less active clerks. This difference was not present when the men were first hired for their respective jobs. No significant differences were apparent in the diastolic blood pressure recordings. Kang et al.[60] found similar results in Korean divers as compared to less active controls. Miall and Oldham[61] compared 60 heavy workers with 180 light workers and found that the former had significantly lower systolic and diastolic pressures. The differences could not be explained by social class standing. Karvonen et al.[62] showed that Finnish lumberjacks had lower systolic and diastolic blood pressures than did less active countrymen, and Morris[63] likewise had similar findings in comparing active and inactive London transportation workers. In the Seven Countries study,[64] the more active men were not only leaner but also had lower systolic and diastolic blood pressures as compared to the less active men.

On the other hand, Chiang et al.[65] compared 100 pedicabmen with 1,346 less active Chinese. Although the former were leaner, there were no blood pressure differences between the two groups. Similarly, no differences were shown between the blood pressure of active and less active YMCA members,[66] Chicago utility workers,[67] professional men,[68] and civil servants.[69]

A drawback of many of the above studies is that total active hours (on the job and leisure time) are often not considered. Montoye et al.[70] took this into account in an assessment of habitual physical activity in 1,700 males over age sixteen years. The total energy expenditure was calculated from questionnaire interview data. The least active men had the highest systolic and diastolic blood pressures. This difference persisted even when the men were divided into specific age groups.

Considerable data has accumulated to indicate a modest blood pressure lowering effect of exercise both in normals[71] and in postcoronary patients.[25] Mann et al.[24] found a decrease in both systolic and diastolic levels after physical training, as did Boyer and Kasch.[72] In the latter study, the mean systolic blood pressure fell 13.5 mm Hg in 23 essential hypertensive patients who participated in a six-month exercise program. The mean diastolic pressure fell 11.8 mm Hg. Although the normotensive exercise group had no significant change in mean systolic blood pressure, there was a mean decrease of six mm Hg in the diastolic blood pressure. Mellerowicz[73] noted that trained sportsmen had an average systolic blood pressure of 20 mm Hg lower than the control group. Although Naughton et al.[74] and Clausen et al.[23] found a significant decrease in systolic blood pressure in 9 cardiac patients who underwent four to six weeks of physical training, other investigators have reported no basic change in arterial pressure.[40, 57, 75]

The evidence to date suggests that exercise therapy can produce reductions in systolic and diastolic pressures in both hypertensive and normotensive persons. Similar changes probably occur in coronary patients, although additional data is needed.

CIGARETTE SMOKING

Fox and Skinner[76] indicated in a 1964 review that no adequate investigations have been conducted to determine whether physical exercise diminishes the desire for smoking. Such studies would indeed be difficult to substantiate, as multiple variables are involved. For instance, all patients in our coronary rehabilitation program are strongly advised to give up cigarette smoking and are educated as to the deleterious effects of cigarettes on the cardiovascular system. Their response to such urging may be delayed and consequently falsely attributed to a subsequent exercise program.

One study that bears mention is the randomized evaluation of exercise training in coronary-prone Finnish males.[77] One hundred seventy-eight men were placed into two groups after matching for variable of serum cholesterol, age, systolic blood pressure, S-T segment depression in postexercise ECG, and smoking habits. One group remained as a control, while the other engaged in physical training for an eighteen-month period. While psychological testing showed improvements in the exercise group, there were no definite differences with regard to changes in smoking habits. In another Finnish study, however, Kentala[78] found that regular attendance in a postinfarction exercise class was associated with an enhanced success rate in cessation of cigarette usage.

CARBOHYDRATE INTOLERANCE

In 1924, Levine et al.[79] reported that physical exercise was usually accompanied by a fall in the blood sugar level. In 1945, Blotner[80] noted improvement of glucose tolerance after exercise. Despite reports by Davidson et al.[81] (based on only 5 subjects) that very intense physical training impairs glucose tolerance, clinical experience indicates that diabetic patients require less insulin when more physically active. However, well-controlled studies on physical training and insulin requirements are lacking. Nevertheless, Mann et al.[24] showed that fasting blood sugar level could be significantly decreased after a six-month exercise program (involving 62 men); however, the glucose tolerance did not change. There was no change in the fasting blood sugar level of exercising cardiac patients according to Frick and Katila,[75] but the group was small (7 men) and the frequency (three times per week) and duration of physical training (one to two months) was mild.

Glucose intolerance in adult Eskimos living in western Alaska seems to be on the rise in the past decade.[82] The increased use of such labor-saving devices as chain saws, snowmobiles, and fuel oil (instead of gathered wood) may be a contributing factor to this, and to the 6 percent increase in those overweight.

PHYSICAL INACTIVITY—OVERWEIGHT

Doctor Jean Mayer,[83] nutritional consultant to the President, has commented that the reason many people are obese is not because they always eat more but because they often exercise less than nonobese persons. Nelson et al.[84] at the Mayo Clinic recently reported physiologic studies which indicated that one does not necessarily have to overeat to become obese, for as one ages, basal metabolic requirements decrease. If exercise habits remain the same or decrease in frequency, obesity can develop even if there is some reduction of food intake.

In comparisons of active and inactive population groups, the degree of body fatness is generally less in the former group. This pertains to London transportation workers,[63] middle-aged men in the Seven Countries study,[64] American railroad workers,[59] Chinese pedicabmen,[65] and civil servants.[69]

Significant weight loss in normal and obese persons has been noted in response to prolonged physical training.[24, 71, 85, 86, 87] Analysis of studies reporting no change or a weight gain during exercise therapy frequently reveal appreciable increases in caloric intake.[88] Perhaps the most representative study is that by Mann et al.,[24] wherein a small but significant weight loss and loss of subcutaneous fat was recorded in the exercise group but not in the controls or dropouts. It is important to note the effect of physical training on body composition rather than upon body weight. While the training experience might increase lean body mass, Boileau et al.[89] noted that the percentage of body weight as fat tends to decrease.

Regarding cardiac patients in exercise programs, Naughton et al.[74] found no weight change over an eight-month period of observation, although Hellerstein[22] recorded an average weight reduction of five pounds in a total of 158 men over a longer follow-up period (thirty-three months).

DIET-HEREDITY-PERSONALITY AND BEHAVIOR PATTERNS

Although exercise per se has no direct effect on the type of diet that is consumed or on hereditary factors, it has been shown to cause changes in personality and behavior patterns.[90] Most of the latter are subjective, however, although there are scattered reports containing more objective evaluations. Ismail and Trachtman[91] evaluated the effects of physical training on the personality traits on 60 middle-aged Purdue University faculty members, using the Cattell 16 Personality Factor Questionnaire. They found that the high fitness group were more imaginative, self-sufficient, emotionally mature, and self-satisfied of conquering a certain goal.

In exercised cardiac patients, Hellerstein[92] was able to show a lessening of fatigue and an improvement in sleeping ability in addition to improvements in the depression scale on the Minnesota Multiphasic Personality Inventory (MMPI). Naughton et al.[93] found no significant change in the MMPI of a smaller group but also noted the subjective improvements in sleep patterns and stress relationships. Hellerstein and Friedman[94, 95] found that improved physical fitness had a favorable effect on sexual activity in postcoronary patients. An increase in sexual tension, along with anxiety and alterations in sleep patterns, was found in fourteen college students during a thirty-day period of exercise deprivation.[96]

ELECTROCARDIOGRAPHIC ABNORMALITIES

Electrocardiographic abnormalities, namely voltage criteria for left ventricular hypertrophy[3] premature ventricular beats,[97] and nonspecific T wave changes,[98] are additional coronary risk factors. Persons with left ventricular hypertrophy have an increased risk of death during an initial episode of myocardial infarction than do those without this finding.[99]

Strenuous physical activity may actually result in voltage criteria for left ventricular hypertrophy. Of twenty-one marathon runners studied, sixteen had voltage criteria suggesting this diagnosis.[100] While the hypertrophied ventricle of cardiac patients is felt to operate on the depressed Frank-Starling curve, this does not seem to apply to the hypertrophy of exercise.[101]

Hellerstein et al.[102] were able to show a disappearance of premature ventricular beats in four persons who underwent physical training. Blackburn et al.[103] noted similar lessening of ventricular ectopic activity after an exercise training regimen. Since ventricular ectopic activity may spontaneously subside, and since multiple factors can be operational, it is difficult to say with certainty that physical training alone was therapeutic. In the study by Pyorala et al.[77] (Finland), statistically significant increases in T wave amplitudes were seen in the exercise group but not in the matched controls. It is doubtful that such a change has any impact on future coronary risk.

DISORDERS IN BLOOD COAGULATION

In a review of the literature in 1962, Burt[104] noted a definite correlation between whole blood clotting time and occupational status. Those who performed more active physical work had the longest clotting times. He also noted that physical training could result in prolongation of both the prothrombin time and the blood clotting time. While ingestion of a meal high in fat tends to inhibit fibrinolysis and to accelerate clotting, these effects can be altered by postprandial exercise. MacDonald and Fullerton[105] studied a group of young men after breakfast of eggs, bacon, and buttered toast. Provided they remained inactive, the blood collected three and one-half hours after breakfast clotted more rapidly than it did before breakfast. The enhanced clotting was not seen if the men went for a brisk walk after breakfast. Warnock et al.[106] walked chickens instead of men and found that those who walked four times per week had longer clotting times than did those who remained in cages.

Although unaccustomed strenuous exercise can actually result in increased blood clotting and thrombus formation,[107, 108] regular exercise in general will enhance fibrinolysis and consequently prolong blood clotting.[107, 109, 110] Forty-four college men[104] exercised on the treadmill until exhaustion. Eighty-nine percent showed acceleration of the blood clotting time, and all displayed accelerated fibrinolytic activity. Astrup and Brakman[111] have commented that increased blood fibrinolytic activity may be the explanation as to the beneficial effects of exercise in preventing thrombosis. They surmised that persons who failed to show this response to exercise training might be prone to coronary thrombosis.

In assessing the effects of exercise on fibrinolytic activity, one needs to take into consideration the levels of obesity, for overweight subjects have reduced fibrinolytic activity (perhaps relating to their more sedentary living habits).[112] Patients with coronary disease have less of an exercise-related fibrinolytic response than do those without this disease.[113] Since the fibrinolytic response varies with the intensity of exercise, patients whose exercise tolerance is severely limited due to angina pectoris may show no significant effects on their fibrinolytic activity.[114]

Other risk factors can interact with the coagulation mechanism; for instance, several studies in addition to the one mentioned above have shown the accelerating effect on blood clotting by the development of hyperlipemia.[115, 116] Such interactions need to be sorted out, and additional studies of a significant number of patients and controls are warranted to further assess the interesting relationship between exercise and coagulation.

ELEVATION IN BLOOD URIC ACID

Mann et al.[24] noted an increase in blood uric acid in exercising individuals. This may account for the cases of gout which developed for the first time in 7 persons exercising under the supervision of Harris et al.[71] Mann et al.[24] postulated that episode hyperlactemia might interfere with urate excretion.

Although Montoye et al.[117] found that high school athletes had significantly higher uric acid levels than nonathletes, these levels tended to decrease during the active season for the particular athlete. This suggested a possible beneficial effect of exercise. Bosco et al.[118] revealed that serum uric acid levels were reduced from 0.3 to 3.2 mg% in 16 of 20 men who exercised over an eight-week period. The decrease was greatest in those with the highest initial serum uric acid levels and in those who underwent the most strenuous exercise. Calvy et al.[40] were unable to detect any significant changes in serum uric acid in marine corps recruits. More data is obviously needed to settle the relationship between exercise and serum uric acid levels.

PULMONARY FUNCTION ABNORMALITIES

A decreased vital capacity as a coronary risk factor was noted in the Framingham study.[119] Rechnitzer et al.[120] demonstrated an average increase in vital capacity of 570 cc in 4 coronary patients who exercised over a twelve-week period. No changes in vital capacity or in forced expiratory volumes were seen in 16 other postcoronary patients,[75,121] although the duration of physical training was not as long (four to eight weeks). Exercise training was recently reported as promising in patients with chronic obstructive pulmonary disease. Lefcoe and Paterson[122] summarized four series, consisting of 38 subjects. Beneficial effects included significant increases in maximal oxygen uptake, ventilation, and work load. In a recent editorial review, Barach and Petty[123] observed that (with the exception of one study) the exercise tolerance of patients with chronic lung disease was appreciably enhanced by physical training.

A summary of the present knowledge concerning the effects of exercise on the coronary risk factors can be seen in Table 4-I. Beneficial effects are indicated with plus (+), adverse effects with minus (−), and no effect with (NE). In other instances, exercise is either unrelated (u) to the factor or there is insufficient evidence (IE) to indicate a positive or negative effect. One could certainly argue that the left ventricular hypertrophy of exercise may not be an "adverse" effect, as such findings are commonplace in the elite athletes from various nations.

A recent cross-sectional study of nearly 3000 men[124] showed inverse correlations between physical fitness levels (based on oxygen uptake analysis) and selected coronary risk factors. In comparing the various fitness groups the following trends were noted:

Fitness Group	Cholesterol	Triglyceride	Glucose	Uric Acid	BP Syst.	Diast.	%Body Fat
Very poor	229.9*	176.8†	111.0†	6.7*	127.6†	83.4	26.1†
Poor	232.9†	163.8†	107.3†	6.8†	124.9	82.4	25.3†
Fair	226.9	138.7†	105.6	6.7*	124.4	83.2	24.0†
Good	225.1	118.9†	105.3	6.5	123.4	81.9	22.4†
Excellent	221.1	98.3	103.4	6.4	122.9	81.4	20.8

*$p<.05$ when compared with the excellent fitness group
†$p<.01$ when compared with the excellent fitness group

TABLE 4-I
EFFECTS OF EXERCISE ON CORONARY RISK FACTORS

Risk Factor	Effect of Exercise
1. Blood lipids	
a. Cholesterol	IE
b. Triglycerides	+
2. Blood pressure	
a. Systolic	+
b. Diastolic	+
3. Cigarette smoking	u
4. Blood sugar	
a. Fasting blood sugar	+
b. Glucose tolerance test	NE
5. Physical inactivity	+
6. Overweight	+
7. Diet	u
8. Heredity	u
9. Personality and behavior patterns	IE
10. EKG abnormalities	
a. Premature ventricular contractions	+
b. Left ventricular hypertrophy	—
11. Blood clotting	IE
12. Blood uric acid	IE
13. Pulmonary function	
a. Vital capacity	IE
b. Forced expiratory volume	IE

+ = beneficial effects; u = unrelated; IE = insufficient evidence; NE = no effect;
— = adverse effects.

REFERENCES

1. Dawber, T.R., and Kannel, W.B.: Susceptibility to coronary heart disease. *Mod Concepts Cardiovasc Dis, 30:*671-676, 1961.
2. Doyle, J.T.: Etiology of coronary disease: Risk factors influencing coronary disease. *Mod Concepts Cardiovasc Dis, 35:*81-86, 1966.
3. Stamler, J., Berkson, D.M., Lindberg, H.A., et al.: Coronary risk factors: Their impact and their therapy in the prevention of coronary heart disease. *Med Clin N Am, 50:*229-254, 1966.
4. Ostrander, L.D., Jr.: Alternations of factors predisposing to coronary heart disease. *Ann Intern Med, 68:*1072-1077, 1968.
5. Rosenman, R.H., Friedman, M., Straus, R., et al.: A predictive study of coronary disease. *JAMA, 189:*15-22, 1964.
6. Trulson, M.F., Clancy, R.E., Jessop, W.J., et al.: Comparisons of siblings in Boston and Ireland. *J Am Diet Assoc, 45:*225-229, 1964.
7. Mann, G.V., Shaffer, R.D., and Rich, A.: Physical fitness and immunity to heart disease in Masai. *Lancet, 2:*1308-1310, 1965.
8. McDonough, J.R., Hames, C.G., Stubb, S.C., et al.: Coronary heart disease among Negroes and Whites in Evans County, Georgia. *J Chronic Dis, 18:*443, 1965.
9. Shaper, A.G., and Jones, K.W.: Serum-cholesterol in camel-herding nomads. *Lancet, 2:*1305-1307, 1962.
10. Cantwell, J.D.: Coronary heart disease in young prisoners. Unpublished data.
11. Walker, W.J., and Gregoratos, G.: Myocardial infarction in young men. *Am J Cardiol, 19:*339-343, 1967.
12. Keys, A.: Coronary heart disease in seven countries. *Circulation, 41: Suppl 1:*1-198, 1970.
13. Dolder, M.A., and Oliver, M.F.: Myocardial infarction in young men: Study of risk factors in nine countries. *Br Heart J, 37:*493-503, 1975.
14. Fredrickson, D.S., Levy, R.I., and Lees, R.S.: Fat transport in lipoproteins—An integrated approach to mechanisms and disorders. *N Engl J Med, 276:*215-225, 1967.
15. Myasnikov, A.L.: Influence of some factors on development of experimental cholesterol atherosclerosis. *Circulation, 17:*99-113, 1958.
16. Kobernick, S.D., Niawayama, G., and Zuehlewski, A.C.: Effect of physical activity on cholesterol atherosclerosis in rabbits. *Proc Soc Exp Biol Med, 96:*623, 1957.
17. Montoye, H.J.: Summary of research on the relationship of exercise to heart disease. *J Sports Med, 2:*35-43, 1962.
18. Gollnick, P.D.: Cellular adaptation to exercise. In Shephard, R.J. (ed.): *Frontiers of Fitness,* Springfield, Thomas, 1971, p. 122.
19. Watt, E.W., Foss, M.L., and Block, W.D.: Effects of training and detraining on the distribution of cholesterol, triglyceride, and nitrogen in tissues of Albino Rats. *Circ Res, 31:*908-914, 1972.

20. Dalderup, L.M., Voogd, N. de, Meyknecht, E.A., et al: The effects of increasing the daily physical activity on the serum cholesterol levels. *Nutr Dieta,* (Basel), *9:*112-123, 1967.

21. Hoffman, A.A., Nelson, W.R., and Goss, F.A.: Effects of an exercise program on plasma lipids of senior air force officers. *Am J Cardiol, 20:*516-524, 1967.

22. Hellerstein, H.K.: The effects of physical activity: Patients and normal coronary-prone subjects. *Minn Med, 52:*1335-1341, 1969.

23. Clausen, J.P., Larse, N.O.A., and Trap-Jensen, J.: Physical training in the management of coronary artery disease. *Circulation, 40:*143-154, 1969.

24. Mann, G.V., Garrett, H.L., Farhi, A., Murray, H., and Billings, F.T.: Exercise to prevent coronary heart disease. An experimental study of the effects of training on risk factors for coronary disease in men. *Am J Med, 46:*12-27, 1969.

25. Siegel, W., Blomqvist, G., and Mitchell, J.H.: Effects of a quantitated physical training program on middle-aged sedentary men. *Circulation, 41:*19-29, 1970.

26. Campbell, D.E.: Effect of controlled running on serum cholesterol of young adult males of varying morphological constitutions. *Res Q Am Assoc Health Phys Educ, 39:*47-53, 1968.

27. Berkson, D., et al.: Experience with a long-term supervised ergometric exercise program for middle-aged sedentary American men. *Circulation, 36:Suppl 2*67, 1967.

28. Mann, G.V., et al.: Exercise and coronary risk factors: *Circulation, 36:Suppl 2:*181, 1967.

29. Golding, L.A.: Effects of exercise training upon total serum cholesterol levels. *Res Q Am Assoc Health Phys Educ, 33:*499, 1961.

30. Johnson, T.F., et al.: The influence of exercise on serum cholesterol, phospholipids, and electrophoretic serum protein patterns in college swimmers. *Fed Proc, 18:*77, 1959.

31. Karvonen, M.J., et al.: Serum cholesterol of male and female champion skiers. *Ann Med Int Fenn, 47:*75, 1958.

32. Chailley-Bert, Libignette, P., and Fabre-Chevalier: Contribution a L'Tude des variations du cholesterol sanguin au corns des activities physique. *La Presse Medicale, 63:*415-416, 1955.

33. Rochelle, R.H.: Blood plasma cholesterol changes during a physical training program. *Am Assoc Health Phys Educ, 32:*838, 1961.

34. Phillips, L.: Physical fitness changes in adults attributable to equal periods of training, non-training, and re-training. Doctoral Dissertation, University of Illinois, 1960.

35. Daniel, B.J.: The effects of walking, jogging and running on the serum lipid concentration of the adult Caucasian male. Doctoral Dissertation, University of Southern Mississippi, 1969.

36. Pollock, M.L., et al.: Effects of frequency of training on serum lipids,

cardiovascular function, and body composition. In Franks, B. Don (Ed.): *Exercise and Fitness*, Chicago, Athletic Institute, 1969, p. 161.

37. Konttinen, A.: Frysinen Akstiviteeti ja Seerumia Lipidit. *Sotiaslaatietillinen Aikakauslchti, 35:*169, 1960.

38. Pohndorf, R.H.: Improvements in physical fitness on two middle-aged adults. Doctoral Dissertation, University of Illinois, 1957.

39. Metivier, J.G.: The effects of five different physical exercise programs on the blood serum cholesterol of adult women. Doctoral Dissertation, University of Illinois, 1960.

40. Calvy, G.L., Cady, L.D., Mufson, M.A., Nierman, J., and Gertler, M.M.: Serum lipids and enzymes. Their levels after high-caloric, high-fat intake and vigorous exercise regimen in marine corps recruit personnel. *JAMA, 183:*1-4, 1963.

41. Holloszy, J.O., Skinner, J.S., and Toto, G.: Effects of a six-month program of endurance exercise on the serum lipids of middle-aged men. *Am J Cardiol, 14:*753-760, 1964.

42. Karvonen, M.W.: Effects of vigorous exercise on the heart. In Rosenbaum, F.F., and Belknap, E.L. (Eds.): *Work and the Heart.* New York, Paul B. Hoebner, Inc., 1959, p. 190.

43. Skinner, J.S.: The effect of an endurance exercise program on the serum lipids of middle-aged men. Doctoral Dissertation, University of Illinois, 1963.

44. Olson, H.W.: The effect of supervised exercise program on the blood cholesterol of middle-aged men. *Physical Education, 15:*135, 1958.

45. Brumbach, W.B.: Changes in the serum cholesterol levels of male college students who participated in vigorous physical exercise program. Doctoral Dissertation, University of Oregon, 1959.

46. Zauner, C.W., and Swenson, E.W.: Physical training performance in relation to blood lipid levels and pulmonary function. *Am Correct Ther J, 21:*159, 1967.

47. Rochelle, R.: Blood plasma cholesterol changes during a physical training program. *Res Am Assoc Health Phys Educ, 32:*538, 1961.

48. Romanova, D., and Barbarin, P.: The influence of physical exercises on the content of serum protein, lipoprotein and total cholesterol in persons of middle and elderly age with symptoms of atherosclerosis. *Kardiologiia, 1:*36, 1961.

49. Mirkin, G.: Labile serum cholesterol values. *N Engl J Med, 279:*1001, 1968.

50. Wood, P.D., Klein, H., Lewis, S., et al.: Plasma lipoprotein concentrations in middle-aged male runners (Abstr). *Circulation, (Suppl III), 49* and *50:*111-115, 1974.

51. Rhoads, G.G., Gulbrandsen, C.L., and Kagan, A: Serum lipoproteins and coronary heart disease in a population study of Hawaii Japanese men. *N Engl J Med, 294:*293, 1976.

52. Castelli, W.P., Doyle, J.T., Gordon, T., et al.: HDL cholesterol and other lipids in coronary heart disease. *Circulation, 55:*767-772, 1977.
53. Oscai, L.B., Patterson, J.A., Bogard, D.L., et al.: Normalization of serum triglycerides and lipoprotein electrophoretic patterns by exercise. *Am J Cardiol, 30:*775-780, 1972.
54. Nikkila, E.A., and Konttinen, A.: Effect of physical activity on postprandial levels of fats in serum. *Lancet, 1:*1151-1154, 1962.
55. Cohen, H., and Goldberg, C.: Effect of physical exercise on alimentary lipaemia. *Br Med J, 5197:*509-511, 1960.
56. Lampman, R.M., Santinga, J.T., Hodge, M.F., et al.: Comparative effects of physical training and diet in normalizing serum lipids in men with type IV hyperlipoproteinemia. *Circulation, 55:*652-658, 1977.
57. Varnauskas, E., Bergman, H., and Houk, P.: Haemodynamic effects of physical training in coronary patients. *Lancet, 2:*8-12, 1966.
58. Goode, R.C., Firstbrook, J.B., and Shephard, R.J.: Effects of exercise and cholesterol-free diet on human serum lipids. *Can J Physiol Pharmacol, 44:*575-580, 1966.
59. Taylor, H.L.: Occupational factors in the study of coronary heart disease and physical activity. *Can Med Assoc J, 96:*825-831, 1967.
60. Kang, B.S., Song, S.J., Suh, C.S., et al.: Changes in body temperature and basal metabolic rate. *Am J Appl Physical, 18:*483-488, 1963.
61. Miall, W.E., and Oldham, P.D.: Factors influencing arterial blood pressure in the general population. *Clin Sci, 17:*409-444, 1958.
62. Karvonen, M.J., Rantaharun, P.M., Orma, S., et al.: Cardiovascular studies on lumberjacks. *J Occup Med, 3:*49-53, 1961.
63. Morris, J.N.: Epidemiology and cardiovascular disease of middle age: Part II. *Mod Concepts Cardiovasc Dis, 30:*633-638, 1960.
64. Keys, A., Aravanis, C., Blackburn, H.W., et al.: Epidemiological studies related to coronary heart disease: Characteristics of men aged 40-59 in Seven Countries. *Acta Med Scand, Suppl,* 460, 1966.
65. Chiang, B.N., Alexander, E.R., Bruce, R.A., et al.: Physical characteristics and exercise performance of pedicab and upper socioeconomic classes of middle-aged Chinese men. *Am Heart J, 76:*760-768, 1968.
66. Doan, A.E., Peterson, D.R., Blackman, J.R., et al.: Myocardial ischemia after maximal exercise in healthy men. *Am J Cardiol, 17:*9-19, 1966.
67. Berkson, D.M., Stamler, J., Lindberg, H.A., et al.: Socioeconomic correlates of atherosclerotic and hypertensive heart disease. *Ann NY Acad Sci, 84:*835-850, 1960.
68. Raab, W., and Krzywanek, H.J.: Cardiovascular sympathetic tone and stress response related to personality patterns and exercise habits. *Am J Cardiol, 16:*42-53, 1965.
69. Rose, G.: Physical activity and coronary heart disease. *Proc R Soc Med, 62:*1183-1188, 1969.
70. Montoye, H.J., Metzner, H.L., Keller, J.B., et al.: Habitual physical activity and blood pressure. *Med Sci Sports, 4:*175-181, Winter, 1972.

71. Harris, W.E., Bowerman, W., McFadden, R.B., et al.: Jogging, An adult exercise program. *JAMA, 201:*759-761, 1967.
72. Boyer, J.L., and Kasch, F.W.: Exercise therapy in hypertensive men. *JAMA, 211:*1668-1671, 1970.
73. Mellerowicz, H.: Vergleichende Untersuchungen uber das Oknomie-prinvip in Arbeit and Leistung des trainierten Kreislaufs and seine Bedeutung fur die preventive and rehabilitive Medizi. *Arch Kreislauf-forsch, 24:*70, 1956.
74. Naughton, J., Shanbour, K., Armstrong, R., McCoy, J., and Lategola, M.T.: Cardiovascular responses to exercise following myocardial infarction. *Arch Int Med* (Chicago), *117:*541-545, 1966.
75. Frick, M.H., and Katila, M.: Hemodynamic consequences of physical training after myocardial infarction. *Circulation, 37:*192-202, 1968.
76. Fox, S.M. III, and Skinner, J.S.: Physical activity and cardiovascular health. *Am J Cardiol, 14:*731-746, 1964.
77. Pyorala, K., Karava, R., Punsar, S., et al.: A controlled study of the effects of 18 months physical training in sedentary middle-aged men with high indexes of risk relative to coronary heart disease. In Larsen, O. Andree, and Malmborg, R.D. (Eds.): *Coronary Heart Disease and Physical Fitness.* University Park Press Munksgaard, 1971, p. 261.
78. Kentala, E.: Physical fitness and feasibility of physical rehabilitation after myocardial infarctions in men of working age. *Ann Clin Res, 4:Suppl 9:*1-84, 1972.
79. Levine, S.A., Gordon, B., and Derick, C.L.: Some changes in the chemical constituents of the blood following a marathon race with special reference to the development of hypoglycemia. *JAMA, 82:*1778-1779, 1924.
80. Blotner, H.: Effect of prolonged physical inactivity on tolerance of sugar. *Arch Intern Med, 75:*39-44, 1945.
81. Davidson, P.C., Shane, S.R., and Albrink, M.J.: Decreased glucose tolerance following a physical conditioning program. *Circulation, 34:Suppl 3:*7, 1966.
82. Mouratoff, G.J., and Scott, E.M.: Diabetes mellitus in Eskimos after a decade. *JAMA, 226:*1345-1346.
83. Mayer, J.: Some aspects of the problem of regulation of food intake and obesity. *N Engl J Med, 274:*662-673, 1966.
84. Nelson, R.A., Anderson, L.F., Gastineau, C.F., et al.: Physiology and natural history of obesity. *JAMA, 223:*627-630, 1973.
85. Frick, M.H.: The effect of physical training in manifest ischemic heart disease. *Circulation, 40:*433-435, 1969.
86. Skinner, J.S., Holloszy, J.O., and Cureton, T.K.: Effects of a program of endurance exercises on physical work. *Am J Cardiol, 14:*747-752, 1964.
87. Rechnitzer, P.A., Yuhasz, M.S., Pickard, H.A., et al.: Effects of 24-week exercise program on normal adults and patients with previous myocardial infarction. *Br Med J, 1:*734-735, 1967.

88. Morris, J.N., Heady, J.A., Raffle, P.A.B., et al.: Coronary heart disease and physical activity of work. *Lancet, 2:*1053-1057, 1953.
89. Boileau, R.A., Buskirk, E.R., Horstman, D.H., et al.: Body composition changes in obese and lean men during physical conditioning. *Med Sci Sports, 3:*183-189, 1971.
90. McPherson, B.D., Paivo, A., Yuhasz, M.S., et al.: Psychological effects of an exercise program for post-infarction and normal adult men. *J Sports Med, 7:*3, 1967.
91. Ismail, A.H., and Trachtman, L.E.: Jogging the imagination. *Psychology Today, 7:*79-82, 1973.
92. Hellerstein, H.K.: Exercise therapy in coronary disease. *Bull NY Acad Med, 44:*1028-1047, 1968.
93. Naughton, J., Bruhn, J.G., and Lategola, M.T.: Effects of physical training on physiological and behavioral characteristics of cardiac patients. *Arch Phys Med, 49:*131, 1968.
94. Hellerstein, H.K., and Friedman, E.H.: Sexual activity and the post coronary patient. *Medical Aspects of Human Sexual, 3:*70, 1969.
95. Hellerstein, H.K., and Friedman, E.H.: Sexual activity and the postcoronary patient. *Arch Intern Med, 125:*987-999, 1970.
96. Baekeland, F.: Exercise deprivation. *Arch Gen Psychiat, 22:*365-369, 1970.
97. Chiang, B.N., Perlman, L.V., Ostrander, L.D., and Epstein, F.H.: Relationship of premature systoles to coronary heart disease and sudden death in the Tecumseh epidemiologic studies. *Ann Intern Med, 70:*1159-1166, 1969.
98. Rotman, M., Colvard, M.D., Ruskin, J., et al.: Nonspecific T-wave changes. *Arch Intern Med, 130:*895-897, 1972.
99. Kannel, W.B., Gordon, T., Castelli, W.P., et al.: Electrocardiographic left ventricular hypertrophy and risk of coronary heart disease. *Ann Intern Med, 72:*813-822, 1970.
100. Smith, W.G., Cullen, K.G., and Thorburn, I.O.: Electrocardiograms of marathon runners in 1962 Commonwealth games. *Br Heart J, 26:*469-476, 1964.
101. Spann, J.F., Jr., Mason, D.T., and Zelis, R.F.: Recent advances in the understanding of congestive heart failure. *Mod Concepts Cardiovasc Dis, 39:*73-78, 1970.
102. Hellerstein, H.K., Hirsch, E.Z., and Cumber, W., et al.: Reconditioning of the coronary patient: A preliminary report. In Likoff, W., and Moyer, J.G. (Eds.): *Coronary Heart Disease.* New York, Grune & Stratton, 1963, pp. 448-454.
103. Blackburn, H.W., Taylor, H.L., and Keys, A.: Prognostic significance of the postexercise electrocardiogram: Risk factors held constant. *Am J Cardiol, 25:*85, 1970.
104. Burt, J.J., et al.: The effects of exercise on the coagulation-fibrinolysis equilibrium. U.S. Naval Medical Field Research Laboratory, Camp LeJune, N.C., 1962.

105. MacDonald, G.A., and Fullerton, H.W.: Effects of physical activity on increased coagulation of blood after ingesting high-fat meal. *Lancet,* 2:1006, 1971.

106. Warnock, N.H., et al.: Effects of exercise on blood coagulation time and atherosclerosis of cholesterol-fed cockerels. *Circ Res, 5:*478, 1957.

107. Iatridis, S.G., and Ferguson, J.H.: Effects of physical exercise on blood clotting and fibrinolysis. *J Appl Physiol, 18:*337-344, 1963.

108. Egeberg, O.: The effect of exercise on the blood clotting system. *Scand J Clin Lab Invest, 15:*8-13, 1963.

109. MacDonald, G.A., and Fullerton, H.W.: Comparison of animal and vegetable fats in increasing blood coagulability. *Lancet, 2:*598-599, 1958.

110. Guest, M.M., and Celander, D.R.: Fibrinolytic activity in exercise. *Physiologist, 3:*69, 1960.

111. Astrup, T., and Brakman, P.: Responders and non-responders in exercise-induced blood fibrinolysis. In Larsen, O.A., and Malmborg, R.D. (Ed.): *Coronary Heart Disease and Physical Fitness.* Baltimore, University Park Press, 1971, p. 130.

112. Danlievicious, Z.: Fibrinolytic activity, obesity, and coronary heart disease (Editorial). *JAMA, 224:*1288, 1973.

113. Khanna, P.K., Seth, H.N., Balasubramanian, V., et al.: Effect of submaximal exercise on fibrinolytic activity in ischaemic heart disease. *Br Heart J, 37:*1273-1276, 1975.

114. Redwood, D.R., Rosing, D.R., and Epstein, S.E.: Circulatory and symptomatic effects of physical training in patients with coronary-artery disease and angina pectoris. *N Engl J Med, 286:*959-965, 1972.

115. Buzina, R., and Keys, A.: Blood coagulation after a fat meal. *Circulation, 14:*854-858, 1956.

116. McDonald, L., and Edgill, M.: Coagulability of the blood in ischemic heart disease. *Lancet, 2:*457-460, 1957.

117. Montoye, H.J., Howard, G.E., and Wood, J.H.: Observations of some hemochemical and anthropometric measurements in athletes. *J Sports Med, 7:*35-44, 1967.

118. Bosco, J.S., Greenleaf, J.E., and Kaye, R.L.: Reduction of serum uric acid in young men during physical training. *Am J Cardiol, 25:*46-52, 1970.

119. Dawber, T.R.: Identification of excess cardiovascular risk. A practical approach. *Minn Med, 52:*1217-1221, 1969.

120. Rechnitzer, P.A., Yuhasz, M.S., Pickard, H.A., et al.: The effects of a graduated exercise program on patients with previous myocardial infarction. *Can Med Assoc J, 92:*858-860, 1965.

121. Clausen, J.P., Larse, N.O.A., and Trap-Jensen, J.: Physical training in the management of coronary artery disease. *Circulation, 40:*143-154, 1969.

122. Lefcoe, N.M., and Paterson, N.A.M.: Adjunct therapy in chronic obstructive pulmonary disease. *Am J Med, 54:*343-349, 1973.
123. Barach, A.L., and Petty, T.L.: Is chronic obstructive lung disease improved by physical exercise? (Editorial). *JAMA, 234:*854-855, 1975.
124. Cooper, K.H., Pollock, M.L., Martin, R.L., et al.: Physical fitness levels vs selected coronary risk factors. *JAMA, 236:*166-169, 1976.

Chapter 5

EXERCISE STRESS TESTING—A REVIEW

HISTORICAL ASPECTS

Feil and Siegel[1] were perhaps the first to point out the electrocardiographic changes of exercise-induced angina. Their study was reported in 1928, fourteen years after Doctor Paul Dudley White brought his first electrocardiographic apparatus to this country from Europe. There was little enthusiasm for using exercise to evaluate cardiac performance until the following year (1929), when Master and Oppenheimer[2] described a "simple tolerance test for circulatory efficiency." This test, later to be known throughout the world as the Master 2-step test, paved the way for future studies and advances in the field of exercise testing. As early as 1932, Goldhammer and Scherf[3] were able to effectively induce electrocardiographic changes in over half of their patients with angina pectoris.

The past forty years have witnessed the evolution of exercise testing from the simple step test approach to some involving interrupted or continuous bicycle ergometry and treadmill activity. The former has achieved tremendous popularity in various parts of Europe, particularly in the Scandanavian countries. This has largely been attributed to the prolific work and writing of Astrand.[4] In the United States, many medical centers are relying on treadmill testing with oxygen collection at the peak workload. The bicycle ergometer has been less popular, probably due to the fact that Americans are less accustomed to bicycle activity than their European counterparts. The advantages of the bicycle and the treadmill lie in the feasibility of greater workloads, constant electrocardiographic monitoring during and postexercise, and the collection of expired air to quantitate oxygen uptake and ventilation. The disadvantages

72

include equipment costs and lack of a standard-
ized exercise protocol, as many centers use their own regimen.

The reasons for stress testing are multiple. Perhaps the main
reason in the field of cardiology is the search for electrocardiographic signs of subtle coronary disease in the form of intra– and
post-exercise-induced S-T segment depression. One also looks
for exercise-related cardiac rhythm disorders and the repro-
duction of chest symptoms during the stress of exercise,
particularly those symptoms which are hard to assess by history
alone. Still another reason for exercise testing is to quantitate the
tolerance for exercise. At times, it is difficult by history alone to
judge a patient's ability to perform physical work. By directly
observing the patient with valvular or other forms of heart
disease on the bicycle or the treadmill, one can get a better idea
of his functional classification. Exercise testing also gives one a
means of measuring the response to a certain type of therapy, be
it in the form of a drug, an open-heart operation, or an exercise
program. The physiologist has long used exercise testing to
quantitate the aerobic capacity of man by analysis of oxygen
uptake during peak workloads. One of the first to do such
studies using treadmill techniques was Edward Smith in the
mid-1800s.[5]

METHODS OF TESTING

The Master 2-step

What form of testing is applicable to the practicing physician?
The Master 2-step[6] is by far the simplest, cheapest, and safest of
all. For a patient with no cardiac symptoms, the presence of a
physician in the exercise room itself is not necessary (although
s/he should be within twenty feet of the exercise room). Cohen et
al.[7] feel that this test is indicated in the initial evaluation of the
patient. If the "augmented" test regimen (15% more steps than
the basic 2-step test) is negative or uninterpretable, one can then
move on to bicycle or treadmill testing. Although the pulse rate
during Master testing is said to reach 74 percent of the

age-adjusted maximum rate, Cohen et al.[7] considered 20 percent of their tests on 305 patients "uninterpretable" because the pulse rates were less than 110 beats per minute.

Since time is a factor not only to the patient but also to the physician and the technician, a single initial test that is safe and vigorous enough is warranted. For this reason, we prefer the treadmill. The variety of available testing protocols make it as applicable to the trained athlete as it is to the severely limited cardiac patient.

Treadmill Testing: Georgia Baptist Hospital

At our hospital, we employ a regimen in which the speed is fixed at 2 mph and the treadmill slope is increased 2½ percent every two and one-half minutes, starting from the level (Table 5-I). We find the speed to be easily tolerated by most subjects and that there is less emotional overlay in testing if the speed is not progressively increased along with the slope. Patients without definite cardiac disease are urged to walk to the point of heart rate elevation to approximately 85 percent of the normal maximal rate adjusted for the patient's age. Additional end points include severe fatigue or dyspnea, anginal pain,

TABLE 5-I

GEORGIA BAPTIST PROTOCOL FOR TREADMILL STRESS TESTING

Stage	Speed (mph)	Grade (%)	Duration (min)	Total Time Elapsed (min)
1	2	0	2.5	2.5
2	2	2.5	2.5	5.0
3	2	5.0	2.5	7.5
4	2	7.5	2.5	10.0
5	2	10.0	2.5	12.5
6	2	12.5	2.5	15.0
7	2	15.0	2.5	17.5
8	2	17.5	2.5	20.0
9	2	20.0	2.5	22.5
10	2	22.5	2.5	25.0

arrhythmias, S-T segment depression greater than 2.0 mm for duration of .08 seconds, or systolic blood pressure elevation to 240 mm Hg. A physician or physician's assistant and nurse are in constant communication with the patient, and the patient is urged to describe any functional and/or physical symptoms that develop as the testing progresses. At the end of the test, the patient is instructed to sit in a chair on the treadmill while immediate, one–, two–, and three-minute postexercise blood pressure recordings and rhythm strips are made. If there are any symptoms or signs of near-syncope, dizziness, or postural hypotension, the subject is placed in a supine position until stable. A direct current defibrillator as well as emergency cardiac drugs are available in the room.

Over the past eighteen months, 250 patients have been evaluated by this method.[8] These include both outpatients and inpatients who were referred by their private physicians. Reasons for referral included chest discomfort (152 patients), clinical suspicion of ischemic heart disease based upon the presence of multiple coronary risk factors (48 patients), abnormal electrocardiograms (23 patients), history of arrhythmias (9 patients), and a variety of symptoms including dizziness, syncope, and dyspnea (18 patients). The ages ranged from 14 to 75 years, with the average age of 47.6 years. There were 176 male patients and 74 female patients; 6 subjects were black. The range of test time duration was 45 seconds to 31 minutes, the average being 14.3 minutes. The range of maximum heart rate attained was from 80 beats per minute to 180 beats per minute, with an average for the entire group of 142.4 beats per minute.

Testing results revealed that 27 of 250 patients (10.8%) had S-T segment depression of 0.5 mm or more and were considered to have abnormal results highly suggestive of, or compatible with, ischemic heart disease. Thirty-two of 240 patients (12.8%) had the development of, or an increase in, premature ventricular beats, and 20 of 250 patients (8.0%) developed supraventricular arrhythmias (premature atrial beats, premature nodal beats, or supraventricular tachycardia). Of this group of 250 patients, 2 (with histories of undocumented tachycardia) developed paroxysmal atrial tachycardia during exercise to document the arrhythmia; another, with a previous supraventricular tachycardia that required cardioversion, developed frequent premature nodal beats during exercise to further document a suspected abnormality to explain his tachyarrhythmia.

Further evaluation of the resting electrocardiogram in the 250 patients revealed that 17 of the 176 male patients (9.6%) and 22 of the 75 females (29.7%) had nonspecific S-T segment and T wave abnormalities as interpreted by two independent electrocardiographers. This difference in incidence (increase in the females) is significant statistically at the $p < .01$ level of probability. Of these patients with abnormal resting electrocardiograms (S-T segment and T wave variations), 17 of 22 males (77.3%) and 13 of 17 females (76.4%) had positive ischemic changes on exercise testing, compared to the male patients in whom only 2 of 17 (11.8%) had positive ischemic changes with exercise testing. Of the 20 patients on digitalis therapy, 3 had positive tests for ischemic heart disease. (These 3 tests, however, had to be considered false positive because of the inherent difficulty in interpreting electrocardiograms when digitalis effect was present.) Of these 3 patients, however, 2 had classical symptoms of angina pectoris at the time of the ischemic electrocardiographic changes. Of the other 17 patients on digitalis therapy, 1 developed ventricular premature beats with exercise; none of these had angina pectoris or electrocardiographic changes.

No one in the group developed hypertension (above 240 mm Hg systolic), syncope, or extreme dizziness. No one fell, although 1 emotionally labile subject stepped off the treadmill unexpectedly. The postexercise recovery periods were uneventful.

Follow-up in this group of 250 patients was made by personal contact with the private physician and by reviewing their records for an eighteen-month period following exercise testing. These results are seen in Table 5-II. Of the 152 subjects referred for chest pain of undetermined cause, 100 (65%) returned to work. Ten of these subjects returning to work or to a more active physical status had abnormal exertional responses suggestive of ischemic heart disease; of these, 7 were treated with coronary vasodilators. Of the other 52 patients referred for undiagnosed chest discomfort, 12 had decreased activity and each of these 12 had abnormal tests for ischemic heart disease. Forty patients had no follow-up after eighteen months.

Of the 52 subjects in whom arrhythmias developed or increased during testing, only 7 (13%) received specific treatment. However, all but 3 of the 52 returned to more activity with no clinical problems.

The Bruce Method of Treadmill Testing

In the Preventive Cardiology Clinic, we employ the Bruce method[9] of multistage treadmill testing since we deal primarily with the cardiopulmonary fitness evaluation of young executives, airline pilots, and amateur and professional athletes. The Bruce method (Table 5-III) begins at a slope of 10 percent and a speed of 1.7 miles per hour. At three-minute intervals, the slope is increased by 2 percent increments and the speed by 0.8 to 0.9 mph increments. Few nonathletes progress beyond the fourth stage (twelve minutes).

Bruce and colleagues[10] have recently reported the results of the third annual test of maximal exercise in 186 middle-aged men who were drawn from physical education classes, the

TABLE 5-II
FOLLOW-UP DATA ON 250 SUBJECTS UNDERGOING SUBMAXIMAL
TREADMILL EXERCISE TESTING AT GEORGIA BAPTIST HOSPITAL

Reason for Referral	Patients returning to increased activity	Patients with no change or decreased activity	Patients with no follow-up
Undiagnosed chest discomfort	100	12	40
High incidence of risk factors	39	3	6
Abnormal resting ECG	4	1	18
Syncope, dyspnea, dizziness	6	4	8
Arrhythmias	7	1	1

TABLE 5-III

THE BRUCE PROTOCOL FOR TREADMILL STRESS TESTING

Stage	Speed (mph)	Grade (%)	Duration (min)	Total Time Elapsed (min)
1	1.7	10	3	3
2	2.5	12	3	6
3	3.4	14	3	9
4	4.2	16	3	12
5	5.0	18	3	15
6	5.5	20	3	18
7	6.0	22	3	21

Seattle YMCA, and the Boeing Aircraft Company. Of these, 155 men (83.4%) had negative electrocardiographic responses to exercise on three successive tests, using 1.0 mm of S-T segment depression as the criteria for any abnormal test. Ten men (5.3%) had three successive positive tests for ischemia. Of the remaining 21 men (11.3%), the results were variable. Seven with initially negative tests subsequently became positive on retesting. Six men were positive on two successive tests, only to become negative on the third. Seven men were negative on first testing, positive on the second testing, and reverted back to negative again on the third annual treadmill test. Such changes may represent reversibility of myocardial ischemia or random variations in the test procedure. Bruce found that interobserver differences in exercise electrocardiogram interpretation occurred in 5 percent of the tracings, adding another variable to contend with.

The Spangler-Fox Method of Treadmill Testing

Spangler et al.[11] devised a treadmill exercise test protocol for screening high risk population groups. The test was devised with the goal of achieving near-maximal heart rates without inducing physical exhaustion. The protocol involves alterations of both treadmill speed and slope, as seen in Table 5-IV.

In this study, 362 asymptomatic men were tested by the above method after first having performed a double Master 2-step test. The men ranged in age from twenty-eight to sixty-six years, with a mean age of forty-four years. Only 3 men were unable to complete the test because of fatigue. Three others were stopped because of positive S-T segment changes, 8 because of frequent premature ventricular beats, and 1 because of paroxysmal atrial tachycardia. For men in the thirty– to thirty-four-year-old age group, the mean peak heart rate was 167 beats per minute or 91 percent of the predicted maximum. For the fifty-five– to fifty-nine-year-old age group, the mean peak heart rate during exercise was 162 beats per minute, which was 99 percent of the predicted maximum. Five of the 362 men (1.3%) had unequivocally positive tests, while 8 others (2.2%) had borderline positive tests during or postexercise. Two of the men with positive exercise tests had normal postexercise tracings and would have been undiagnosed without the benefit of continuous electrocardiographic monitoring. The mean peak heart rate during Master 2-step testing was 124 beats per minute, a rate achieved at the end of only the third stage of treadmill testing.

One advantage of the Spangler-Fox test is that patients could complete the six stages without having to jog, thereby causing less monitor-lead artifact from running movements.

The Ellestad Method of Treadmill Testing

Using a fixed treadmill machine with variable speeds (Table 5-V), Ellestad and associates[12] have performed maximal stress tests on 4,028 patients.

No deaths occurred while testing by this method, although there were 2 instances of nonfatal myocardial infarctions temporally related to the test and 9 instances of transient ventricular tachycardia. Only 1 of the latter required specific therapy.

Criteria for a positive test for ischemia include the following:
1. An S-T segment depression 2 mm below the isoelectric line lasting at least 0.08 seconds from the J-point.

TABLE 5-IV
THE SPANGLER-FOX PROTOCOL FOR TREADMILL STRESS TESTING

Stage	Speed (mph)	Grade (%)	Duration (min)	Total Time Elapsed (min)
1	1.5	0	2	2
2	3.0	0	1	3
3	3.0	4	3	6
4	3.0	8	3	9
5	3.0	12	3	12
6	3.0	16	3	15

TABLE 5-V
THE ELLESTAD PROTOCOL FOR TREADMILL STRESS TESTING

Stage	Speed (mph)	Grade (%)	Duration (min)	Total Time Elapsed (min)
1	1.7	10	3	3
2	3.0	10	2	5
3	4.0	10	2	7
4	5.0	10	3	10

2. An upsloping S-T segment which is at least 2 mm below the isoelectric line at a point 0.08 seconds after the J-point. Of 284 apparently normal executives who were tested on the treadmill, 30 (11%) had S-T segment changes of ischemia and 10 (3 to 5%) had equivocal changes.

Of 236 other patients with positive exercise tests for ischemia, only 37 percent developed accompanying chest pain.

In a recent report, Ellestad and Wan[13] described the findings in 2700 subjects who underwent maximal stress testing. Of the subjects with positive responses for ischemia (≥ 1.5 mm of S-T depression), the annual incidence of new coronary events was 9.5 percent, as compared to only 1.7 percent in the negative responders. This annual incidence rose to 15 percent if one considered tests that became positive for ischemia within the first three minutes of exercise (at a work load of ≤ 4 METS). Patients with a history of a prior myocardial infarction and a positive exercise test for ischemia had twice the incidence of new coronary events as those with no prior infarction and an abnormal stress test. Increased risk of new coronary events existed in the presence of a slower-than-expected pulse rate response to exercise, an equivocal test for ischemia (0.5-1.4 mm S-T depression), and frequent or multiform ventricular premature beats in the test. Within a four-year follow-up period after a positive exercise test in this patient population, 40 percent experienced either progression of angina pectoris, myocardial infarction, or death. In the positive responders with a history of a prior myocardial infarction, the incidence of these events was 70 percent over four years.

The reproducibility of this test was impressive in a group of 25 men, ages forty to sixty-eight years, who were retested within one to ninety days. As regards treadmill duration time, 90 percent of the men finished the repeat test with less than one minute variation from the initial test. Of the 25 men, 22 had clinical coronary heart disease, and all had positive initial tests for ischemia. On the retest, 68 percent of the men developed ischemic S-T segment changes at the identical time interval as on the initial test, and 27 percent developed ischemic S-T segment changes within one minute of the initial test onset.

The Modified Balke-Ware Treadmill Test

In this protocol,[14] the speed is constant at 3.3 mph. The treadmill is level to begin with, and the grade is increased 1 percent each minute. After twenty-five minutes of test duration, the speed is increased 0.2 mph every minute. In the past six years, 15,136 such tests have been conducted by Cooper and colleagues (in Dallas), with 82.9 percent being normal, 7.8 percent equivocal, and 9.3 percent abnormal. There were 4 cardiovascular complications (2 episodes of myocardial infarction and 2 of ventricular fibrillation) during the testing, but no deaths occurred. This test is obviously safe and provides a very gradual increment in work load between each stage. The length of the test is a disadvantage to a busy clinician, as is the need to change the slope every minute.

The USAFSAM Treadmill Test

Froelicher and associates[42] have used this protocol in testing Air Force personnel. The speed is constant at 3.3 mph, with the slope increasing by 5 percent (starting on the level) every three minutes.

The increment in oxygen costs, as one progresses from stage to stage, is more uniform in this protocol than in the Bruce test.

The National Exercise Project Treadmill Test

Naughton, Fox, and Hellerstein have recently devised a treadmill protocol (Table 5-VI) which is to be used in the HEW controlled exercise study on post-myocardial-infarction patients. The protocol has one major advantage in that each stage of the test is one MET unit greater than the previous stage, allowing for easy conversion of treadmill work performance into MET unit values. Disadvantages include the lack of reported studies using this method for a busy clinic practice.

Each stage of the various tests is quantitated as to estimated oxygen uptake and MET units of work. Clinical status and functional classifications are also provided. This chart is

TABLE 5-VI
THE NATIONAL EXERCISE PROJECT PROTOCOL FOR TREADMILL
STRESS TESTING*

Stage	Speed (mph)	Grade (%)	Duration (minutes)	MET (unit)	Physiological Functional Class
1	2.0	0	3	2	III
2	2.0	3.5	3	3	
3	2.0	7.5	3	4	II
4	2.0	10.5	3	5	
5	2.0	14.0	3	6	
6	2.0	17.5	3	7	I
7	3.0	12.5	3	8	
8	3.0	15.0	3	9	
9	3.0	17.5	3	10	
10	3.0	10.4	3	11	

* Naughton, Hellerstein, Fox

extremely useful in comparing results from laboratories who use different methods of testing. For those who cannot afford the luxury of oxygen analysis equipment, it provides a means of estimating the oxygen uptake for a given individual.

Comparison of Step and Treadmill Energy Costs

Fox et al.[15] have published a chart comparing the approximate energy requirement of some step test and treadmill protocols.

Exercise Stress Testing Using the Bicycle Ergometer

The Europeans have long favored the bicycle ergometer as an instrument for evaluating physical work capacity. They cite certain advantages such as the low cost, lack of need of electrical power, and relative immobility of the chest and arms (permitting artifact-free exercise electrocardiograms). Astrand[16] notes that within certain limitations, the mechanical efficiency of the ergometer is independent of body weight. Furthermore, he points out that the oxygen uptake can be predicted with greater accuracy than on any other type of exercise test.[17] A protocol for bicycle ergometric testing is shown in Table 5-VII, along with the predicted oxygen uptake for each stage. Women generally begin at a load of 300 kpm/minute, while men begin at a setting

TABLE 5-VII
PROTOCOL FOR BICYCLE ERGOMETER TESTING

Men Stage	Work load (kpm/min)	Time (min)	Predicted O₂ uptake (L/min)	Women Stage	Work load (kpm/min)	Time (min)	Predicted O₂ uptake (L/min)
1	600	0–6	1.5	1	300	0–6	0.9
2	900	6–12	2.1	2	450	6–12	1.2
3	1200	12–18	2.8	3	600	12–18	1.5
				4	750	18–24	1.8

kpm = kilopond meter
L/min = liters per minute

of 600 kpm/minute. Each stage is six minutes long; at the end of each stage, the workload is increased by 150 kpm/minute for women and 300 kpm/minute for men.

We prefer the treadmill device, particularly for maximal stress testing, since higher values of oxygen uptake can be achieved before leg fatigue and exhaustion set in. Americans are less familiar with bicycle riding than their European counterparts and often have difficulty keeping up with the metronome. We have not had difficulty in obtaining optimal exercise electrocardiograms when proper attention is given to skin preparations and lead attachment. Moreover, we are impressed with the data of Bruce et al.,[18] in which high correlations were shown between the duration of treadmill test time and the predicted oxygen uptake. Pollock et al.[19] likewise found good correlation between treadmill time and maximal oxygen consumption for the Bruce, Ellestad, and Balke tests (r values of 0.88, 0.90, and 0.92 respectively). However, Froelicher et al.[20, 21] exercised 79 men by the Balke protocol and 77 by the Bruce method and concluded that there was no precise correlation between treadmill test time and oxygen uptake.

LEAD SYSTEMS

The lead systems used in most exercise testing centers are of three types: (1) modified or conventional twelve-lead systems, (2) bipolar chest leads, and (3) vector (Frank) lead systems. Most bipolar systems place the positive electrode at the V_5 position. The negative electrode may be placed in variable sites. Some prefer the V_5R position, but others use the high anterior chest region or the right inferior scapular border. The latter is felt by some to offer a vertical component.

Mason et al.[22] use a lead system wherein the right arm electrode is placed in the right subclavicular area and the left leg electrode to the left midclavicular line halfway between the iliac spine and left costal margin. This is the system we prefer. Hellerstein et al.[23] have used a system wherein the right arm electrode is placed on the forehead, the left arm electrode over the ensiform process, the left leg electrode at the V_6 position, the chest lead at the V_4 position, and the right leg at the V_4R position. Redwood and Epstein[24] favor a lead system which combines a CM_5 bipolar lead with a vertical lead (third electrode placed on the sacrum), feeling that inferior wall changes might be detected that otherwise would have been missed on the transverse lead alone.

In comparative studies, Froelicher et al.[25] found that presently accepted criteria for an abnormal S-T segment response to exercise in lead V_5 may not apply to other leads, such as CM_5, nor do J-junctional changes (with upsloping S-T segment) have the same meaning in different leads. These authors caution that CM_5 is less sensitive than V_5 or CC_5 when using standard criteria (≥ 1.0 S-T segment depression) for an abnormal exercise response.

TARGET HEART RATES

For maximal treadmill testing, one can use the 90 percent of maximal target heart rate of Sheffield et al.,[26] the Myrtle Beach guidelines[27] for age-adjusted target heart rates (aiming at 80 to 90 percent maximum aerobic effect—see Table 5-VIII), or the National Exercise and Heart Disease (NEHDP) guidelines. We prefer the latter, striving to get the individual to ≥ 85 percent of maximum (in the absence of sympton-limiting endpoints).

In testing normal middle-aged males, we do not find the Myrtle Beach target rates sufficiently stressful. Most patients in this category are able to progress an additional two to four minutes on the Bruce test before generalized fatigue comes on. By stopping the test at the target heart rate in these persons, one would not get a true reading of oxygen uptake at maximum work. A reason for pushing beyond the 85 percent maximum heart rate level in normal persons is evidenced by the recent report of Cumming.[28] This study subjected 510 men, forty to sixty-five years of age and having no evidence of underlying cardiovascular disease, to maximum stress testing on a bicycle ergometer. Criteria for a positive test included S-T segment

TABLE 5-VIII
TARGET HEART RATES FOR EXERCISE STRESS TESTING

Sheffield Target Rates 90% of Maximal Heart Rate		Myrtle Beach Target Rates 80 to 90% of Maximal Heart Rates		NEHDP	
Age		Age		85%	100%
20	177	20-29	170	165	194
25	175	30-39	160	160	188
30	173	40-49	150	155	182
35	172	50-59	140	150	176
40	170			145	171
45	168			140	165
50	166			135	159
55	164			130	153
60	162				
65	160				
70	158				
75	157				

depression of 1.0 mm or greater with a horizontal or downsloping segment. For those with minor ST-T abnormalities at rest, a further S-T segment depression of at least 1.0 mm during or postexercise was considered a positive response, as was functional S-T segment depression of over 2.0 mm with the ascending slope being either 1.0 mm below the isoelectric point at the onset of the T-wave or having a rate of ascent less than 10 mm/sec. The yield of positive tests in the 510 men was 63 (12%). Of persons under age forty-five, the yield was 4 percent, whereas it was 37 percent in those over age sixty years. Half of the abnormal responses developed after the exercise heart rate had exceeded 85 percent of the maximum heart rate. That is to say that had the test been stopped at the 85 percent maximum target rate, half of the abnormal responses would have been missed. This study, though provocative, needs documentation in other centers.

PREVALENCE AND PREDICTIVE VALUE OF EXERCISE TESTING

In 1931, Wood and Wolferth[29] suggested that electrocardiographic abnormalities which developed after exercise in patients with angina pectoris were an unfavorable omen. Thirty-one years later, Mattingly[30] reported the prognostic value of the Master 2-step test in 871 men, many of whom had symptoms suggestive of coronary heart disease. Of 145 with positive tests, 13.8 percent developed myocardial infarctions within the next three years and 38 percent did so within ten years. Of 726 men with negative Master tests, 1.2 percent developed myocardial infarctions within the next three years and 4.7 percent did so within ten years following the test.

At the Greenbrier Clinic, Brody[31] performed double Master tests on 756 business executives, ranging in age from twenty-three to seventy-four years (mean of fifty-four years). None of the men had a prior history or symptoms suggestive of coronary heart disease. Positive exercise tests (0.5 mm S-T segment depression) were recorded in 23 of the men (3%). Of the latter,

70 percent developed clinical coronary heart disease over a three– to ten-year follow-up period.

Doyle and Kinch[32] performed a prospective epidemiological study with 2,437 men. Like the group above, none of the men had known coronary disease. A twenty-minute treadmill test was used in which the speed was fixed at 3 mph and the grade at 5 percent. The electrocardiogram was obtained immediately postexercise and at the three-minute recovery period; no tracings were made during exercise. All tracings were interpreted by a single reader and subsequently reviewed in a blind fashion with repeatability of 96 percent. Seventy-five of the men (3.6%) had positive exercise tests. Over a five-year period of follow-up, 45 percent of this positive group developed other evidence of coronary disease such as angina pectoris or a myocardial infarction.

Bruce's group (Seattle) evaluated 186 healthy men with maximal treadmill stress tests. The interobserver variation in ECG reading among the four physicians conducting the study was 5 percent. Hence, the concurrence of ECG observations was 95 percent. Ten of the men (5.3%) had consistently positive tests on annual repeats. Twenty-one of the men (11%) exhibited variable responses (13 with initially positive tests reverted to negative on retesting). In the three-year follow-up period, none of those with initially positive tests developed clinical evidence of coronary disease. However, at the five-year period, 13.6 percent of the initial positive responders developed such clinical evidence. Only 1 percent of those who initially had normal maximal treadmill tests developed clinical signs or symptoms of coronary heart disease. This study brings out two important points: (1) The use of a maximal stress test with electrocardiographic monitoring during as well as postexercise did not appreciably increase the yield of positive tests in normal middle-aged men (from 3 to 3.5 percent in Master 2-step testing to 5.3 percent for the Bruce test). However, if one counts the patients in the Bruce study who were positive initially but were negative on retesting, the initial yield by this method would be 11 percent. (2) In view of the 13 men who converted from a positive to a negative result on retesting, this phenomena needs to be looked for in all future studies in which prognostic implications are made. In other words, the prognosis in those with variable test results needs to be compared with those who are either consistently negative or consistently positive.

In the Seattle Heart Watch Project, Bruce et al.[33] found horizontal or downsloping S-T segment depression with exercise in 16.8 percent of 1,275 apparently healthy men. This increased to 28.1 percent if one included those with upsloping S-T segment depression. Of 97 patients with a prior myocardial infarction, 18.9 percent had an abnormal S-T segment response to exercise.

Beard et al.[34] performed double Master 2-step tests on 1,375 persons (1169 men and 206 women). Although none of the group had a classical history of angina pectoris, 42 percent had some form of nonspecific chest pain; hence, they cannot be considered as completely normal. Of the total group, 106 (8%) had positive Master tests. During an average follow-up period of thirty months 60 percent of the positive responders developed coronary heart disease by clinical criteria, 10 percent died, and the remaining 30 percent were essentially well. Of the 1,269 persons (92%) with negative stress tests, only 2 percent developed coronary heart disease during the follow-up period and only 1 percent died.

Kattus et al.[35] studied 314 male insurance underwriters, some of whom had symptoms suggestive of ischemic heart disease. A near-maximal treadmill test was utilized. Thirty men (9.5%) had positive stress tests, and the latter finding showed significant correlation with the serum cholesterol level and the nondiagnostic abnormalities on the resting electrocardiogram. There were no significant differences between the positive and negative treadmill responders regarding smoking habits, level of blood pressure, degree of physical inactivity, and family history of coronary disease. Over a 2.5-year follow-up period, 3 of the 30 positive responders developed a nonfatal myocardial infarction, angina pectoris, or had significant abnormalities on coronary arteriography.

In the Seven Countries study, Blackburn et al.[36] reported post-step-test electrocardiograms on 12,770 men, ages forty to fifty-nine years. Persons with ischemic S-T segment responses had a threefold risk of developing manifest coronary heart disease within five years, even when other risk factors were held constant by means of the multiple logistics equation.

Robb and Marks[37] obtained Master 2-step tests on 2,224 men, half of whom had a history of chest pain but only 3.6 percent of whom gave a classical story for angina pectoris. The age range was forty to sixty-five years. Thirteen and one-half percent of the men had positive electrocardiographic responses, (using the extreme criteria of 0.1 mm horizontal or downsloping S-T segment depression, persisting for 0.08 seconds duration). In a follow-up period that extended to fifteen years and averaged 5.6 years, the mortality rate could be correlated to the degree of S-T segment depression as follows:

S-T Segment Depression	*Mortality*
0.1—0.9 mm	↑ 2.5 times
1.0—1.9 mm	↑ 3.7 times
≥ 2.0 mm	↑15.8 times

Robb and Seltzer[38] reported a nine-year average follow-up on 3325 men who had Master 2-step tests as part of life insurance applications. While half of the men had chest pain, the latter was nonspecific in 80 percent. The authors used three grades of ischemic response:

Grade 1—0.1—0.9 mm of S-T depression
Grade 2—1.0—1.9 mm of S-T depression
Grade 3— ≥ 2.0 mm of S-T depression.

The prevalence of ischemic response was 13.5 percent, two-thirds of which were grade 1, one-fifth grade 2, and one-tenth grade 3. The positive responders had a mortality rate of 24.7 per 1000 person years, over three times the rate of negative responders. The mortality rate from coronary disease was five times higher in the positive responders. The authors concluded that a nonischemic response practically excluded individuals at risk for premature death from coronary disease. They also felt that even slight ischemic changes (0.1 mm of S-T depression) were significant and that ischemic changes in multiple leads suggested widespread coronary disease.

Bellet et al.[39] performed double Master 2-step tests of 795 male employees of the Bell Telephone Company. The age range was twenty-five to sixty-five years, and none of the men had evidence of coronary disease. Criteria for a positive test included either ischemic S-T segment depression of 1.0 mm or more or the development of multiple premature ventricular beats. Positive stress tests were noted in 11.9 percent of the men. During the three-year follow-up period, clinical coronary disease was diagnosed in 13 of the 95 positive responders (13.7%) and in 10 of the 700 negative responders (1.4%). Hence, the group of positive responders had an incidence of subsequent coronary symptoms more than ten times greater than the negative group.

Aronow[40] recently reported a thirty-month follow-up in 100 normal subjects who underwent maximal treadmill stress testing and a double Master step test. Using 1.0 mm of horizontal S-T segment depression or greater as a positive test, 4 of 100 (4%) were considered to have abnormal Master 2-step test. These 4 plus 9 others (13 of 100 or 13%) had a positive ECG test for ischemia on treadmill testing. Of the 13 positive treadmill responders, 3 (23.1%) developed other manifestations of coronary disease in the follow-up period. Of 96 persons with a normal double Master test, 3 (3.1%) developed ischemic heart disease within thirty months. Only 1 of 87 (1.1%) normal treadmill responders developed coronary disease within the thirty-month follow-up.

Froelicher et al.[41] followed 1390 asymptomatic men for a mean of 6.3 years. The probability of developing the "hard" end points of coronary disease (angina, sudden death, myocardial infarction) was 20 percent in those with a positive exercise test. The risk ratio of developing any of the aforementioned end points was fourteen times greater in those with positive stress tests as compared to those with negative tests.

In a study[42] of 298 asymptomatic aircrewmen who had coronary arteriograms because of abnormal ECGs, the predictive value of an abnormal exercise stress test for an abnormal arteriogram was 30.6 percent.

At this point, it may be appropriate to make sure the reader clearly understands several key terms and the concept of Bayes' law:

> Predictive Value = the percentage of patients with an abnormal exercise test who will develop coronary disease on follow-up.

It can be expressed as follows:

$$= \frac{\text{True Positives (TP)}}{\text{True Positives (TP)} + \text{False Positives (FP)}} \times 100$$

False positive rate = 100 − predictive value

Relative Risk (or Risk Ratio) = the percentage of persons with a positive exercise test who will manifest coronary disease

the percentage of subjects with a normal exercise test who will manifest coronary disease on follow-up

$$= \frac{\dfrac{TP}{TP + FP}}{\dfrac{FN}{TN + FN}}$$

In a review of several studies, the predictive value of the exercise test varied from 13.6 percent to 46 percent. In other words, 13.6 to 46 percent of those with positive exercise tests developed coronary disease on follow-up. This leaves 54 to 86 percent who did not (the so-called "false positive rate"), but logic tells us that if the follow-up period is carried out long enough (say to ten years), this "false positive rate" may dwindle as more and more subjects manifest coronary disease.

In several studies, the relative risk has ranged from ten to fourteen. That is to say, if an asymptomatic individual has a positive exercise test, he will then have a ten– to fourteen-fold risk of developing coronary disease on follow-up compared with the negative responders.

The predictive value, the false positive rate, and the relative risk are all influenced by Bayes' rule,[43] which states that the diagnostic value of any test is dependent upon the incidence of the disease to be diagnosed within the population studied. As Froelicher has shown,[44] given an exercise test with a sensitivity of 60 percent and a specificity of 90 percent, one sees the following variable results, depending upon the prevalence of coronary disease in the population studied:

Prevalence of Coronary Disease in the Study Population	Relative Risk	Predictive Value	False Positive Rate
1%	12.7	5.7%	94.3%
5%	10.4	24%	76%
10%	8.5	40%	60%
50%	2.8	85.7%	14.3%

A summary of the prognostic value of exercise testing can be seen in Table 5-IX. The variable results may reflect differences in testing techniques, along with Bayes' law.

SENSITIVITY AND SPECIFICITY OF EXERCISE TESTING

The true measure of any noninvasive study is how well it stands up against the most sensitive reference study, in this situation the invasive technique of coronary angiography. Before reviewing the literature dealing with this correlation, it is advisable to review two additional definitions:

$$\text{Sensitivity} = \frac{\text{True Positives}}{\text{True Positives} + \text{False Negatives}}$$

$$\text{Specificity} = \frac{\text{True Negatives}}{\text{True Negatives} + \text{False Positives}}$$

A *true positive* for our purpose is a patient who has both a positive ECG stress test and significant abnormalities on coronary angiography. A *false negative* is a patient who has a normal exercise stress test but an abnormal coronary angiogram. A *true negative* is one with no abnormalities in either stress testing or coronary angiography. On the other hand, a *false*

TABLE 5-IX
PROGNOSTIC VALUE OF EXERCISE STRESS TESTING

Author	Number	Follow-up (years)	Type of Test	% + Test	CHD Mortality	CHD Morbidity
Mattingly	871	10	Master	2% (of 300)	↑4.8x	38%
*Brody	756	3-10	Master	3%		70%
*Doyle	2003	5	Treadmill	3.6%		45%
*Bruce	186	5	Treadmill	5.3%		13.6%
Kattus	314	2.5	Treadmill	9.5%	10%	23%
Beard	1375	2.5	Master	8.0%		60%
*Blackburn	12,770	5	Step			↑3.0x
Robb & Marks	2224	up to 15 (average 5.6)	Master		↑15.8x for 2mm ST dep.	
*Bellet	795	3	Master	11.9%		13.7%
*Aronow	100	2.5	Master	4%		25%
			Treadmill	13%		23.1%

*Denotes completely asymptomatic persons from a cardiovascular standpoint.
CHD = coronary heart disease
dep = depression

positive is a patient with an abnormal stress test but a normal coronary angiogram.

For a noninvasive test to be highly useful, the sensitivity and specificity should both be as close to 100 percent as possible. Unfortunately, this is rarely possible, and one is faced with using a specific test or a set of criteria by which the greatest number of "true positives" can be identified within a population without a high rate of "false positives."

With this in mind, let us review the available studies in which various types of stress tests (2-step, treadmill, bicycle) and diagnostic criteria (S-T segment depression of 0.5 mm, 1.0 mm, etc.) are compared with the findings on coronary arteriography. One must realize before doing so that the latter test is by no means infallible; when compared with postmortem examination of the coronary arteries, the arteriogram often underestimates the extent and degree of disease, particularly that involving the main left coronary artery, the proximal half of the left circumflex artery, and the intermediate portion of the right coronary artery.

Mason et al.[45] compared the results of exercise stress testing on an ergometer (bicycle or escalator) with the findings of coronary arteriography in 84 patients. The sensitivity (true positives) was 77 percent. In other words, of 100 patients with significant obstructions on coronary arteriography, 77 would be picked up on exercise testing and 23 would be missed. The specificity (true negatives) was 88 percent. Thus, for 100 persons who had normal coronary arteriograms, 88 likewise have normal tests while 12 would be given a false positive diagnosis of coronary disease.*

McConahay et al.[46] compared the Master 2-step test with coronary arteriography in 100 patients who were evaluated at the Mayo Clinic. Using the criteria of 0.5 mm S-T segment depression as an abnormal exercise response, 63 percent of those with abnormal coronary arteriograms were detected on

---

*at least "false" in the sense that there was no large coronary vessel disease. This, of course, does not exclude small vessel disease and abnormal myocardial metabolic factors which perhaps could result in an abnormal electrocardiographic response to stress.

the step test. If the criteria of ≥ 1.0 S-T segment depression was employed, the sensitivity was reduced, as only 35 percent of persons with abnormal coronary arteriograms were detected on the postexercise electrocardiograms. Although there were no false positive responders (specificity of 100%) when the latter S-T segment criteria was used, the marked diminution in sensitivity offset this. McConahay collaborated with Martin in doing a similar study involving maximal treadmill testing.[47] Again, 100 patients were evaluated. The criteria for a positive exercise test was ≥ 1.0 mm S-T segment depression (horizontal or downsloping). The criteria for an abnormal coronary arteriogram was ≥ 50 percent obstruction of a major coronary vessel. The sensitivity was 62 percent, similar to the Master 2-step data, while the specificity of 89 percent was 6 percent better than that of the step test (when ≥ 0.5 mm S-T segment criteria was used).

Lewis and Wilson[48] found that the treadmill test uncovered more coronary artery disease (as defined by angiography) than did the Master 2-step test. Using S-T segment criteria of 1.0 mm or more for both exercise tests, 16 of 26 patients (61%) had positive double Master tests. The same 16 patients plus an additional 5 (81% sensitivity) had positive treadmill tests.

Cohn et al.[7] favor the retention of the 2-step test as a screening procedure after validating it with coronary arteriography in 244 patients. They point out that the test is simple, inexpensive, and safe, and at the same time provides a relatively high sensitivity rate (84%). It should be noted, however, that the false positive rate was relatively high (27%), thereby showing a specificity (true negative reading) of only 73 percent. Moreover, their original group was 305 patients, but 61 had "uninterpretable" postexercise electrocardiograms since the heart rates were less than 110 beats per minute. An S-T segment depression of 2.0 mm had ominous implications in this study, as 70 percent of these responders had three-vessel coronary disease.

McHenry et al.[49] quantitated the S-T segment response to treadmill exercise by digital computer in 85 patients. All patients had angina pectoris and were shown to have at least 75 percent obstruction of one or more major coronary arteries on cineangiography. A modified bipolar V_5 lead system was used. The digital computer averaged the S-T segment responses of twenty-five consecutive beats from the immediate and the three-minute recovery periods. Seventy patients had an abnormal S-T segment response either during or postexercise, a sensitivity of 82 percent. Of the 16 patients with a negative response, 12 had disease confined to a single vessel. The right coronary artery or the left circumflex vessel was involved in 11 of the 12 cases. In another group of 80 patients with chest pain and normal coronary arteriograms, the specificity was 95 percent (there were 5 percent with a false positive S-T segment response to exercise testing).

Most et al.[50] evaluated the results of Master 2-step testing in 65 patients wth angina pectoris and angiography-documented coronary atherosclerosis. The sensitivity was 58 percent, indicating that 42 out of every 100 patients with documented coronary disease would not be detected on the stress test. More disturbing was the finding that 12 of 39 patients with widespread three-vessel disease had normal postexercise electrocardiograms. On the other hand, 13 of the 39 patients (33%) with three-vessel disease had at least 2.0 mm of S-T segment depression postexercise.

Roitman et al.[51] used maximal treadmill testing in 46 patients with a sensitivity of 80 percent and a specificity of 87 percent. They concluded that if one could exclude a variety of clinical signs,* a normal maximal treadmill test will be associated with a false negativity of only 4 percent when compared with coronary angiography.

Although we generally reflect upon S-T segment depression during exercise, Fortuin and Friesinger[52] have recently called attention to the significance of exercise-induced S-T segment elevations. The patients were exercised on a stairway ergometer with constant electrocardiographic monitoring using a multiple lead system. Eight patients had S-T segment elevations during or postexercise in the anterior precordial leads. Coronary

---

*aortic and mitral valve disease, bundle branch block, hypertension, digitalis usage, LVH, and S-T segment abnormalities on the resting ECG.

arteriography in these patients indicated complete or near-complete occlusion of the left anterior descending vessel in 7 of the 8 cases. Four other patients developed S-T segment elevations in the inferior limb leads upon exercise testing. Each of the 4 was shown to have almost total occlusion of the right coronary artery on arteriography. Hence, it would appear from this small series that S-T segment elevation in the exercise electrocardiogram might predict the anatomic location of significant coronary disease with relatively high accuracy. More studies of this nature are needed to substantiate this.

There are at least thirteen studies to date in which an attempt to validate exercise testing with coronary arteriography has been made. Table 5-X lists pertinent details of each study, including the sensitivity and specificity values. The data can be broken down into each type of test, permitting one to compare the validity of one type of exercise test with another as follows:

Type of Test	Number of Patients	Sensitivity	Specificity
Bicycle	225	69%	84%
2-step	652	68%	79%
Treadmill	259	74%	90%

The treadmill method scores the highest in validity, with a false positive rate of 10 percent (versus 21% for the Master test). The false negative rates for all the test methods (26 to 32%) is sizeable and accounts for the continued striving to enhance the yield of exercise testing in coronary heart disease.

Borer et al.[53,54] stirred considerable controversy[55,56] by questioning the validity of exercise stress testing in a study of 89 persons with type II hyperlipoproteinemia. They divided the patients into three groups and compared the results of submaximal bicycle testing. *Group one* consisted of 43 patients with a history of prior myocardial infarction or angina pectoris. Of the 43, 39 had greater than 50 percent occlusion of at least one major coronary artery on angiography. In spite of the latter, two-thirds had negative stress tests. One wonders what the results might have been if maximal treadmill testing had been used. Since many of these patients had old myocardial infarctions, the low yield of positive tests might not be unusual if

TABLE 5-X

SENSITIVITY AND SPECIFICITY OF EXERCISE STRESS TESTING

Author	No. Cases	Exercise Test	Criteria for + ET	Criteria for Abnormal Coronary Angiogram	Sensitivity	Specificity
Mason	84	Bicycle	1.0 mm S-T dep.	≥50% narrowing	77%	88%
Likoff	74	Bicycle	1.0 mm S-T dep.	≥50% narrowing	58%	68%
Martin and McConahay	100	Treadmill (maximal)	1.0 mm S-T dep.	≥50% narrowing	62%	89%
McHenry	86	Treadmill	1.0 mm S-T dep.	≥75% narrowing	82%	Not Applicable
McConahay	100	Master 2-Step	a) 0.5 mm S-T dep. b) 1.0 mm S-T dep.	≥50% narrowing ≥50% narrowing	63% 35%	89% 100%
Fitzgibbon	87	Master 2-Step	0.5 mm S-T dep.	Special index (approximately 50% obstruction)	67%	84%
Lewis	26	a) Master 2-Step b) Treadmill (Bruce)	1.0 mm S-T dep.		61% 81%	91% 100%
Roitman	46	Treadmill (maximal)	1.0 mm S-T dep.	≥50% narrowing	80%	87%
Most	65	Master 2-Step	1.0 mm S-T dep.	≥50% narrowing	58%	Not Applicable
Cohn	244	Master 2-Step	0.5 mm S-T dep.	≥50% narrowing	84%	73%
Kassebaum	67	Bicycle	0.5 mm S-T dep. 1.0 mm S-T dep.	≥50% narrowing	73% 71%	97% 97%
Demany	75	Master 2-Step	1.0 mm S-T dep.	≥50% narrowing	43%	69%
Hultgren	55	Master 2-Step	1.0 mm S-T dep.	≥50% narrowing	60%	100%

ET = exercise test

the nonscarred myocardium was not ischemic. *Group two* consisted of 5 patients with atypical angina, all of whom had greater than 50 percent occlusion of at least one coronary artery. Of these 5, 2 had negative exercise tests. The sparse number of subjects in this group makes the results difficult to critique. *Group three* was comprised of 30 asymptomatic subjects, all of whom had positive exercise tests; only 1 of the 30 had greater than 50 percent occlusions on coronary angiography, so the remaining 29 were considered to have false positive tests. This low specificity was not in keeping with multiple other studies and must be interpreted in this context.

DIAGNOSTIC CRITERIA

Most exercise electrocardiographers consider a horizontal or downsloping S-T segment depression of 1.0 mm or more, lasting for 0.08 seconds, as indicative of a "positive" exercise response for ischemia. In addition to the depth of S-T segment response, one should also look at the S-T configuration (downsloping, horizontal, or upsloping), the time of onset of S-T response, and the duration of response. In the study of Goldschlager et al.[57] (in 269 patients with angiography-proven coronary disease), 87 percent of those with downsloping S-T segment depression in the first three minutes had two– to three-vessel disease, while 90 percent had similar findings if the S-T abnormality persisted for eight minutes or longer in the recovery phase.

An upsloping S-T junctional depression during exercise has been looked at in a critical fashion in a six-year follow-up study of 438 patients, 90 percent of whom had been referred for evaluation of possible angina pectoris. Those with an upsloping S-T segment that was 1 to 2 mm below the baseline (0.08 seconds after the J-point) had the same annual incidence rate of coronary events (death, myocardial infarction, onset or progression of angina) as did those with 2 mm of horizontal S-T depression:[58]

S-T Response	Annual Incidence of Coronary Events
2 mm downslope	13%
2 mm horizontal	9%
2 mm upslope	9%
1 mm upslope	9%
Normal	1.8%

In addition, those with 1 to 2 mm of upsloping S-T depression had a similar prevalence of two- to three-vessel coronary disease on angiography as those with horizontal S-T segment depression (57% versus 60%). Froelicher feels that such J-junctional changes need to be interpreted with caution, for they may not have the same meaning in lead CM_5 as in lead V_5. In Goldschlager's series,[57] an upsloping S-T response was associated with an increased number of false positives (32%). McHenry and Fisch[59] feel that a slow upsloping S-T response is reliable only during or immediately postexercise, not in the recovery phase.

How valid is the stress test in women? In the 56 cases of Sketch et al.,[60] 15 had positive tests; two thirds of these were considered false positive in view of normal angiograms. Cumming et al.[61] claimed a high false positive rate in 357 women with negative histories for coronary disease but did not have coronary angiographic data, used less strict criteria for positive responses (0.06 second duration of S-T segment depression), and did not clearly discuss influence of drugs, hyperventilation, and postural factors. On the other hand, Linhart et al.[62] performed exercise tests and coronary angiograms on 98 female patients and found a reasonable sensitivity (71%) and specificity (78%) if drug effects were considered.

The effect of digitalis and nonspecific baseline ST-T changes on the exercise electrocardiogram has been looked at in several recent studies.[63-66] In considering those with an additional S-T depression of 0.1 mV or more with exercise, the sensitivity ranged from 63 to 92 percent and the specificity from 75 to 95 percent.

False positive tests for ischemia may occur in 38 percent of patients in the presence of left ventricular hypertrophy;[67] the abnormal result may reflect imbalances in myocardial oxygen supply and demand, however.

Some have claimed that an additional 1.5 mm of S-T segment depression with exercise is highly suggestive of significant coronary disease in the presence of baseline left bundle branch block.[68] This particular series was too small (10 patients, half of whom did not have coronary arteriograms) to make this assumption.

An elevation of the S-T segment on exercise testing may be indicative of significant underlying coronary disease with associated left ventricular aneurysm formation. Chahine et al.[69] found S-T elevation in 29 of 840 exercise tests (3.5%). Of those 29, 25 (85%) had an old anterior wall myocardial infarction. Angiograms were done in 21 and revealed a significant left anterior descending lesion in 19 (90%) and left ventricular aneurysm formation in 18 (86%). Looking at the data another way, of 113 patients with old anterior wall infarctions, 25 (or 22%) had exercise-induced S-T segment elevation. Of 104 patients with critical lesions of the proximal left anterior descending coronary artery, 19 (18%) had S-T elevations with exercise; of 28 patients with angio-proven left ventricular apical aneurysms, 18 (64%) had S-T segment elevation with exercise. The authors conclude that the latter may be more a reflection of abnormal myocardial wall motion than of myocardial ischemia per se.

In the face of a strongly positive test, ≥ 2 mm S-T segment depression, one should think of left main coronary disease or multivessel disease. Although DeMots et al.[70] observed this response in only 2 of 14 patients with left main lesions, this could reflect the type of test they employed, namely supine bicycle ergometry. Cohen et al.,[71] using a double Master test, noted this response in 34 of 42 (81%) of their series. In another study,[72] of 45 patients with > 2 mm of S-T segment depression with exercise, three fourths had critical lesions (such as a left main, a left main equivalent, or a 90% high left anterior descending artery occlusion). All 11 patients in this series with left main lesions had greater than 2 mm of S-T segment depression.

RISKS OF EXERCISE TESTING

In a survey of 170,000 exercise tests from 73 medical centers, the mortality rate was only 1 per 10,000 tests, while the combined mortality-morbidity rate was only 4 per 10,000 tests.[73] In the experience of Detry et al.,[74] involving over 10,000 tests, there was 1 episode of ventricular fibrillation per 1000 tests. All subjects were successfully defibrillated.

A recent death occurred after a normal near-maximal treadmill test in a fifty-six-year-old man. An autopsy report showed that hemorrhage into an intimal atherosclerotic plaque produced total occlusion of the LAD coronary artery.[75]

Patients who develop ventricular tachycardia or ventricular fibrillation on the treadmill may have severe underlying coronary disease; in one series of three cases, aortocoronary saphenous vein bypass grafting produced excellent results over a two-year period of follow-up.[76]

RECENT ADVANCES IN STRESS TESTING

While future modifications are likely in the selection of test protocols and in the electrocardiographic criteria utilized, it might be that ancillary noninvasive techniques will be required to supplement the exercise test in hopes of enhancing the sensitivity. One such ancillary technique is that of recording the *systolic time intervals* pre– and postexercise. By simultaneously recording the carotid pulse, the electrocardiogram, and the phonocardiogram, one can derive the left ventricular ejection time (LVET) the Q-S_2 interval, and the preejection period (PEP). Weissler et al.[77] have recently emphasized the use of these measurements to appraise ventricular performance. As left ventricular performance decreased, characteristic changes were noted in the rate-corrected systolic time intervals. The PEP, an index of the rate of rise of the left ventricular pressure plus electromechanical delay, is shown to lengthen, while the LVET tends to shorten in patients with left ventricular dysfunction. The result is a significant increase in the PEP/LVET ratio.

Hemodynamic studies have shown a close correlation between this ratio and measured cardiac index and stroke volume index.[78] Inotropic influences, such as digitalis administration, tend to shorten both the PEP and the LVET, thereby shortening the overall measurement of electromechanical systole ($Q-S_2$).

Pouget et al.[79] made comparisons between 20 normals and 20 patients with angina pectoris, matching the groups according to age. The angina patients had a slightly longer PEP and a shorter LVET at rest, but the overlap was considerable between the patients and the normal controls. Repeat measurements of the systolic time intervals after two– to four-minute exercise sessions tended to separate the two groups. The normals showed a slight shortening of the PEP and LVET postexercise. The angina patients shortened their PEP and lengthened their LVET. The latter, a seemingly paradoxical response, may have been due to the inability of the Frank-Starling mechanism and catecholamine-mediated increased contractility to offset the delay in LVET induced by the temporary decrease in left ventricular performance associated with exercise.

Whitsett and Naughton[80] studied four groups of individuals (sedentary healthy, active healthy, post-myocardial-infarction sedentary, and post-myocardial-infarction reconditioned). In the postinfarction inactive group, the LVET lengthened after treadmill testing, comparable to the data of Pouget et al. In the coronary active group (conditioned), the LVET was significantly shortened, suggesting an improvement in left ventricular performance due to physical training.

McConahay et al.[81] compared resting and postexercise systolic time intervals in 33 normal subjects and 32 age– and sex-matched patients with coronary heart disease. At rest, the coronary group showed a longer rate-corrected PEP, a shorter rate-corrected LVET, and a larger PEP/LVET ratio than the normals with significance at the $p < .01$ level. Postexercise values showed the same significant difference. Both groups (normals and coronary patients) had significant decreases in the rate-corrected PEP, increases in the LVET, and lessening of the PEP/LVET ratio postexercise.

Gilbert and Cantwell[82] studied 29 normal sedentary persons,

13 normal trained persons, and 21 persons with well-documented coronary heart disease. The data from this study was in accord with previous investigators showing the postexercise increase in LVET in coronary patients. The postexercise LVET seemed of value as another objective means of assessing the physical training effect. Although there were no significant differences at rest between the rate-corrected LVET of normal sedentary and normal trained persons, significant differences ($p < .05$) did develop on the two-minute postexercise tracings. As previously mentioned in another study, the postexercise shortening of the LVET might also be useful in determining a similar training effect in coronary patients who are engaged in physical training programs.

A brief summary of the systolic time interval data is noted in Table 5-XI.[3]

TABLE 5-XI
SYSTOLIC TIME INTERVALS AFTER EXERCISE STRESS TESTING

Pouget, et al.	*PEP after acute exercise*	*LVET after acute exercise*
Normals	↓	↓
Angina patients	↓ ↓	↑
Whitsett and Naughton		
Normals (inactive)	↓	sl ↓
Normals (active)	↓	↓
Coronary patients (inactive)	↓ ↓	sl ↑
Coronary patients (active)	↓ ↓	↓
Gilbert and Cantwell		
Normal (inactive)	↓	↓
Normal (active)	↓	↓ ↓
Coronary patients (inactive)	↓	↑

PEP = pre-ejection period
LVET = left ventricular ejection time
sl = slightly

Another noninvasive technique which has been utilized in conjunction with exercise stress testing is *phono– and apex-cardiography.* Benchimol and Dimond[83] were among the first to study the effect of Master 2-step exercise on the latter in normal subjects and in patients with coronary heart disease. They found that the a wave ratio (a/e-o) was significantly greater in the coronary patients. Aronow et al.[84] found significant differences in the postexercise a wave ratios between normal subjects who had an abnormal maximal treadmill test and normal subjects who had a normal treadmill test. The postexercise a wave ratio was 19.7 percent in the former and 12.8 percent in the latter, the significance being at the $p < .001$ level. Over half of the so-called normals with abnormal treadmill tests had postexercise a wave ratios of 20 percent as compared to only 9 percent of the normal subjects with normal treadmill tests. The mechanism behind the augmented a wave is probably related to the increased resistance of a left ventricle that becomes ischemic during or postexercise. Because of the added resistance, the left ventricular end-diastolic pressure rises, necessitating a more vigorous left atrial contraction to achieve adequate ventricular filling.

Aronow et al.[84] also compared resting and postexercise (Master 2-step) phonocardiograms in 100 normal subjects and 100 patients with angina pectoris. On the resting recording, fourth heart sounds were present in 14 percent of the normals and in 43 percent of the coronary patients. After exercise, 94 percent of the patients and 29 percent of the normals had fourth heart sounds. Third heart sounds were recorded at rest in 1 percent of the normals and in 15 percent of the angina patients. Following exercise testing, 60 percent of the angina patients had third heart sounds, versus 11 percent of the normals. Of the 11 normal subjects who developed third heart sounds following double Master tests, 4 (36%) had abnormal maximal treadmill stress tests and 7 (64%) had normal treadmill responses. The incidence of both third and fourth heart sounds was significantly greater in the normal subjects having abnormal maximal treadmill stress tests than in the normal subjects who had normal treadmill tests.

A noninvasive technique that has stimulated great interest

within the past few years is *echocardiography*. This technique of cardiac examination by reflected ultrasound was first introduced in 1954. Although there are no reports on pre– and postexercise echocardiograms, there may be some merit in looking into this. By using ultrasound to measure the distance between the interventricular septum and an area of the posterior left ventricular wall, one can assess the left ventricular systolic and diastolic volumes.[85] With the former figures, the stroke volume and ejection fraction can be estimated with reasonable accuracy. A measure of stroke volume change after treadmill, bicycle, or step testing could be an important clue to cardiac function in normal subjects and in coronary patients, both trained and untrained.

Zaret et al.[86] recently described the use of radioactive potassium injections followed by myocardial perfusion scanning both pre– and postexercise. Sixteen of nineteen patients with angina pectoris showed regions of decreased ^{43}K accumulations during exercise that were not present at rest. The zones of decreased radioactivity corresponded to abnormalities noted at coronary arteriography.

Myocardial stress perfusion scintigraphy, using markers such as Thallium-201 and Rubidium-81, has shown definite promise.[87, 88, 89, 90] In a study of 56 patients (35 with anginalike pain and 21 with atypical chest pain), the validity of stress scans and stress electrocardiograms was compared, using coronary arteriography as the reference test. The results were as follows:[90]

Test	Sensitivity	Specificity
Stress ECG	79%	61%
Stress Scan	91%	91%

EXERCISE TESTING FOR EVALUATION AND DETECTION OF CARDIAC RHYTHM DISTURBANCES

In addition to its use in detecting repolarization abnormalities, exercise stress testing is also of diagnostic aid in assessing cardiac rhythm and conduction disturbances. The arrhythmia-prone person can sometimes be spotted on submaximal or maximal exercise testing. In addition, the stability and significance of a rhythm disorder can sometimes be demonstrated by this method. An example of the latter is as follows.

A fifty-two-year-old woman was referred to a cardiologist because of a history of palpitations which dated back twenty years or more. The cardiopulmonary examination was normal. The resting electrocardiogram was unremarkable except for frequent premature ventricular beats (Fig. 5-1), at times occurring in trigeminy. The patient underwent treadmill testing by the Bruce method, attaining a maximal heart rate of 167 beats per minute. As soon as the heart rate exceeded a rate of 80/minute, the patient had no further premature beats (Fig. 5-2). There were no ischemic changes on the electrocardiogram during or after exercise.

The normal response to maximal exercise and the complete cessation of ventricular ectopic beats made it highly likely that the ventricular ectopy at rest was of a relatively benign nature, even though recent findings may question the "benign" nature of exercise-related cessation of ectopic beats.[91]

Gooch[92] has perhaps the most extensive experience of anyone in this field, having performed exercise tests to record changes in rhythm and conduction in over 3000 subjects over a five-year period. His findings can be summarized as follows:

1. Premature ventricular beats occur frequently during exercise stress testing and do not by themselves necessarily indicate underlying cardiac disease unless they occur in bigeminy or in paroxysms of multifocal ventricular beats.

2. Atrial arrhythmias are fairly common after exercise, occurring both in normal subjects and in those with known cardiac disease. Brief paroxysms of supraventricular tachyarrhythmias are not unusual during exercise.

3. Exercise testing might be of help in identifying the inadequately digitalized patient with atrial fibrillation (who will develop enhanced A-V conduction). On the other hand, rhythm suggesting digitalis intoxication can sometimes be brought out by exercise stress testing.

4. Complete bundle branch block (left or right) can be induced

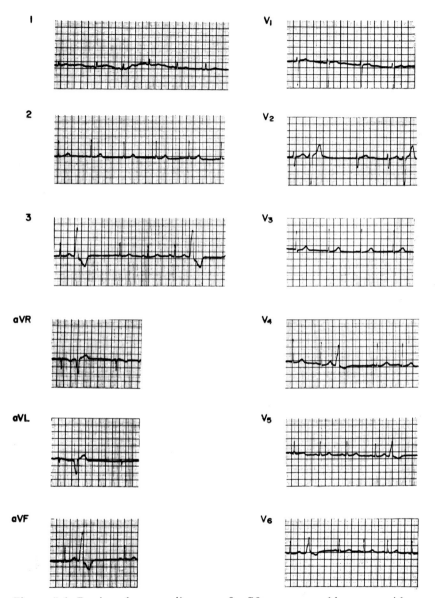

Figure 5-1. Resting electrocardiogram of a fifty-two-year-old woman with a chronic history of frequent ventricular premature beats.

by exercise, most likely as a result of the "critical rate" phenomenon.

5. If A-V block is present on the resting electrocardiogram, it is difficult to predict the response to exercise, i.e. the condition may either improve, stay the same, or worsen.

Exercise stress testing has been of value in separating the patient with congenital complete heart block from the one with acquired complete heart block. The ventricular rate of the former usually increases significantly during exercise, while that of the latter often shows very little rate increase.

The following is an example of the use of treadmill testing to assess the significance of recently acquired bifascicular conduction disturbances.

A thirty-two-year-old very athletic physician was seen by Doctor Cantwell in consultation. Over a five-year period he had developed left anterior hemiblock and incomplete right bundle branch block (Fig. 5-3). The patient advanced to the fifth stage

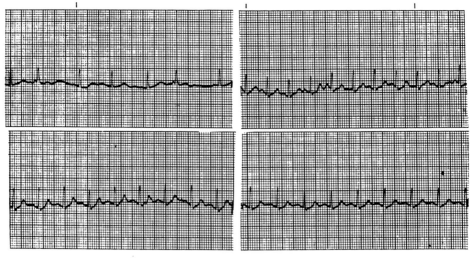

Figure 5-2. Suppression of ventricular premature beats during exercise in the patient described in Figure 5-1. Upper left tracing shows the ventricular premature beats which appeared on the resting electrocardiogram. There is suppression during exercise (upper right), immediately postexercise (lower left), and two minutes postexercise (lower right).

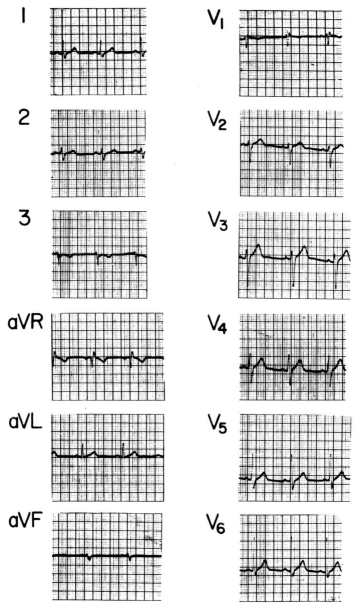

Figure 5-3. Resting electrocardiogram of a thirty-two-year-old physician and distance runner, showing left anterior hemiblock and incomplete right bundle branch block.

of the Bruce treadmill test with no evidence of myocardial ischemia and no increase in the degree of block (Fig. 5-4). His oxygen uptake was 55 ml/kg/minute, placing him in the very high category for his group. He was advised to continue his active ways and to undergo resting and exercise electrocardiography at six– to twelve-month intervals.

Vedin et al.[93] correlated exercise-induced ventricular ectopic beats to several coronary risk factors (elevated blood pressure and fasting blood glucose, cardiac enlargement on x-ray, ischemic exercise electrocardiogram changes) in the Goteborg study of men born in 1913. Two of the men who had frequent ventricular premature beats precipitated by exercise died suddenly and unexpectedly, raising the possibility that this finding might be an important predictor of high risk for future sudden death.

Exercise stress testing has been of help in evaluating patients with pacemakers. Singer et al.[94] discovered various types of arrhythmias in 75 percent of 27 patients with permanent pacemakers, including 5 instances of ventricular tachycardia. As

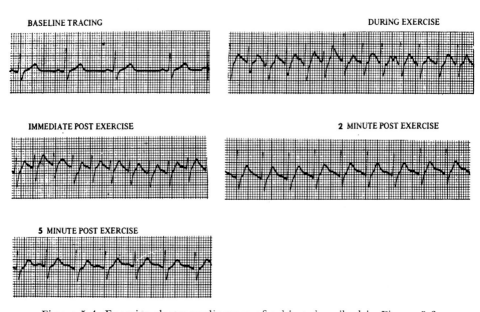

Figure 5-4. Exercise electrocardiogram of subject described in Figure 5-3.

patients developed new rhythms during testing, it became possible to assess the type of pacemaker (fixed-rate or demand) and how well the sensing mechanism of the latter was functioning.

MISCELLANEOUS ASPECTS OF EXERCISE TESTING

Exercise testing is highly adaptable and extremely flexible. It may be used to evaluate peripheral vascular insufficiency[95] or to help in the assessment of a new surgical procedure such as aortocoronary saphenous vein graft operations.[96] An arm ergometer test may be employed in amputees.[97] Patients with Prinzmetal's (or "variant") angina may need to start at higher initial work loads, as the warm-up phenomenon may obscure the electrocardiographic findings.[98]

Caution should be used in avoiding the overinterpretation of the exercise electrocardiogram. Murray[99] will consider an exercise electrocardiogram positive based on the magnitude of S-T segment junctional depression alone. If the S-T (J) depression is 1.0 mm or greater, the S-T slope (mv/sec.) is subtracted from it. If the result is less than zero, the test is considered abnormal. The S-T slope is calculated (Fig. 5-5) by drawing a line along the S-T segment and extending it to a point three seconds distal on the electrocardiogram paper (point D). The distance from point D to the isoelectric line (point C) is the S-T slope. Although such additional calculations might increase the sensitivity of exercise testing, this remains to be proven. Moreover, long-term follow-up data on patients with junctional S-T segment changes alone is lacking. Recent studies suggest that false positive readings may be commonplace in the presence of left ventricular hypertrophy.[100] They may also be noted after glucose ingestion.[101]

SUMMARY

A brief historical review of exercise stress testing has been presented. The various methods of testing are described,

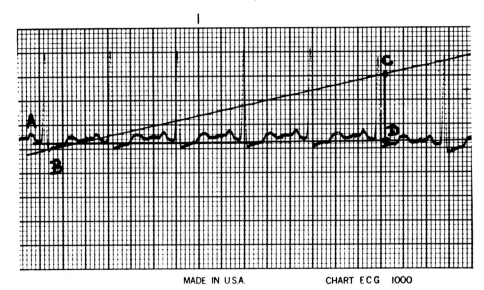

Figure 5-5. Calculation of the S-T segment slope of the exercise electrocardiogram shown in Figure 5-4.

including specific test protocols, lead systems, target heart rates, and criteria for positive tests. The predictive value of exercise testing, along with the sensitivity and specificity of such testing, is reviewed in detail. A discussion of noninvasive measures which may complement exercise stress testing (such as systolic time intervals, apex and phonocardiography, and echocardiography) is provided. The use of exercise testing to assess cardiac rhythm and conduction is reviewed. It would appear that exercise stress testing plays a significant role in our armamentarium against coronary heart disease. In spite of obvious limitations, such as false negative readings of 25 percent and an inability to predict the extent and locations of coronary disease,[102] it is a safe, simple, and relatively inexpensive way to quantitate cardiovascular performance and to detect subclinical coronary disease or tendencies for such. There are at least eight indications for its use:

1. To quantitate levels of physical fitness
2. To screen for possible significant underlying coronary disease in asymptomatic individuals

3. To assess exercise-related chest pain
4. To screen for exercise-related cardiac dysrhythmias
5. To screen candidates for cardiac rehabilitation programs
6. To evaluate exercise-related leg cramps
7. To detect labile hypertension and to assess antihypertensive therapy
8. To measure the response to medical or surgical therapy

REFERENCES

1. Feil, H., and Siegel, M.L.: Electrocardiographic changes during attacks of angina. *Am J Med Sci, 175:*256, 1928.
2. Master, A.M., and Oppenheimer, E.T.: A simple tolerance test for circulatory efficiency with standard tables for normal individuals. *Am J Med Sci, 177:*223-242, 1929.
3. Scherf, D., and Goldhammer, S.: Zur Fruhdiagnose der Angina Pectoris mit Helfe des Eletrokarkograms. *Z Klin Med, 124:*111, 1933.
4. Astrand, P.O., and Rodahl, K.: *Textbook of Work Physiology.* New York, McGraw-Hill, 1970.
5. Smith, E.: Inquiries into the quantity of air inspired throughout the day and night, and under the influence of exercise, food, medicine and temperature. *Proc Roy Soc Med, 8:*451-456, 1857.
6. Master, A.M.: Exercise testing for evaluation of cardiac performance. *Am J Cardiol, 30:*718-721, 1972.
7. Cohen, P.F., Vokonas, P.S., Most, A.S., et al.: Diagnostic accuracy of two-step post-exercise ECG. Result in 305 subjects studied by coronary arteriography. *JAMA, 220:*501-506, 1972.
8. Fletcher, G.F.: Submaximal treadmill exercise evaluation in patients with symptoms of cardiovascular disease. *Chest, 63:*153-158, 1973.
9. Doan, A.E., Peterson, D.R., Blackman, J.R., et al.: Myocardial ischemia after maximal exercise in healthy men. A method for detecting potential coronary heart disease? *Am Heart J, 69:*11-21, 1965.
10. Most, A.S., Hornstein, T.R., Hofer, V., et al.: Exercise S-T changes in healthy men. *Arch Intern Med, 121:*225-229, 1968.
11. Spangler, R.D., Horman, M.J., Miller, S.W., et al.: A submaximal exercise electrocardiographic test as a method of detecting occult ischemic heart disease. *Am Heart J, 80:*752-758, 1970.
12. Ellestad, M.H., Allen, W., Wan, M.C., et al.: Maximal treadmill stress testing for cardiovascular evaluation. *Circulation, 39:*517-522, 1969.
13. Ellestad, M.H., and Wan, M.K.C.: Predictive implications of stress testing. Follow-up of 2700 subjects after maximal treadmill stress testing. *Circulation, 51:*363-369, 1975.

14. Balke, B., and Ware, K.: An experimental study of physical fitness of Air Force personnel. *US Armed Forces Med J, 10:*675-688, 1959.
15. Fox, S.M., III, Naughton, J.P., and Haskell, W.L.: Physical activity and the prevention of coronary heart disease. *Ann Clin Res, 3:*404-432, 1971.
16. Astrand, P.O., and Rodahl, K.: *Textbook of Work Physiology.* New York, McGraw-Hill, 1970, pp. 362-363.
17. Shepard, R.V., Aleen, C., Benade, A.V.S., et al.: The maximal oxygen intake. An international reference standard of cardiorespiratory fitness. *Bull WHO, 38:*757, 1968.
18. Bruce, R.A., Kusumi, F., and Hosmer, D.: Maximal oxygen intake and nomographic assessment of functional aerobic impairment in cardiovascular disease. *Am Heart J, 85:*546-562, 1973.
19. Pollock, M.L., Bohannon, R.L., Cooper, K.H., et al.: A comparative analysis of four protocols for maximal treadmill stress testing. *Am Heart J, 92:*39-46, 1976.
20. Froelicher, V.F., Jr., and Lancaster, M.C.: The predictors of maximal oxygen consumption from a continuous exercise treadmill protocol. *Am Heart J, 87:*445-450, 1974.
21. Froelicher, V.F., Jr., Thompson, A.J., Jr., Noguera, I., et al.: Predictors of maximal oxygen consumption. Comparison of the Bruce and Balke treadmill protocol. *Chest, 68:*331-336, 1975.
22. Mason, R.E., and Likar, I.: A new system of multiple-lead exercise electrocardiography. *Am Heart J, 71:*196-205, 1966.
23. Hellerstein, H.K., Hornstein, T.R., Goldbarg, A.W., et al.: The influence of active conditioning upon coronary atherosclerosis. A progress report. In Brest, A.N., and Moyer, J.H., (Eds.): *Atherosclerotic Vascular Disease.* New York, Appleton-Century-Crofts, 1967, p. 115.
24. Redwood, D.R., and Epstein, S.E.: Uses and limitations of stress testing in the evaluation of ischemic heart disease. *Circulation, 46:*1115-1131, 1972.
25. Froelicher, V.F., Jr., Wolthius, R., Keiser, N., et al.: A comparison of two bipolar exercise electrocardiographic leads to lead V5. *Chest, 70:*611-616, 1976.
26. Sheffield, L.T., Roitman, D., and Reeves, T.J.: Submaximal exercise testing. *J SC Med Assoc, 65:Suppl 1:*18-25, 1969.
27. Summation of guidelines on exercise. *J SC Med Assoc, 65:*92, 1969.
28. Cumming, G.R.: Yield of ischemic exercise electrocardiograms in relation to exercise intensity in a normal population. *Br Heart J, 34:*919-923, 1972.
29. Wood, P.C., and Wolfeth, C.C.: Angina pectoris; clinical and electrocardiographic phenomena of attack and their comparison with effects of experimental temporary coronary occlusion. *Arch Intern Med, 47:*339, 1931.

30. Mattingly, T.W.: The post-exercise electrocardiogram. *Am J Cardiol, 9:*395-409, 1962.
31. Brody, A.J.: Master two-step exercise test in clinically unselected patients. *JAMA, 171:*1195-1198, 1959.
32. Doyle, J.T., and Kinch, S.H.: The prognosis of an abnormal electrocardiographic stress test. *Circulation, 41:*545-553, 1970.
33. Bruce, R.A., Gey, G.O., Cooper, M.N., et al.: Seattle Heart Watch: Initial clinical, circulatory and electrocardiographic responses to maximal exercise. *Am J Cardiol, 33:*459-468, 1974.
34. Beard, E.F., Garcia, E., Burke, G.E., et al.: Postexercise electrocardiogram in screening for latent ischemic heart disease. *Dis Chest, 56:*405-408, 1969.
35. Kattus, A.A., Jorgensen, C.R., Worden, R.E., et al.: S-T-segment depression with near-maximal exercise in detection of preclinical coronary heart disease. *Circulation, 44:*585-595, 1971.
36. Blackburn, H.W., Taylor, H.L., and Keys, A.: Prognostic significance of the postexercise electrocardiogram: Risk factors held constant. *Am J Cardiol, 25:*85, 1970.
37. Robb, G.P., and Marks, H.H.: Postexercise electrocardiogram in arteriosclerotic heart disease: Its value in diagnosis and prognosis. *JAMA, 171:*1195, 1959.
38. Robb, G.P., and Seltzer, F.: Appraisal of the double two-step exercise test. *JAMA, 234:*722-727, 1975.
39. Bellet, S., Roman, L.R., Nichols, G.J., et al.: Detection of the coronary-prone subjects in a normal population by radioelectrocardiographic exercise test: Follow-up studies. *Am J Cardiol, 19:*783-787, 1967.
40. Aronow, W.S.: Thirty-month follow-up of maximal treadmill stress test and double Master's tests in normal subjects. *Circulation, 47:*287-290, 1973.
41. Froelicher, V.F., Jr., Thomas, M.M., Pillow, C., et al.: Epidemiologic study of asymptomatic men screened by maximal treadmill testing for latent coronary artery disease. *Am J Cardiol, 34:*770-776, 1974.
42. Froelicher, V.F., Jr., Thompson, A.J., Wolthius, R., et al.: Angiographic findings in asymptomatic aircrewmen with electrocardiographic abnormalities. *Am J Cardiol, 39:*32-38, 1977.
43. Jelliffe, R.W.: Quantitative aspects of clinical judgement. *Am J Med, 55:*431-433, 1973.
44. Froelicher, V.F., Jr.: Data presented at the Fourth Annual Cardiac Rehabilitation Workshop. Georgia Baptist Hospital, September, 1976, Atlanta, Georgia.
45. Mason, R.E., Likar, I., Biern, R.O., et al.: Multiple-lead exercise electrocardiography: Experience in 107 normal subjects and 67 patients with angina pectoris, and comparison with coronary cinearteriography in 84 patients. *Circulation, 36:*517-525, 1967.

46. McConahay, D.R., McCallister, B.D., and Smith, R.E.: Postexercise electrocardiography: Correlations with coronary arteriography and left ventricular hemodynamics. *Am J Cardiol, 28:*1, 1971.
47. Martin, C.M., and McConahay, D.R.: Maximal treadmill exercise electrocardiography: Correlations with coronary arteriography and cardiac hemodynamics. *Circulation, 46:*956-962, 1972.
48. Lewis, W.J., and Wilson, W.J.: Correlation of coronary arteriograms with Master's test and treadmill test. *Rocky Mt Med J, 68:*30-34, 1972.
49. McHenry, P.L., Phillips, J.F., and Knoebel, S.B.: Correlation of the computer-quantitated treadmill exercise electrocardiogram with arteriographic location of coronary artery disease. *Am J Cardiol, 30:*747-752, 1972.
50. Most, A.S., Kemp, H.G., and Gorlin, R.: Postexercise electrocardiography in patients with arteriographically documented coronary artery disease. *Ann Int Med, 71:*1043-1049, 1969.
51. Roitman, D., Jones, W.B., and Sheffield, L.T.: Comparison of submaximal exercise ECG test with coronary cineangiocardiogram. *Ann Intern Med, 72:*641-647, 1970.
52. Fortuin, N.J., and Friesinger, G.C.: Exercise-induced S-T segment elevation. *Am J Med, 49:*459-464, 1970.
53. Borer, J.S., Brensike, J.F., Redwood, D.R., et al.: Limitations of the electrocardiographic response to exercise in predicting coronary artery disease. *N Engl J Med, 293:*367-371, 1975.
54. Redwood, D.R., Borer, J.S., and Epstein, S.E.: Whither the ST segment during exercise? (editorial). *Circulation, 54:*703-706, 1976.
55. Sheffield, L.T., Reeves, T.J., Blackburn, H., et al.: The exercise test in perspective (Editorial). *Circulation, 55:*681-683, 1977.
56. McHenry, P.L.: The actual prevalence of false positive ST-segment responses to exercise in clinically normal subjects remains undefined (Editorial). *Circulation, 55:*683-685, 1977.
57. Goldschlager, N., Selzer, A., and Cohn, K.: Treadmill stress as indicators of presence and severity of coronary artery disease. *Ann Intern Med, 85:*277-286, 1976.
58. Stuart, R.J., Jr., and Ellestad, M.H.: Upsloping S-T segments in exercise stress testing. *Am J Cardiol, 37:*19-22, 1976.
59. McHenry, P.L., and Fisch, C.: Clinical application of the treadmill exercise test. *Mod Concepts Cardiovasc Dis, 46:*21-25, 1977.
60. Sketch, M.H., Mohiuddin, S.M., Lynch, J.D., et al.: Significant sex differences in the correlation of electrocardiographic exercise testing and coronary arteriograms. *Am J Cardiol, 36:*169-173, 1975.
61. Cumming, G.R., Dufresne, C., and Sammon, J.: Exercise ECG changes in normal women. *Can Med Assoc J, 109:*108-111, 1973.
62. Linhart, J.W., Lamus, J.G., and Satinsky, J.D.: Maximum treadmill exercise electrocardiography in female patients. *Circulation, 50:*1173-1178, 1974.

63. Cohn, P.F., Vokonas, P.S., Herman, M.V., et al.: Post-exercise ECG in patients with abnormal resting electrocardiograms. *Circulation,* *43:*648, 1971.

64. Linhart, J.W., and Turnoff, H.B.: Maximal treadmill exercise test in patients with abnormal control electrocardiograms. *Circulation,* *49:*667, 1974.

65. Nasrallah, A., Garcia, E., Beuresy, J., et al.: Treadmill exercise testing in the presence of non-specific ST-T changes or digitalis effect (Abstr). *Am J Cardiol, 35:*160, 1975.

66. Kansal, S., Roitman, D., and Sheffield, L.T.: Stress testing with ST-segment depression at rest. *Circulation, 54:*636-639, 1976.

67. Harris, C.N., Aronow, W.S., Parker, D.P., et al.: Treadmill stress test in left ventricular hypertrophy. *Chest, 63:*353-357, 1973.

68. Cooksey, J.D., Parker, B.M., and Bahl, O.P.: The diagnostic contributions of exercise testing in left bundle branch block. *Am Heart J, 88:*482-486, 1974.

69. Chahine, R.A., Raizner, A.E., and Ishimori, T.: The clinical significance of exercise-induced ST-segment elevation. *Circulation, 54:*209-213, 1976.

70. DeMots, H., Bonchek, L.I., Rosch, J., et al.: Left main coronary artery disease. *Am J Cardiol, 36:*136-141, 1975.

71. Cohne, M.V., Gorlin, R.: Main left coronary artery disease. *Circulation, 52:*275-285, 1975.

72. Cheitlin, M.D., Davia, J.E., de Castro, C.M., et al.: Correlation of "critical" left coronary artery lesions with positive submaximal exercise tests in patients with chest pain. *Am Heart J, 89:*305-310, 1975.

73. Rochmis, P., and Blackburn, H.: Exercise tests. A survey of procedures, safety, and litigating experience in approximately 170,000 tests. *JAMA, 217:*1061-1066, 1971.

74. Detry, J.M.R., Mengeot, P., and Rousseau M.F.: Maximal exercise testing in variant angina (Letter). *Br Heart J, 38:*655-656, 1976.

75. Lintgen, A.B.: Death from myocardial infarction after exercise test with normal result. *JAMA, 235:*837-839, 1976.

76. Bryson, A.L., Parisi, A.F., Schechter, E., et al.: Life-threatening ventricular arrhythmias induced by exercise. *Am J Cardiol, 32:*995-999, 1973.

77. Weissler, A.M., Harris, W.S., and Schoenfeld, C.D.: Systolic time intervals in heart failure in man. *Circulation, 37:*149-159, 1968.

78. Garrard, C.L., Jr., Weissler, A.M., and Dodge, H.T.: Relationship of alterations in systolic time intervals to ejection fraction in patients with cardiac disease. *Circulation, 42:*455, 1970.

79. Pouget, J.M., Harris, W.S., Myron, B.R., et al.: Abnormal responses of the systolic time intervals to exercise in patients with angina pectoris. *Circulation, 43:*289-298, 1971.

80. Whitsett, T.L., and Naughton, J.: The effect of exercise on systolic time

intervals in sedentary and active individuals and rehabilitated patients with heart disease. *Am J Cardiol, 27:*352-358, 1971.

81. McConahay, D.R., Martin, C.M., and Cheitlin, M.D.: Resting and exercise systolic time intervals. Correlations with ventricular performance in patients with coronary artery disease. *Circulation, 45:*592-601, 1972.

82. Gilbert, C.G., and Cantwell, J.D.: The response of systolic time intervals following exercise in patients with coronary atherosclerotic heart disease (Abstr). *Med Sci Sports, 4:*56-57, 1972.

83. Benchimol, A., and Dimond, E.G.: The apexcardiogram in normal older subjects and in patients with arteriosclerotic heart disease. Effect of exercise on the "a" wave. *Am Heart J, 65:*789-801, 1963.

84. Aronow, W.S., Uyeyama, R.R., Cassidy, J., et al.: Resting and postexercise phonocardiograms and electrocardiograms in patients with angina pectoris and in normal subjects. *Circulation, 43:*273-278, 1971.

85. Feigenbaum, H.: Clinical applications of echocardiography *Prog Cardiovasc Dis, 14:*531-558, 1972.

86. Zaret, B.L., Strauss, H.W., Martin, N.D., et al.: Noninvasive regional myocardial perfusion with radioactive potassium. *N Engl J Med, 288:*809-812, 1973.

87. Klein, G.J., and Kostuk, W.J.: Diagnostic accuracy of noninvasive stress myocardial perfusion imaging (Abstr). *Circulation, 54: Suppl II:*II-207, 1976.

88. Peterson, K., Tsuji, J., Schelbert, H., et al.: Improved diagnosis of coronary artery disease during exercise test using a computer-processed Thallium-201 image (Abstr). *Circulation, 54: Suppl II:*II-207, 1976.

89. Bailey, I.K., Griffith, L.S.C., Ronleau, J., et al.: Thallium-201 myocardial perfusion imaging at rest and during exercise. *Circulation, 55:*79-87, 1977.

90. Stvinick, E.H., Shames, D.M., Gershengorn, K.M., et al.: Myocardial stress perfusion scintigraphy with Rubidium-81 versus stress electrocardiogram. *Am J Cardiol, 39:*364-370, 1977.

91. Goldschlager, N., Cake, D. and Cohn, K.: Exercise-induced ventricular arrhythmias in patients with coronary heart disease. Their relation to angiographic findings. *Am J Cardiol, 31:*434-440, 1973.

92. Gooch, A.S.: Exercise testing for detecting changes in cardiac rhythm and conduction. *Am J Cardiol, 30:*741-746, 1972.

93. Vedin, J.A., Wilhelmsson, C.E., Wilhelmsen, L., et al.: Relation of resting and exercise-induced ectopic beats to other ischemic manifestations and to coronary risk factors. *Am J Cardiol, 30:*25-31, 1972.

94. Singer, E., Gooch, A.S., and Morse, D.: Exercise-induced arrhythmias in patients with pacemakers. *JAMA, 224:*1515-1518, 1973.

95. Garrison, G.E., Floyd W.L., and Orgain, E.S.: Exercise in the physical

examination of peripheral arterial disease. *Ann Int Med, 66:*587-593, 1967.

96. Siegel, W., Attar, O.A., Proudfit, W.L., et al.: Acute hemodynamic and clinical effects of direct coronary revascularization (Abstr). *Am J Cardiol, 31:*158, 1973.

97. Kavanagh, T.: Application of exercise testing to elderly amputee. *Can Med Assoc J, 108:*314-318, 1973.

98. Mac Alpin, R.N., Kattus, A.A., and Alvaro, A.B.: Angina pectoris at rest with preservation of exercise capacity. Prinzmetal's variant angina. *Circulation, 47:*956, 1973.

99. Murray, J.A.: Exercise testing in the diagnosis of coronary artery disease. Luncheon Panel #9, American College of Cardiology, Washington, D.C., Feb. 4, 1971.

100. Harris, C.N., Aronow, W.S., Parker, D.P., et al.: Treadmill stress test in left ventricular hypertrophy. *Chest, 63:*353-357, 1973.

101. Riley, C.P., Oberman, A., and Sheffield, L.T.: Electrocardiographic effects of glucose ingestion. *Arch Intern Med, 130:*703-707, 1972.

102. Kaplan, M.A., Harris, C.N., Aronow, W.S., et al.: Inability of the submaximal treadmill stress test to predict the location of coronary disease. *Circulation, 47:*250-255, 1973.

Chapter 6

GUIDELINES TO
EXERCISE TRAINING

PRIOR TO COMMENCING any physical conditioning program, it is absolutely essential that certain medical requirements be met. The *apparently healthy person under age thirty years* needs only to have a complete medical history and physical examination within the preceding year. For those *between ages thirty and forty,* the examination should be done within three months of the starting date and should include a resting electrocardiogram. Those *between the ages of forty-one and fifty-nine* years should also have an exercise electrocardiogram, using either the bicycle or treadmill technique. For the apparently healthy person *over age fifty-nine,* the physical examination needs to be done within two weeks of starting the fitness program and should include a resting and an exercise electrocardiogram. The person with *known coronary heart disease* should be at least two months postinfarction before starting a long-range conditioning program involving other than walking. If such a program is limited to walking, it can be performed without medical supervision, provided a screening examination does not detect heart failure or serious cardiac rhythm disturbances. The patient should be taught to check his own radial or carotid pulse rate and should limit the intensity of walking to that producing a pulse rate of less than 120 beats per minute. He should be instructed to wait two hours after a meal before walking, to avoid walking in extremes of weather, and to stop promptly if he experiences any chest discomfort.

Postcoronary patients who wish to undergo more strenuous forms of conditioning, including jogging and swimming, should do so under the direct supervision of medical or highly skilled paramedical personnel, and in the presence of emergency resuscitation equipment (including a defibrillator). We prefer a defibrillator which has "print-out paddles" and frequently spot-check cardiac rates and rhythm by this method. The ten absolute contraindications to such forms of activity are as follows:

1. Moderate to severe aortic outflow obstruction (supravalvular, valvular, subvalvular)
2. Congestive heart failure
3. Acute infectious disease, including active myocarditis
4. Rapidly progressive angina pectoris
5. Acute myocardial infarction
6. Dissecting aortic aneurysms
7. Thrombophlebitis
8. Poorly controlled supraventricular rhythm disorders (as rapid atrial fibrillation), serious ventricular rhythm disorders (as paroxysmal tachycardia, multifocal premature beats, or uniform premature beats occurring in pairs or at a frequency of more than 6/minute), and fixed-rate cardiac pacemakers
9. Severe systemic arterial hypertension (systolic pressure 200 mm Hg, diastolic pressure > 110 mm Hg)
10. Cyanotic congenital heart disease

There are a number of relative contraindications to exercise training in which the possible benefits of exercise must be carefully weighed against the risks involved. These relative contraindications include pulmonary hypertension, ventricular aneurysms, poorly controlled metabolic diseases such as diabetes mellitus or thyroid disorders, and toxemias of pregnancy. In addition, special consideration should be given to patients with cardiac pacemakers, congenital heart disease other than the cyanotic variety, and any form of chronic disease that might make it difficult to achieve a training effect. Such diseases include chronic renal or hepatic disorders, arthritis and musculoskeletal problems, and neuropsychiatric disorders. The cardiac exercise class should not be permitted to become a "catch-all" for severe cardiac problems in which there is no other form of therapy. Patients with severe angina pectoris, three-vessel coronary disease on angiography, and an akinetic myocardium on ventriculography are not candidates for coronary bypass surgery and neither are they candidates for a progressive exercise rehabilitation program.

Upon entering the exercise program, the patient must be advised to adhere to the exercise prescription. Unless this is done, patients have a tendency to keep up with advanced members of the group and to see how many repetitions of one exercise can be performed without serious sequelae. The group supervisors must be on the lookout for such instances and should report them immediately to the physician in charge. We make it a routine practice before each exercise session of asking each participant whether s/he has experienced chest pain within the past twenty-four hours. Several of our participants, after having been up most of the night before with prolonged chest pain, will report to the gym and try to "work the pain out." It requires patient education (and reeducation), daily questioning, and careful supervision to keep such instances from occurring. In our program, patients are not permitted to exercise if they have experienced any unusual type of recent chest pain. They are advised instead to promptly get in touch with their personal physician.

There are several basic rules that exercise participants are expected to adhere to. They are advised against exercising within two hours of a large meal and to refrain from coffee, tea, cigarettes, and alcohol during the same time segment. They should warm up for five minutes before the inception of exercise and should cool down for the same period of time after exercise before showering. The latter should be done using lukewarm water. The "buddy" system is used in the dressing room so that no individual is alone in the shower or dressing room. The doors on the toilets should not be locked from the inside, for in one program a patient suffered a cardiac arrest while straining during defecation.

The rules are applied in an inconspicuous manner. One does not wish for the participants to look upon the exercise class as an extension of the coronary care unit but rather as a place to enjoy meaningful and pleasurable activity and social exchange. There are several ways to enhance the program and thereby to improve the patient adherence. One is for the physician and paramedical team members to actually participate with the class. This not only makes it easier to know each member, but it emphasizes that the medical staff practices what it preaches. It is important for the medical staff to know the names of all class members and for the members to learn the names of each other. Periodic group photographs, with an accompanying name list, help in this direction, as do names on the back of T-shirts (Fig. 6-1). New members should be introduced to at least several of the veterans so that they feel more comfortable in the initial phases of the program, the period in which the drop-out rate tends to be the highest. The patient's spouse is encouraged to also participate in the program, (Fig. 6-2), provided that she obtains permission from her personal physician. In some instances, children are

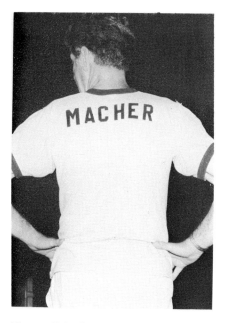

Figure 6-1. Gym shirt with patient's name printed on the back helps in identification.

likewise permitted to exercise with their parents. This enhances adherence, emphasizes the use of exercise as a preventive health measure, and can lead to stronger family ties. By including coronary-prone members in the same class with the postcoronary patients, one can impress upon the former the importance of preventive cardiology. When asked in the locker room when he had his "event," one coronary-prone member promptly replied that he had not had one "yet." After collecting his thoughts, he indicated that hopefully his participation in the rehabilitation program might considerably decrease his chances of ever having one.

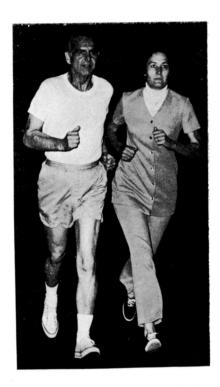

Figure 6-2. A post-myocardial-infarction patient and his wife jog together in the gymnasium exercise program.

Chapter 7

CORONARY RISK FACTOR DETECTION AND EXERCISE PRESCRIPTION IN A PREVENTIVE CARDIOLOGY CLINIC

A LTHOUGH AN ASSOCIATION for the "prevention and relief" of heart disease was started in 1920,[1] the practice of preventive cardiology has long been neglected, prompting Doctor Irvine Page to make the following statement: "Someday we may even realize that it is vastly more important, if not glamorous, to prevent atherosclerosis rather than repair the damage after it is done."[2] In an attempt to fulfill a need in this area, the Preventive Cardiology Clinic was formed in July, 1972. It is a highly specialized center with a staff that includes an attending cardiologist, an exercise physiologist, dieticians, and nursing personnel. A local and national committee of physicians and physiologists assist the clinic in providing the broad professional competency necessary to meet the objectives of preventive cardiology. The latter includes (1) detection of early signs of coronary heart disease, (2) identification and modification of known risk factors that predispose a person to this disease, and (3) determination of an individual's physical work capacity (the physiological evaluation of the oxygen transport system).

Each complete evaluation includes the following:

1. A comprehensive medical, physical activity, and dietary history, using the problem-oriented method of medical record keeping.
2. A biochemical profile, including serum cholesterol, triglyceride, and high-density lipoprotein
3. Body composition analysis (determination of lean body mass and percent body fat), using the skinfold caliper technique and sampling at ten sites

127

4. Pulmonary function testing
5. Personality-behavior pattern testing, using a modified Rosenman-Friedman questionnaire and structured interview
6. A resting electrocardiogram
7. A submaximal or maximal exercise stress test with continuous electrocardiographic monitoring and maximal oxygen uptake determination.

METHODS OF QUANTITATING CORONARY RISK

Several methods of quantitating coronary risk can be utilized. A simple method entails the completion of a risk factor questionnaire at the initial clinic visit (Table 7-I). The points for various positive factors are totaled, and the patient is placed in one of five categories (Table 7-II). While this provides a rough

TABLE 7-I
CORONARY RISK FACTOR QUESTIONNAIRE

RISK FACTOR	*POINTS*
1. Cigarette Smoking	
(a) 2 packs/day	7
(b) 1-2 packs/day	6
(c) ½-1 pack/day	5
2. Hypertension (systolic bp > 150 or diastolic bp > 90)	5
3. Elevated serum cholesterol	
(a) 350	7
(b) 300-350	6
(c) 250-300	5
(d) 225-250	3
4. Family history of coronary disease before age 55	4
5. Overweight > 15%	3
6. Elevated serum triglyceride	
(a) > 300	5
(b) 150-300	3
7. Diabetes mellitus	3
8. Type A personality	2
9. Abnormal EKG	2
10. Enlarged heart on chest X-ray	2
11. Low aerobic capacity	3
(no regular (3x week) endurance as swimming, jogging or bicycling)	
12. Abnormal exercise stress test	17

TABLE 7-II
CORONARY RISK CATEGORIES

I. Very Low	(<6 points)
II. Low	(6–10 points)
III. Average	(11–15 points)
IV. Above average	(16–20 points)
V. Very high	(>20 points)

index of risk, there are certain obvious limitations. The main limitation is the lack of statistical support for the relative significance of each factor. For instance, it is arbitrary to say that the relative risk of a serum cholesterol level of 350 mg % is the same as a cigarette intake in excess of two packs per day.

A more specific clinical index of coronary artery disease is that used by Cohn et al.[3,4,5] at the Peter Bent Brigham Hospital. These investigators obtained multiple clinical parameters on a series of 100 persons who were suspected of having underlying coronary heart disease. Coronary arteriograms were normal in 38 percent and abnormal, i.e. greater than 75 percent occlusion of one major artery, in 62 percent. Chemical parameters of statistical significance between the two groups included age, sex, history of ischemic episodes, resting electrocardiograms (pathologic Q waves and ST-T abnormalities), postexercise electrocardiograms, serum lipoprotein and glucose levels, and graphic recordings (third and fourth heart sound recordings, apexcardiogram, left ventricular ejection time). Multiple discriminant analysis was used, and each factor was given a numerical coefficient. The product of the latter times the coded value of each risk factor produced a numerical clinical index. Of 62 patients with coronary artery disease documented on arteriography, 69 (97 percent) had clinical index values above 100 points. Of the 38 patients with normal coronary arteriograms, 34 (89 percent) had clinical indices below 100 points. There were no false negatives in those patients whose clinical index was less than 80 points; that is, there were no significant abnormalities on coronary angiography in these patients. On the other hand, false positive results were seen in only 10 percent of those with indices ranging from 100 to 120 points and less than 5 percent in those with indices above 120 points.

The practicality and simplicity of the clinical index point system can be seen in the following example.

A fifty-year-old executive with vague chest pain unrelated to exertion was evaluated at the clinic. His resting electrocardiogram revealed ST-T abnormalities. The maximal treadmill stress test showed down-sloping S-T segment depression of 1.0 mm. The lipoprotein electrophoresis indicated a type IV pattern. A two-hour postprandial blood sugar was normal. A fourth heart sound was noted clinically and recorded during phonocardiography. His clinical index was calculated as seen in Table 7-III.

This patient's point total would make him likely to have significant (greater than 75 percent) obstruction of at least one major coronary vessel.

TABLE 7-III
CLINICAL INDEX FOR CORONARY DISEASE DETECTION

Variable	Coded value of variable	Numerical Coefficient	Points
1. age	years	0.7	0.7 x 50 = 35
2. sex	0 = Female	24	1 x 24 = 24
	1 = Male		
3. history of ischemia	0 = atypical angina	16	16 x 0 = 0
	1 = typical angina		
	3 = documented myocardial infarction		
4. resting ECG	0 = normal	2	2 x 1 = 2
	1 = ST-T abnormalities		
	3 = pathologic Q waves		
5. stress test ECG	0 = negative	14	14 x 2 = 28
	2 = positive		
6. lipoprotein and glucose	0 = normal	16	16 x 1 = 16
	1 = type II or IV lipoprotein and blood glucose abnormalities		
7. graphic recordings (apex- and phonocardiography and external carotid pulse tracings)	0 = normal	8	8 x 1 = 8
	1 = S4 and/or S3 sounds; abnormal "a" wave on apex; decreased left ventricular ejection time		
	3 = combinations of above		
	Total		113 points

The original study of Cohn et al.[3] was done in retrospective fashion. A prospective series, also on 100 patients, revealed similar results. Of 34 persons with clinical indices below 100 points, 31 (91%) had normal coronary arteriograms. Of 66 patients with clinical indices above one hundred points, 61 (92%) had significant abnormalities on coronary angiography, including 49 (74%) with multivessel disease.

A more complex method of assessing future coronary risk is that of Keys et al.[4] which involves the use of a programming calculator. The probability of developing future coronary disease was estimated by the multiple logistic equation using characteristics of age, serum cholesterol, cigarette smoking habits, body mass index, and systolic blood pressure. Of 11,132 men, ages forty to fifty-nine years, who were followed for five years, 615 developed heart disease. There was high correlation between the number of predicted cases and the number of observed cases. Since the actual number of cases among American men was underpredicted, risk factors which were not measured or possibly not yet identified are implied.

A new booklet on risk factor quantitation has recently been published by the American Heart Association (Fig. 7-1). Based on the Framingham data, it is easy to use and is of assistance to the practicing physician. The booklet deals with five risk factors (in addition to age and sex):

1. serum cholesterol level
2. glucose tolerance (as two-hour postprandial blood sugar)
3. cigarette usage
4. systolic blood pressure
5. left ventricular hypertrophy (on resting electrocardiogram).

For example, a forty-five-year-old man who smokes cigarettes, has a systolic blood pressure of 180 mm Hg, normal glucose tolerance, a cholesterol level of 310 mg/dl, and does not have left ventricular hypertrophy on the electrocardiogram has a 16.9 percent probability of developing coronary disease in six years, a fourfold increased risk compared to the average man of this age. Similarly, a fifty-year-old woman with glucose intolerance, a history of cigarette smoking, an electrocardio-

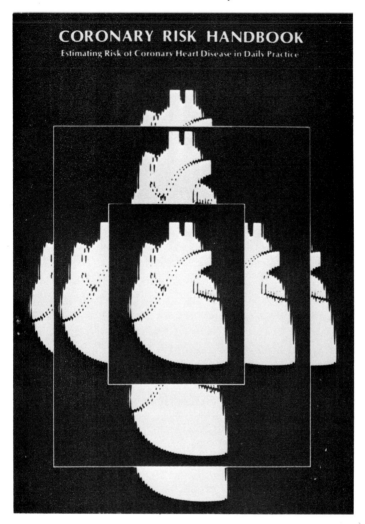

Figure 7-1. Coronary risk factor booklet used in clinical practice.

gram positive for left ventricular hypertrophy, a systolic blood pressure of 180 mm Hg, and a cholesterol level of 335 mg/dl has a 15.5 percent probability of developing coronary disease within the next six years, a seven– to eightfold increased risk compared to the average woman this age.

Salel et al.[5] used this risk factor handbook in 158 consecutive

WHITE MALE AGE 40-44

Rank	Cause of Death	Chance in 100,000 of the individual dying from this cause	
		68	60
1	Arteriosclerotic Heart Disease	1861	1877
2	Motor Vehicle Accidents	339	285
3	Cirrhosis	304	222
4	Malig. Neoplasms Of The Lung	291	202
5	Suicide	253	264
6	Vascular Lesions Affecting C.N.S.	209	222
7	Pneumonia	114	111
8	Malig. Neopl. Of Lg. Int. & Rectm.	88	111
9	Homicide	87	—
10	Rheumatic Heart Disease	87	167

Figure 7-2. Leading threats to health and life in a middle-aged man.

patients (117 men, 41 women, mean age 43 years) prior to coronary arteriography. Significant coronary lesions were subsequently observed in 105 of the 158. A probability index for coronary disease was calculated from the booklet data by dividing the patient's numerical risk by the average risk in his/her age group. The index was 1.52 for patients later shown to have significant coronary disease and 1.08 for those who did not. Moreover, there was a linear relationship between the probability index and the extent of coronary disease.

Another booklet that we find of great use is the *Probability Tables of Deaths In the Next Ten Years From Specific Causes* (Health Hazard Appraisal, Methodist Hospital of Indiana). This gives the patient a clear understanding of the leading threats to health and life for their particular age group. For example, a forty-two-year-old white male has the risks listed in Figure 7-2. Since cancer of the large bowel and rectum is number 8, the individual is encouraged to have a proctoscopic examination and stool guaiac sampling.

THE EXERCISE PRESCIPTION

Since many of the clinic patients are young executives, airline pilots, and various professional people, a major interest and emphasis of the center is exercise testing and prescribing an exercise program that is specifically tailored to an individual's needs and desires.

At the consultation session, the cardiologist and physiologist review the accumulated data on coronary risk and fitness classification with the patient. The latter is taught that he has a maximum pulse rate based on age and degree of present physical conditioning, that this rate can be predicted from a chart, and that it can be more precisely measured by exercise stress testing. He is further advised that to achieve a training effect he must perform endurance-type activities that will maintain the pulse rate between 70 and 85 percent of the maximum rate for a total of at least 90 to 100 minutes per week. If the person has not participated in any regular exercise program recently, he is advised to build up gradually and is given a schedule to guide him (Table 7-IV).

The exercise prescription is based upon the MET unit system, one MET unit being the amount of energy expended at rest multiplied by a factor of 1.1. If a person's maximum tolerance for work, as measured on the treadmill, is 10 MET units, the exercise prescription is for 70 to 85 percent of this value, (or 7-8.5 MET units). In order to make the endurance exercise more enjoyable, this patient may choose from a list of activities

TABLE 7-IV
CARDIOPULMONARY ENDURANCE EXERCISE SCHEDULE
FOR THE UNTRAINED PERSON

Week 1-2	15 minutes (at the prescribed MET unit level)	3 times/week
Week 3-4	20 minutes	4 times/week
Week 5-6	25 minutes	3 times/week
Week 7-8	25 minutes	4 times/week
Week 9 and beyond	Select one of the following:	
	(1) 20 minutes, 5 days/week	
	(2) 25 minutes, 4 days/week	
	(3) 30 minutes, 3 days/week	

which are comparable to a given number of MET units (Table 7-V). Obviously, if someone strongly dislikes jogging, he is unlikely to adhere to a regimen in which this form of activity is emphasized.

Patients are instructed in the self-determination of pre– and postexercise pulse rates. They are asked to record this on a postcard, along with the frequency of exercise per week, and mail it to the clinic. Repeat treadmill testing is done three months after initial evaluation and at least annually thereafter. The maximal oxygen uptake value is recorded on a graph (Fig. 7-3) in order to better enable a patient to follow his progress and to see how his fitness level compares to others in the same group.

For a baseline maintenance exercise regimen, exercises that can be done alone are stressed. These include brisk walking, jogging, swimming, cycling, rope skipping and bench stepping. Except for swimming, none of these activities require a special facility. A certain amount of skill is required only for swimming, unless one has never ridden a bicycle nor skipped rope as a youth. These activities should constitute the majority of time spent in cardiopulmonary conditioning. As previously mentioned, they should be supplemented by some of the group activities in the cases where that is possible. For example, the businessman who travels extensively could easily pack a jump rope or a pair of walking or jogging shoes. He might swim at a motel pool or perhaps carry a stationary cycle in the trunk of his car. Easier still, he could measure the elevation of a certain object, such as a chair or stool in his room, and use it for bench-stepping exercise. A minimum of time is required, but this is well worth the investment.

The following four case histories best exemplify the nature of the preventive cardiology evaluation and the method of exercise prescription.

Case 1

A forty-five-year-old airline pilot was evaluated for coronary risk and level of physical fitness. The history revealed sporadic

TABLE 7-V

CLASSIFICATION OF ACTIVITY BY MET UNITS*

3-4 METS	6-7 METS (continued)
Walking (3 MPH)	Tennis (singles)
Cycling (6 MPH)	Badminton (competition)
Softball (excluding pitcher)	Swimming (1.6 MPH)
Dancing (moderate)	Step-up (24 steps/minute, 32 cm height)
Pitching horse shoes	7 METS
Golf (pulling cart)	Double Master's test
Volleyball (6-man, not vigorous)	
Badminton (doubles)	*7-8 METS*
Steps (24 steps/minute, 12 cm height)	Jogging (5 MPH)
4 METS	Cycling (12 MPH)
Treadmill (2 MPH, 3.5% grade)	Swimming (side stroke, 1 MPH)
3 METS	Treadmill (3 MPH, 10% grade)
	7 METS
4-5 METS	Basketball (moderate)
Tennis (doubles)	Touch football
Walking (3½ MPH)	Skiing (hard, downhill)
Cycling (8 MPH)	Horseback riding (gallop)
Ping Pong	Mountain hiking (without back pack)
Golf (carrying clubs)	Step-up (24 steps/minute, 35 cm height)
Raking leaves	8 METS
Calisthenics (in general)	
Rowing (noncompetitive)	*8-9 METS*
Dancing (vigorous)	Jogging (5½ MPH)
Step-up (24 steps/minute, 18 cm height)	Cycling (13 MPH)
5 METS	Fencing
Treadmill (2 MPH, 7% grade) 4 METS	Basketball (vigorous)
	Handball
5-6 METS	Paddleball
Walking (4 MPH)	Step-up (30 steps/minute, 28 cm height)
Cycling (10 MPH)	9 METS
Ice Skating	*10-11 METS*
Roller skating	Running (6 MPH) 10 METS
Horseback riding (trot)	Handball (vigorous)
Swim (1 MPH)	Paddleball (vigorous)
Step-up (24 steps/minute, 25 cm height)	Swimming (back stroke, 1.6 MPH)
6 METS	Step-up (30 steps/minute, 36 cm height)
Treadmill (2 MPH, 10.5% grade)	11 METS
5 METS	Treadmill (3.4 MPH, 14% grade)
	10 METS
6-7 METS	
Walking (5 MPH)	*12+ METS*
Cycling (11 MPH)	Running (8 MPH) 13½ METS
Water skiing	Rowing (11 MPH) 13½ METS
Lawn-mowing (hand mower)	Step-up (30 steps/minute, 40 cm height)
Skiing (towing or easy downhill)	12 METS
Square dancing	Treadmill (3.4 MPH, 18% grade)
	12 METS

* From S.M. Fox III et al., Physical activity and the prevention of coronary heart disease, *Annals of Clinical Research, 3:*404-432, 1971.

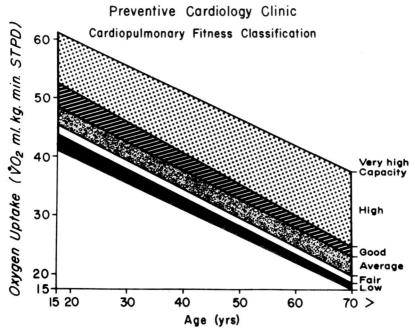

Figure 7-3. Cardiorespiratory fitness, based on oxygen uptake analysis, as plotted on an age-adjusted graph.

jogging in the past and a fatal myocardial infarction in a brother, age fifty-three years. The physical examination indicated mild hypertension and excess body weight. The biochemical profile indicated an elevated fasting blood sugar (144 mg %), serum cholesterol (321 mg %), and serum triglyceride (369 mg %). The resting electrocardiogram was normal. The patient underwent treadmill testing by the Bruce method, reaching a maximum heart rate of 170 beats per minute before onset of fatigue. The S-T segment was depressed 1.0 mm in a horizontal fashion during the latter stages of exercise but was upsloping in the postexercise tracings. The maximum oxygen uptake was 35 ml/kg/min., placing him in an average category for his age group. The personality pattern questionnaire was suggestive of a Type B pattern. Body composition analysis by the skinfold technique indicated that fat constituted 19 percent of his total body weight. A three-day dietary diary was assessed and indicated a daily caloric consumption ranging between 4,000 to 5,000 calories.

A lipoprotein electrophoresis was subsequently obtained and was normal. A two-hour postprandial blood glucose was mildly elevated. Because of the positive exercise test, the patient was placed in the medically supervised exercise class at Georgia Baptist Hospital. His nutritional prescription called for a 1,400-calorie, fat-controlled diet, in which he and his wife were instructed. When retested three months later, the amount of body fat decreased from 19 percent to 16 percent (of total weight). The oxygen uptake was 43.19 ml/kg/min. (vs. 35.9 ml/kg/min. initially). The serum triglyceride showed a 50 percent decrease, while the cholesterol diminished by 25 percent; more significantly, the exercise electrocardiogram showed no evidence of ischemia.

Case 2

A forty-year-old writer was seen for a routine screening evaluation. His father had experienced a myocardial infarction at age sixty-two years, as did a half brother at age forty-seven years. The resting blood pressure was mildly elevated (145/100 mm Hg). The serum cholesterol was 283 mg %, and the triglyceride was 143 mg %. The resting electrocardiogram was normal. The patient completed eight minutes of the Bruce treadmill test, reaching a maximum heart rate of 180 beats per minute. There were junctional S-T segment changes on the electrocardiogram during exercise but no evidence of ischemia. The maximum oxygen consumption of 25 ml/kg/min. was very low. Twenty-one percent of his total body weight was fat, indicating the need to lose twenty pounds of body fat. He was advised of having five coronary risk factors (excess fat, very low aerobic capacity, elevated serum cholesterol, systemic arterial hypertension and a family history of coronary disease).

He was placed on a fat– and calorie-restricted diet and a home jogging program, working up to one-and-one-half miles per day over a six-week period. A friend was instructed in blood pressure recording, and a diary was kept. When retested three months later, he had lost fourteen pounds of fat weight and his oxygen consumption had increased to 31 ml/kg/min., a 16 percent increment. The blood pressure diary showed an average home reading of 130/85 mm Hg. The serum cholesterol had decreased to 258 mg %, a 25 mg % fall.

Case 3

A fifty-seven-year-old company president underwent coronary risk assessment and exercise testing. He had been an Olympic-caliber athlete as a youth and had smoked cigarettes for thirty pack-years, quitting in 1957. Both parents lived beyond their eightieth year. He currently exercised an average of three times per week on a treadmill and on weight-training machines. He had been given clofibrate for hypercholesterolemia two years previously.

The physical examination was normal except for a midsystolic nonejection click at the cardiac apex. The serum cholesterol was moderately elevated at 276 mg %. The resting electrocardiogram was normal as was a chest x-ray. He progressed to the fourth stage of the Bruce treadmill test with a maximum heart rate of 175 beats per minute. The exercise electrocardiogram was normal and the maximum oxygen consumption was 43 ml/kg/min., a very high level for his age group. Since his maximum MET unit of exercise tolerance was 12.3, he was advised to exercise at a level of 9 MET units in hopes of maintaining his excellent level of conditioning. The clofibrate dosage was increased, and nutritional counseling was obtained with the objective of reducing the serum cholesterol level to less than 220 mg %. He was advised to undergo exercise stress testing on an annual basis.

Case 4

A fifty-one-year-old businessman was evaluated because of rather vague anterior chest pain. The history was significant in that his father died at age sixty-one years of a myocardial infarction. The physical examination was unremarkable except for excess body weight and a resting blood pressure of 190/120 mm Hg. On skinfold assessment, the percentage of total weight as fat was 22.5 percent. The cholesterol was moderately elevated (338 mg %), and the triglyceride was significantly elevated (486 mg %). The resting electrocardiogram was normal. The patient completed seven minutes of the Bruce test, attaining a peak pulse rate of 135 per minute and a blood pressure of 190/112 mm Hg. The S-T segment was depressed 2 mm during and immediately postexercise (Fig. 7-4), indicative of ischemia. The maximal oxygen consumption was extremely low at 13.9 ml/kg/min. The patient was advised of the multiple coronary risk factors. In view of the positive exercise electrocardiogram, he was entered in the medically supervised exercise program and started on both antihypertensive and lipid-lowering agents. Six weeks later, while on a golfing vacation, he experienced several bouts of exercise-induced chest pain. An electrocardiogram taken the following day revealed inferior wall injury which subsequently evolved into an extensive anterior and inferior infarction. His two-week hospital course was uneventful, and upon discharge he was begun on the home walking regimen. Two months later, he underwent an evaluation before reentering the outpatient gymnasium program. His body fat had decreased 3 percent. The serum cholesterol had fallen from 388 mg % to 335 mg %; the triglyceride level was now 220 mg %. The exercise electrocardiogram continued to show significant S-T segment depression. He began at a low level of gymnasium exercise and has progressed to brisk walking and slow jogging activities with no adverse signs or symptoms.

We fully concur with the comments of the working party of the British College of Physicians and the British Cardiac Society:[6]

> In the 1960s the average practitioner learned the technique of external cardiac massage; in the late 1970s and 1980s he will also make himself expert on coronary heart disease prevention, the better to advise the coronary prone patient who dislikes the idea of playing Russian roulette with the emergency services.

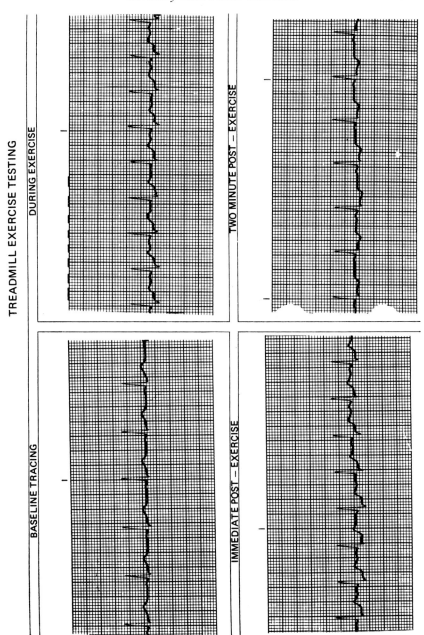

Figure 7-4. A positive exercise stress test on a fifty-one-year-old businessman.

REFERENCES

1. White, P.D.: Tardy growth of preventive cardiology. *Am J Cardiol,* *29:*886-888, 1972.
2. Page, I.H.: Atherosclerosis. A personal overview. *Circulation, 38:*1164-1172, 1968.
3. Cohn, P.F., Gorlin, R., Vokonas, P.S., et al.: A quantitative clinical index for the diagnosis of symptomatic coronary-artery disease. *N Engl J Med, 286:*901-907, 1972.
4. Keys, A., Aravanis, C., Blackburn, H., et al.: Probability of middle-aged men developing coronary heart disease in five years. *Circulation, 45:*815-828, 1972.
5. Salel, A.F., Fong, A., Zelis, R., et al.: Accuracy of numerical coronary profile. *N Engl J Med, 296:*1447-1449, 1977.
6. British College of Physicians: Prevention of coronary heart disease. *Lancet, 1:*783-784, 1976.

Chapter 8

POSTINFARCTION REHABILITATION: HOSPITAL PHASE

U NTIL THE LAST decade, the general consensus among physicians treating patients with coronary heart disease was that physical activity had deleterious effects in the clinical setting of recent myocardial infarction. The treatment was rather stereotyped in that most acute coronary victims could expect up to six to eight weeks of bed rest within the hospital and at home postdischarge. This period of strict bed rest was based upon early studies of Levine and Brown[1] dealing with the duration of the healing process. In 1929, these authors stated that activity too soon postinfarction could lead to mural thrombus formation, aneurysm development, or myocardial rupture. As the maximum healing process, including the formation of scar tissue, took place within six to eight weeks postinfarction, it seemed reasonable to markedly reduce myocardial oxygen demands and cardiac work during this time segment.

With the advent of cardiac catheterization and other refined techniques in hemodynamic assessment, it became obvious that there were certain disadvantages of maintaining a cardiac patient in a recumbent position for prolonged periods of time. Coe[2] found that cardiac work increased 29 percent when normal subjects or cardiac patients were moved from sitting to recumbent positions. The latter position resulted in an augmentation of venous return, increasing contractility through the Frank-Starling mechanism. The failing heart, or the heart with a compromised coronary circulation, could be unduly stressed by prolonged recumbency.

There has been recent controversy, particularly in the British medical literature, as to not only the optimal length of

143

hospitalization postinfarction but also the veracity of hospitalization itself. A randomized study[3] was set up to compare home care by the family doctor and hospital treatment. The latter involved an initial period of observation in a coronary care unit. Participating in the study were 458 English general practitioners who allocated 343 cases at random to the two treatment groups. The groups did not differ significantly with respect to age, prior diagnosis of angina pectoris, previous myocardial infarction, or history of hypertension. The groups were also similar with respect to the prevalence of hypotension when initially examined. Of 169 hospitalized patients, the twenty-eight day mortality rate was 14.2 percent compared to 9.8 percent for the 174 patients who were treated at home. Although the results certainly provide food for thought in an era of super mechanization and medical gadgetry, the study had certain definite drawbacks which bear mentioning. For instance, a number of patients initially treated at home were later transferred to the hospital, clouding the issue considerably since they were still considered to be in the home care group. Moreover, the location and severity of the infarctions were not compared in the two groups, nor was analysis made of the time lapse between the onset of symptoms and the initial call for medical help.

When looking at studies such as this, one needs to be highly critical. It is likewise important for the practitioner to draw upon his past experience and to employ a little common sense. It is certainly not difficult for most practicing physicians to recall numerous instances of life-threatening cardiac arrhythmias which were promptly recognized and treated in the coronary care unit and which probably would have resulted in the patient's demise had they occurred at home.

A more reasonable controversy centers around the question of early versus late mobilization and discharge post-myocardial-infarction. Wenger et al.[4] published the results of a questionnaire as to the current physician practice in managing uncomplicated myocardial infarction patients. The questionnaire was sent to 1200 general practitioners, 1200 internists and 1200 cardiologists. The 69 percent who responded managed

70,000 patients with acute myocardial infarctions during 1970. The responses were similar for the three groups in that 95 percent of the patients were hospitalized for twenty-one days; most were permitted to sit in a chair on the eighth hospital day and to walk in the room on the fourteenth day. Doctor Geoffrey Rose[5] recently made the following statement pertaining to old traditions and modern doubts of inhospital care:

> Physicians have always been very cautious in their management of patients with myocardial infarction. We are less upset if our patient dies in bed than if he dies while walking in the ward or street, for in confining him to bed we feel that at least we did everything possible.

But have we? In 1952, Levine and Lown[6] published the results of armchair rather than bed rest treatment for 73 patients with myocardial infarction, indicating that there were no evident ill effects from such therapy. They also pointed out the various hazards of immobilization, including rapid muscle wasting, decreased pulmonary ventilation, impaired exercise tolerance, and loss of normal postural vasomotor reflexes. The latter was clearly demonstrated by Fareeduddin and Abelmann.[7] They reported that 5 of 10 patients treated for nine to twenty-four days with strict bed rest had transient systemic blood pressure decreases of more than 38 mm Hg during fifteen minutes of passive upright tilt to seventy degrees. This response was abolished after a period of full ambulation and was not observed in eight patients who were treated with modified bed rest. Such a significant fall in blood pressure could be catastrophic to a patient with a compromised myocardial blood supply in that it could lead to reinfarction or to extension of the initial infarction.

Saltin et al.[8] have carried out extensive studies on the effect of a twenty-day period of bed rest on 5 normal subjects, ages nineteen to twenty-one. Two of the subjects were very active physically prior to the study, while the remainder had been essentially sedentary. The maximum oxygen uptake fell from a mean of 3.3 liters/minute before bed rest to 2.43 liters/minute. During supine exercise on a bicycle ergometer at 600 kpm/minute the stroke volume decreased 25 percent and the heart rate increased from an average of 129 beats/minute to 154 beats/minute. An oxygen uptake that could normally be attained at a heart rate of 145 beats/minute now required a rate of 180 beats/minute after bed rest. During maximal treadmill testing the cardiac output fell 26 percent after bed rest (from 20 to 14.8 liters/minute). This was attributed to a reduction in stroke volume, since the maximal arteriovenous oxygen difference and the maximal heart rate was not altered.

Numerous recent reports have dealt with the results of early mobilization and discharge after myocardial infarction. In Northern Ireland, Adgey[9] reported 102 patients who were hospitalized for an average period of thirteen days postinfarction. Over a two-week period after discharge, there was no mortality and no apparent morbidity that might have been prevented by a more prolonged hospital stay. Takkunen et al.[10] in Finland, compared 146 patients who were mobilized after three to seven days in the hospital and discharged between twelve to sixteen days with 108 patients who were bedridden for seven to fourteen days and hospitalized for twenty-one to twenty-eight days. There was no significant difference when the mortality rates were assessed at seven days and again at thirty days postdischarge. This study had the limitations of not being randomized and not including long-term results. Tucker et al.[11] (England) were more aggressive and discharged 89 percent of 289 postinfarction patients by the tenth hospital day. Of this group, 7.6 percent were readmitted during a six-week follow-up period, and 6.7 percent of the discharged patients died. The authors seemed encouraged by this approach and noted that 62 percent of the patients were back at work five months after their infarction. The results and conclusions are, however, a little bothersome for several reasons. First, 38 percent of their patients were still out of work five months postinfarction, a figure which exceeds that in many institutions. Second, in the absence of a randomized control group, the possibility exists that the six-week postdischarge mortality and morbidity rates might exceed that of a group hospitalized for a longer period of time.

Fortunately, there are recent reports of well-controlled studies which may serve as guidelines. Harpur et al.[12] studied 199 patients with uncomplicated myocardial infarctions. All were given seven days of bed rest and then allocated into either Plan A or Plan B. In the former, patients were mobilized on day eight and discharged on the fifteenth hospital day. In Group B, patients were mobilized on day twenty-one and discharged on the twenty-eighth hospital day. All patients were encouraged to return to work one month after discharge. The groups were well matched with respect to previous cardiovascular history, age, sex, interval from onset of pain to admission, and site of infarction. In the first eight months after infarction, the early and late mobilization groups did not differ significantly with respect to cardiac mortality or morbidity, congestive heart failure, serious arrhythmias, or the development of ventricular aneurysm formation. There was a significant difference in the "return to work" rate two months after admission. In the early mobilization group, 41 percent were back at work in two months versus only 17 percent of the late mobilization group. As Rose has pointed out, this study was not entirely free of selection bias in that patients were included in the early mobilization group only if they had been free of hypotension, congestive heart failure, or serious arrhythmias in the preceding five days.

Hutter et al.,[13] at the Massachusetts General Hospital, described a prospective randomized controlled study comparing a two-week and a three-week hospital stay in 138 patients with uncomplicated myocardial infarctions. The groups were comparable for age, sex, prior cardiovascular problems, and location of infarction. During a six-month follow-up period there were no group differences in terms of coronary mortality or morbidity, aneurysm formation, psychological signs and symptoms, congestive heart failure, and number returning to work. The authors concluded that there appeared to be no additional benefit from a three-week hospital course as compared to a two-week period for patients with uncomplicated myocardial infarctions.

Bloch et al.[14] randomly assigned 154 postinfarction patients to an early mobilization group (active physical therapy beginning on day two or three) and a late mobilization group (strict bed rest for at least three weeks). The former had a mean hospital stay of 21.3 days versus 32.8 days for the latter group. Over an average follow-up of 11.2 months, there were no significant group differences in mortality, reinfarction, arrhythmias, heart failure, angina pectoris, aneurysm formation, or exercise test results.

Unlike Bloch's study, Abraham et al.[15] considered early discharge as well as early mobilization in a prospective randomized study of 129 patients who survived for at least five days after a myocardial infarction. The early group was mobilized on day six and discharged after twelve days, while the late group was mobilized on day thirteen and discharged on day nineteen. In a follow-up ranging from six to fifty-two weeks, cardiac complications were more prevalent in the late group than in the early group:

Complication	Early Mobilization and Discharge (64 patients)	Late Mobilization and Discharge (65 patients)
Myocardial ischemia	5	13
Congestive heart failure	2	15
Myocardial infarction	1	8
Pulmonary edema	1	6

Who is a candidate for early discharge? In an analysis of 522 consecutive patients with acute myocardial infarctions at Duke University, McNeer et al.[16] found that in patients having no serious complications through day four, the hospital mortality rate was zero and there were no serious late complications. They suggested studying the feasibility of discharge in the uncomplicated patient after the seventh hospital day, stating that to cut ten or more days off each hospital course would save $2000 to $3000 per patient. Their definition of the "uncomplicated patient" is the individual who in the first four days of hospitalization has none of the following:

1. asystole
2. ventricular tachycardia or fibrillation
3. high-grade heart block
4. pulmonary edema
5. shock
6. extension of infarct
7. persistent sinus tachycardia
8. persistent hypotension

9. supraventricular tachyarrhythmias.

Such a study of very early discharge has been conducted in Belfast.[17] Out of 275 admissions for acute myocardial infarction, 109 (40%) who survived six days were free of the following:

1. sustained sinus tachycardia (>1 hour) within first two days of hospitalization
2. > 2 mm S-T segment elevation in any lead six days after admission
3. the need for morphine analgesia between the second and seventh days postadmission
4. serious rhythm and conduction disturbances between day two and day seven of hospitalization

Sixty-eight percent of those 109 patients who had none of the above complications were discharged by the seventh hospital day, and there were no deaths over a three-month follow-up at home. It was unclear why 32 percent of the so-called uncomplicated patients were not also released on day seven, making the overall results somewhat difficult to interpret.

Rose[5] has summarized the controversies of early versus late mobilization and has offered the following suggested policy:

1. Until further controlled studies are available, the coronary patient free of severe pain or shock may be treated with bed or chair rest for the first seven days of hospitalization. The legs should be exercised daily, and a bedside commode is preferred over a bedpan.
2. Beginning on the eighth hospital day, the "good risk" patient (devoid of persistent pain, congestive heart failure, and ventricular arrhythmias) can be allowed to ambulate in the ward. He can be discharged several days later and can soon return to work.
3. Patients who do not fall in the "good risk" group must be managed on a highly individualized basis. Since this is such a diverse group, fixed rules do not apply.

An ad hoc committee[18] of the American College of Cardiology felt that nine to fourteen days of hospitalization was sufficient if there was no evidence of the following:

1. continuing myocardial ischemia
2. left ventricular failure

3. shock
4. important cardiac arrhythmias
5. conduction disturbances
6. other serious illnesses.

The value of intermediate coronary care (ICC) units has been assessed by several groups.[19-21] Reynell[19] conducted a five-year study (in a district general hospital in England) of 1,000 men, all under age sixty-five, allocating them at random to the ward or to intermediate care areas after release from the coronary care unit. They found no significant differences in mortality between the two groups, although initially successful resuscitation attempts were higher in the intermediate care group (16 of 35) compared to patients randomized to ward care (9 of 41). On the other hand, Vismara et al.[21] noted that potentially serious ventricular ectopy can appear during the second and third weeks of hospitalization of patients whose rhythm while in the coronary care unit was stable. Such dysrhythmias could possibly have been detected if patients had been monitored for additional periods in an intermediate care unit. Friedan and Cooper[20] reported that 18 of 27 patients (67%) who had cardiac arrests while in an ICC were successfully resuscitated and nine of these (50%) were eventually discharged. These figures certainly compare favorably to the 30 percent resuscitation success rate and the 13.3 percent discharge success rate in patients on general medical wards.[22]

At Georgia Baptist Hospital, the cardiac rehabilitation team sees only those patients whose physicians fill out the referral sheet (Table 8-I). The team consists of a physician and nurse coordinators working in conjunction with the physical therapist, dietician, chaplain, social worker, and pharmacologist (Fig. 8-1). The pharmacologist reviews the medication list on all patients, looking for possible adverse interactions, and counsels the patients as to drug mechanisms and potential side effects. The physical therapist follows a modification of the Emory University inpatient activity regimen (Table 8-II). It is similar to the suggestions of Rose in that most patients can be sitting in a chair while still in the coronary care unit. The patients begin to ambulate on the seventh hospital day and prior to discharge at

TABLE 8-I   Cardiac rehabilitation referral sheet, Georgia Baptist Medical Center

Doctor_____   Date_____
Patient_____   Room_____ Age_____

The following services are offered by the Cardiac Rehabilitation Team. Please check the services you desire.

Rehabilitation Services desired

I.   Individual patient and family conferences:
_____ Dietary history, analysis, and instructions.
_____ Risk factors (smoking, diet, exercise, weight, blood lipids).
_____ Instruction concerning current cardiac problems.
_____ Religious counseling (by hospital chaplain).
_____ Psychological testing.

II. Physical activity program (directed by the Cardiac Rehabilitation physician):
_____ Physical therapy.
_____ Progressive daily activities, i.e., self-grooming, chair-walking (a list of these progressive activities is posted on each ward).
_____ Telemetry exercise monitoring _____ with stairs.
_____ Discuss the Outpatient Exercise Program.

III. Recreational therapy program:
_____ Table games, jigsaw puzzles, arts, and crafts.

IV. Patient and family group conferences:
_____ Diet instruction.   _____ Coronary atherosclerotic heart disease.
_____ Risk factors.
_____ Emotional and spiritual implications. _____ Cardiac drugs.

V.   Follow-up:
_____ Home visit.
_____ Return to hospital for group conferences.
_____ Health agency referral.

Signed_____ M.D.

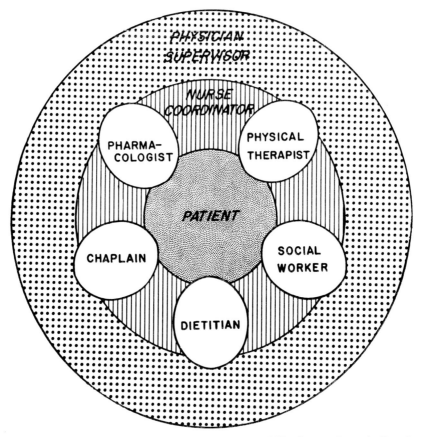

Figure 8-1. The team approach to cardiac rehabilitation at Georgia Baptist Hospital.

day fourteen are walking in the halls and climbing one or two flights of stairs under telemetry monitoring. The patients perform first active assistive (Fig. 8-2) and then active bed exercise under the supervision of the physical therapist (Fig. 8-3A-G). The activities are terminated if the pulse rate is greater than 115 beats/minute or if ectopic beats occur. At Grady Memorial Hospital, the Emory regimen has been used on over 2000 patients[23] with only one mishap, that being an instance of ventricular fibrillation during passive range of motion exercise that was promptly terminated by electrical defibrillation.

TABLE 8-II Cardiac rehabilitation inpatient program/activity-exercise-recreation, Georgia Baptist Medical Center

Where-When	Activity	Exercise	Recreation
Step 1 CCU Day 2	Bedside commode, feed self, self-grooming	Passive range of motion (10 times) to all extremities in bed. Active plantar and dorsiflexion of ankles (10 times) every one to two hours when awake	Conversation with therapist
Step 2 CCU Day 3 and 4	Chair 20 minutes three times a day	Active assistive range of motion (10 times) daily	Reading, conversation with therapist
Step 3 Progressive care Day 5 through 7	Bathe self Chair 30 minutes four times a day Walk to bathroom (if in room) as necessary with assistance	Active range of motion daily (5 times Day 5, 7 times on Day 6, 10 times on Day 7)	Art work, card games, puzzles
Step 4 Ward Day 8 and 9	Walk back and forth in room four times a day. (2 times each Day 8, 4 times each Day 9) Chair 45 minutes four times a day	Minimal resistance to active range of motion (10 times) daily	Noncompetitive or competitive table games.
Step 5 Ward Day 10 and 11	Stand at sink to shave. Walk to bathroom as needed. Chair as needed	Moderate resistance to active range of motion (10 times) twice a day	Noncompetitive or competitive table games.
Step 6 Ward Day 12	Bathe in tub or use shower. Walk 50 yards and climb one flight of stairs (telemetry) Up in chair and room as needed	Add: Standing (a) arm and shoulder (3 times) (b) lateral bend (5 times) (c) knee raise (5 times) Side (a) leg raise (5 times) Unsupervised active range of motion (10 times) twice a day	Initiation of art or craft project (leathercraft, copperwork, etc.).
Step 7 Ward Day 13	Walk length of hall twice a day	Add: Sitting (a) toe touch (4 times) (b) trunk twist (4 times)	Continuation of art or craft project.
Step 8 Ward Day 14 through 21	Up ad lib including walking up and down one flight of stairs.	Add: Standing (a) half knee bends (4 times)	Continuation of previous recreational activity

Any or all stages of Recreation Therapy may include participation by family, friends, or other patients.
CCU = coronary care unit

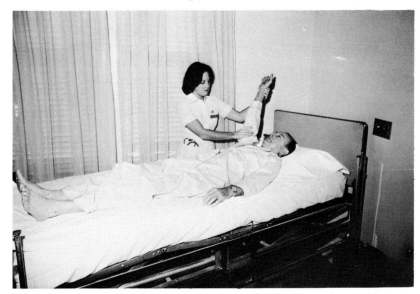

Figure 8-2. *Active-assisted exercise.* With the patient in the supine position, the arm is lifted straight back over the head and then down to the side again.

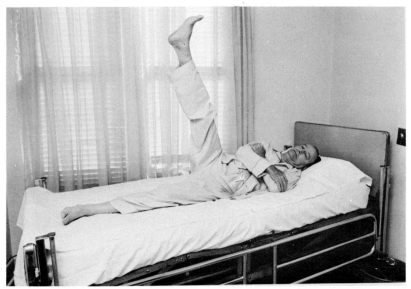

Figure 8-3A. *Side leg raises.* While lying on his side, the patient raises his right leg as high as comfortably possible. He raises the left leg the same number of times.

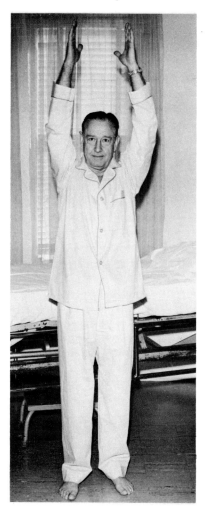

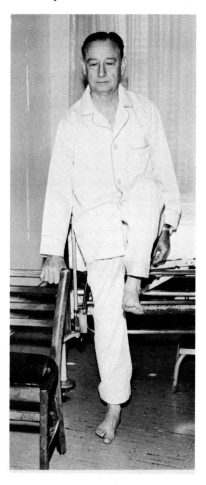

Figure 8-3C. *Knee raise.* The patient, using a stationary object for balance, raises his knee toward his chest and then lowers it to the floor; he should not hold the leg in the raised position. To complete the sequence, he repeats the above with the left leg.

Figure 8-3B. *Arm and shoulder loosening.* With the patient in the standing position, the arms are raised overhead, bringing the palms together. The arms are then lowered to the side, completing the sequence. The patient is instructed to inhale as he raises his arms and to exhale as he lowers his arms to the starting position.

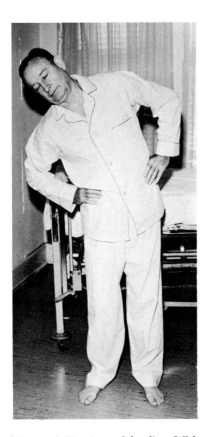

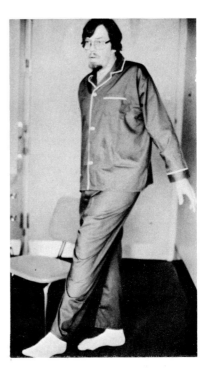

Figure 8-3E. *Leg rotation*. Using a stationary object for balance, the patient brings his left leg in front of his right leg, returns it to the starting position, extends it out to the side, then behind him, and back to the starting position. To complete the sequence, he repeats the above with his right leg.

Figure 8-3D. *Lateral bending*. With the hands placed on the hips, the patient bends laterally at the waist from side to side. He is instructed to exhale while bending and to inhale as he returns to the starting position.

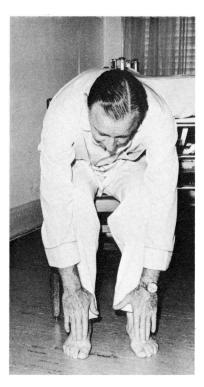

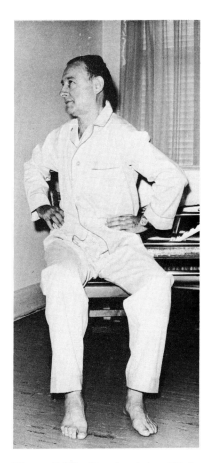

Figure 8-3F. *Reach and touch.* While sitting in a straight-backed chair, the patient bends and touches his toes with his fingertips and then returns to the upright position. He is instructed to exhale as he bends and to inhale as he returns to the starting position.

Figure 8-3G. *Trunk twisting.* While sitting in a straight-backed chair with his hands on his hips, the patient twists his trunk to the right and to the left. He is instructed to exhale as he turns and to inhale as he returns to the starting position.

Patients are encouraged to flex and extend the feet and knees on an hourly basis. To do so on a once– or twice-daily schedule is probably ineffective as suggested by the study of Browse,[24] who measured calf blood flow with venous occlusion plethysmography. The blood flow increased significantly following leg exercises but returned to the resting basal level within one hour of rest. We also encourage the use of elastic stockings which have been known to increase the speed of venous return from ankle to groin as measured by the ^{125}I-labeled Hippuran® injection technique.[25] Other investigators, however, have used the tagged fibrinogen scanning technique in postoperative patients and have demonstrated counts in the lower legs indicative of venous thrombosis in 32 percent of both control and elastic stocking groups;[26] hence, more studies involving postcoronary patients are needed before the true value of this simple form of preventive therapy can be assessed. Multiple studies have shown that minidose subcutaneous heparin, given before surgery and continued for several doses after, is effective in preventing calf vein thrombosis.[27] Handley[28] has shown that this regimen is not effective in patients with acute myocardial infarction, attributing this to the fact that the therapy in these instances is started after the event that initiated the thrombosis. Wray et al.[29] randomly allocated 92 consecutive patients with acute myocardial infarction into a control group and an anticoagulated group. The latter consisted of heparin for the initial forty-eight hours, followed by Coumadin®. Both groups underwent active physiotherapy from the onset of admission and were mobilized to a chair within seven days of the acute event. The groups were well-matched in the severity of cardiac illness as assessed by a coronary prognostic index. All patients were given intravenous injections of labeled fibrinogen, and the lower extremities were scanned daily for evidence of venous thrombosis. Daily chest x-rays were done on both groups, and the last 50 patients in the study all had lung scans on the tenth hospital day. The group receiving the anticoagulants had a 6.5 percent incidence of calf vein thrombosis as compared to a 22 percent incidence in the control group. The thrombosis development occurred remarkedly early in the hospital course, as more than 60 percent developed within seventy-two hours of the clinical onset of infarction. This would suggest that the infarction itself, rather than a period of prolonged immobilization, was the precipitating factor. It is of interest that the thrombi were confined to calf veins in all instances of both control and treatment patients. Moreover, clinically important pulmonary emboli did not occur in either group. It is possible that the active physical therapy and early mobilization regimen played some role in limiting the extension of thrombosis formation. As a result of the study, the authors now reserve anticoagulant therapy for those postinfarction patients who exhibit clinical evidence of deep vein thrombosis and those patients who are confined to bed for more than one week.

At Georgia Baptist Hospital, patients with congestive heart failure are anticoagulated with warfarin at least during the hospital phase of a myocardial infarction. Elastic stockings are commonly utilized in addition to the frequent leg exercises which are performed in the bed.

In addition to the inpatient physical program, there are three other general groups of services which are available to the patient who is referred to the cardiac rehabilitation team. *Group I* consists of individual patient and family conferences, and includes discussion and instructions in diet, coronary risk factors, and current cardiac problems. Religious counseling and psychological testing are done in selected instances. All phases of activities within this group are conducted in the individual patient's room. *Group II* deals with group conferences pertaining to the pathophysiology of coronary atherosclerosis, the psychosocial aspects of coronary disease, diet, and coronary risk factors (Fig. 8-4). These conferences are held in the cardiac rehabilitation office and make use of various audiovisual aids. The conferences are scheduled so that a different discussion is scheduled each week of the month. The patient's spouse and family are strongly urged to attend these sessions.

Group III is the predischarge and follow-up phase. The former includes instructions on a home walking regimen and general guidelines as to "dos" and "don'ts" during the early segment of home care. The topic of sexual activity is brought up by the

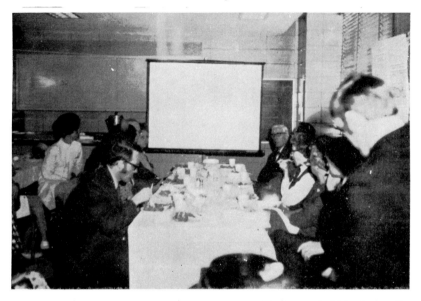

Figure 8-4. Family conference on the coronary risk factors held in the cardiac rehabilitation office.

rehabilitation team, as patients are often embarrassed to initiate such discussion. The energy expenditure during this activity has been studied by Hellerstein and Friedman,[30] who found that the mean pulse rate during intercourse was 117 beats per minute in postinfarction patients. This is approximately the same energy cost of climbing two flights of stairs. Patients who have stable telemetry recordings during inhospital stair climbing are permitted to engage in sexual activities within a week after discharge.

Prior to discharge, patients undergo bicycle ergometry testing (Fig. 8-5), to a target heart rate of 60 percent of their age-predicted maximum. The test is stopped sooner if the patient develops chest pain or ventricular ectopy. The protocol for testing is seen in Table 8-III. To date, we have tested 50 patients by this method with no untoward effects (*Consultant,* July, 1977, pp. 64-68).

Styperek et al.[31] used the bicycle test in 209 postinfarction patients prior to discharge (average of eighteen days postin-

TABLE 8-III
SUMMARY OF TEST PROTOCOL

Stage	Time (minutes)	Work Load*	Blood Pressure	Lead II, AVF, CM_5†
Warm-up	0-3	0 kpm	Initial and 3 min.	Base
I	3-6	150 kpm	6 min.	
II	6-9	300 kpm	9 min.	
III	9-12	450 kpm	12 min.	
IV	12-15	600 kpm	15 min.	Last minute of exercise
Postexercise	1 after through 8 after	rest	immediate and 1,3,5, and 8 after	1,3,5, and 8 after

*speed to remain constant at 10 kph
†Lead CM_5 to be recorded every minute after warm-up stage

farction). The bicycle workload was increased by 300 kpm every sixth minute. The average heart rate increased from 80 to 129 beats per minute and the average systolic blood pressure from 126 mm Hg to 170 mm Hg. There were no serious complications. The reasons for stopping the tests were as follows:

Number of cases	Reason
121	fatigue
24	angina
26	dyspnea
10	arrhythmias
9	significant S-T changes
19	miscellaneous
209	

We feel that such testing is of value in determining the tolerance for a workload that simulates those that may be encountered in the home environment. The latter may range from climbing two flights of stairs to sexual intercourse. If arrhythmias or myocardial ischemia develop during the bicycle test, appropriate drug therapy (such as propranolol, nitrates, etc.), and modification of home activities are carried out. Those who do well on the bicycle test are cleared for the home walking regimen (Table 8-IV).

Group III activities also include the home visit, which is made within the first twenty-four to forty-eight hours after discharge.

TABLE 8-IV
CARDIAC REHABILITATION HOME EXERCISE REGIMEN*
GEORGIA BAPTIST HOSPITAL—ATLANTA MEDICAL CENTER

Week	Activity
1–3	In-hospital exercise regimen
4	Walk 5 minutes at leisurely pace (1/4 mile) once per day
5	Walk 5 minutes at leisurely pace b.i.d. (1/2 mile)
6	Walk 10 minutes at leisurely pace (1/2 mile) once per day
7	Walk 10 minutes at leisurely pace (3/4 mile) once per day
8	Walk 15 minutes at leisurely pace (3/4 mile) once per day
9	Walk 15 minutes at leisurely pace (3/4 mile) once per day
10	Walk 20 minutes at leisurely pace (1 mile) once per day
11	Walk 20 minutes at moderate pace (1 1/3 mile) once per day
12	Walk 30 minutes at moderate pace (2 miles) once per day
13	Begin group activity program—Georgia Baptist Hospital

*For first three months post-coronary-incident   b.i.d. = two times daily

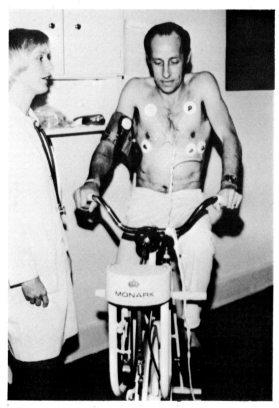

Figure 8-5. Bicycle ergometry testing.

The purpose of this visit is to directly assess the home situation and to consult on any problems that have arisen after discharge. A review of the patient's medications and dietary regimen is made, and a brief cardiopulmonary examination is carried out. After the home visit, a report is written for the rehabilitation files, and a copy is sent to the referring physician. If any problems are encountered which require immediate attention, the private physician is notified by telephone. The home visit provides a certain continuity to the inpatient rehabilitation program. When questions are answered and problems solved at an early point in the rehabilitation phase, the anxiety of the patient and family members is significantly decreased. All patients and family members are encouraged to call the cardiac rehabilitation department at any time they think the various team members might be of assistance.

RESULTS

We published follow-up data on 89 patients who were followed for a mean of 13.5 months after hospitalization (Fig. 8-6).[32] Fifteen percent (14 of 89 patients) were deceased. The following data was compiled from the remaining 75 patients.

Fifty-six per cent (42 of 75 patients) were working; 37 of these 42 held full-time positions and five were working part time. Four per cent (3 of 75) were housewives. Forty per cent (30 of 75) were retired patients; 15 of these were of retirement age and 15 were retired because of medical reasons.

All patients were instructed on the fat-controlled diet. Some were given a second type of diet in combination with the fat-controlled diet. Sixty-six per cent (49 of 75 patients) were following the diets as instructed. Three per cent (2 of 75) decided to follow only the diabetic portion of their diet. Thirty-four per cent (26 of 75) changed their dietary habits from fat-controlled to regular.

All patients were instructed in the proper exercise habits and encouraged to continue an exercise regimen at home. Seventy-seven per cent (58 of 75 patients) had been exercising since discharge from the hospital. Thirty-nine of these were exercising no less than two times each week. Nineteen of 58 exercised once a week or less (periodic).

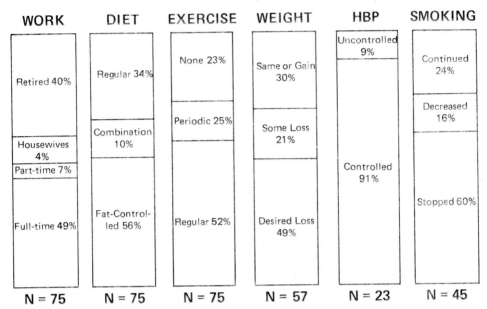

Figure 8-6. Bar graph showing results of inpatient cardiac rehabilitation. Data was acquired at a mean time of 13.5 months after hospitalization. Lower portions of bars display desired effects in each category. From B.L. Johnston, J.D. Cantwell, and G.F. Fletcher, Eight steps to inpatient cardiac rehabilitation: The team effort—methodology and preliminary results, *Heart and Lung, 5,1*.97-111, 1976.

Twenty-three per cent (17 of 75 patients) did not continue an exercise regimen.

Seventy-six per cent (57 of 75 patients) were overweight at the time of infarction. All of these were given a goal to attain in losing the proper amount of weight. The weight goal was assessed according to recommended ideal body weight for a specific height and body frame. Forty-nine per cent (28 of 57 patients) attained this goal, 21 per cent (12 of 57) partially attained their goal, and 30 per cent (17 of 57) failed to attain their goal.

Thirty-one per cent (23 of 75 patients) had a history of high blood pressure prior to infarction. Ninety-one per cent (21 of 23 patients) had their blood pressure controlled and 9 per cent (2 of 23) were not controlled at the time of follow-up. One of these latter two patients had just begun a new antihypertensive drug regimen.

Sixty per cent (45 of 75 patients) were cigarette smokers prior to infarction. Sixty per cent (27 of 45) no longer smoked cigarettes and 16 per cent (7 of 45) had decreased their number of daily cigarettes to one-half their previous smoking rate. However, 24 per cent (11 of 45) continue to smoke on their regular basis.[32]

To summarize, evidence is mounting that the uncomplicated post-myocardial-infarction patient can be mobilized within the first few days of hospitalization and can be discharged after two weeks of hospital care. The latter is enhanced with a team approach to the various facets of the postinfarction state. In small community hospitals, an interested physician and nurse will suffice to guide the patient in secondary prevention measures and to assist in handling the various psychosocial barriers that often accompany coronary disease. The hospital phase of a myocardial infarction can be a frightening experience, particularly to a person who has previously enjoyed good health. The fear of becoming a "cardiac invalid" is always present. The optimistic attitude of the rehabilitation team and the reassurance of returning to an active, productive life has done much to allay the various apprehensions and anxieties of the coronary patient.

REFERENCES

1. Levine, S.A., and Brown, D.L.: Coronary thrombosis: Its various clinical features. *Medicine* (Baltimore), *8:*245, 1929.
2. Coe, W.S.: Cardiac work and the chair treatment of acute coronary thrombosis. *Ann Int Med, 40:*42-48, 1954.
3. Mather, H.G., Pearson, N.G., Read, K.L.Q., et al.: Acute myocardial infarction: Home and hospital treatment. *Br Med J, 3:*334-338, 1971.
4. Wenger, N.K., Hellerstein, H.K., Blackburn, H., et al.: Uncomplicated myocardial infarction. Current physician practice in patient management. *JAMA, 224:*511-514, 1973.
5. Rose, G.: Early mobilization and discharge after myocardial infarction. *Mod Concepts Cardiovasc Dis, 41:*59-63, 1972.
6. Levine, S.A., and Lown, B.: Armchair treatment of acute coronary thrombosis. *JAMA, 148:*1365-1369, 1952.
7. Fareeduddin, K., and Abelmann, W.H.: Impaired orthostatic tolerance after bed rest in patients with myocardial infarction. *N Engl J Med, 280:*345-350, 1969.
8. Saltin, B., Blomqvist, G., Mitchell, J.H., et al.: Response to exercise after bed rest and after training. *Circulation, 38: Suppl 12:*1-55, 1968.

9. Adgey, A.A.J.: Prognosis after early discharge from hospital of patients with acute myocardial infarction. *Br Heart J, 31:*750-752, 1969.

10. Takkunen, J., Huhti, E., Oilinki, O., et al.: Early ambulation in myocardial infarction. *Acta Med Scand, 188:*103-106, 1970.

11. Tucker, H.H., Carson, P.H.M., Bass, N.M., et al.: Results of early mobilization and discharge after myocardial infarction. *Br Med J, 1:*10-13, 1973.

12. Harpur, J.E., Conner, W.T., Hamilton, M., et al.: Controlled trial of early mobilization and discharge from hospital in uncomplicated myocardial infarction. *Lancet, 2:*1331-1334, 1971.

13. Hutter, A.M., Sidel, V.W., Shine, K.I., et al.: Early hospital discharge after myocardial infarction. *N Engl J Med, 288:*1141-1144, 1973.

14. Bloch, A., Maeder, J-P., Haissly, J-C., et al.: Early mobilization after myocardial infarction. *Am J Cardiol, 34:*152-157, 1974.

15. Abraham, A.S., Sever, Y., Weinstein, M., et al.: Value of early ambulation in patients with and without complications after acute myocardial infarction. *N Engl J Med, 292:*719-722, 1975.

16. McNeer, J.F., Wallace, A.G., Wagner, G.S., et al.: The course of acute myocardial infarction. Feasibility of early discharge of the uncomplicated patient. *Circulation, 51:*410-413, 1975.

17. Chaturvedi, N.C., Walsh, M.J., Evans, A., et al.: Selection of patients for early discharge after acute myocardial infarction. *Br Heart J, 36:*533-535, 1974.

18. Swan, H.J.C., Blackburn, H.W., DeSanctis, R., et al.: Duration of hospitalization in "uncomplicated completed acute myocardial infarction." *Am J Cardiol, 37:*413-419, 1976.

19. Reynell, P.C.: Intermediate coronary care. A controlled trial. *Br Heart J, 37:*166-168, 1975.

20. Friedan, J., and Cooper J.A.: The role of the intermediate cardiac care unit. *JAMA, 235:*816-818, 1975.

21. Vismara, L.A., DeMarion, A.N., Hughes, J.L., et al.: Evaluation of arrhythmias in the late hospital phase of acute myocardial infarction compared to coronary care unit ectopy. *Br Heart J, 37:*598-603, 1975.

22. Grossman, J., and Rubin, I.L.: Cardiopulmonary resuscitation. *Am Heart J, 78:*709-714, 1969.

23. Wenger, N.K.: Physical activity, exercise testing, and exercise training programs for patients with myocardial infarction: The state of our knowledge (Editorial). *Acta Cardiol, 28:*13-17, 1973.

24. Browse, N.L.: Effect of bed rest on resting calf blood flow of healthy adult males. *Br Med J, 1:*1721-1723.

25. Makin, G.S., Mayes, F.B., and Holroyd, A.M.: Studies on the effect of "Tubigrip" on flow in the deep veins of the calf. *Br J Surg, 56:*369-372, 1929.

26. Rosengarten, D.S., Laird, J., Jeyasingh, K., et al.: The failure of

compression stockings (Tubigrip) to prevent deep venous thrombosis after operation. *Br J Surg, 57:*296-299, 1970.

27. Kakkar, V.V., Corrigan, T., Spindler, J., et al.: Efficacy of low doses of heparin in prevention of deep vein thrombosis after major surgery: double-blind, randomized trial. *Lancet, 2:*101-106, 1972.

28. Handley, A.J.: Low-dose heparin after myocardial infarction. *Lancet, 2:*623-624, 1972.

29. Wray, R., Maurer, B., and Shillingford, J.: Prophylactic anticoagulant therapy in the prevention of calf-vein thrombosis after myocardial infarction. *N Engl J Med, 288:*815-817, 1973.

30. Hellerstein, H.K., and Friedman, E.H.: Sexual activity and the post-coronary patient. *Arch Intern Med, 125:*987-999, 1970.

31. Styperek, J., Ibsen, H., Kjoller, E., et al.: Exercise-ECG in patients with acute myocardial infarction before discharge from the CCU (Abstr). *Am J Cardiol, 35:*172, 1975.

32. Johnston, B.L., Cantwell, J.D., and Fletcher, G.F.: Eight steps to inpatient cardiac rehabilitation: The team effort—methodology and preliminary results. *Heart and Lung, 5, 1:*97-111, 1976.

Chapter 9

OUTPATIENT EXERCISE THERAPY FOR CORONARY DISEASE—A PRESCRIPTION

OVER THE PAST decade, numerous investigators have expounded the benefits of increased activity and regular exercise for angina pectoris and the post-myocardial-infarction state. The studies dealing with the largest number of patients are those of Hellerstein[1] and Gottheiner.[2] The latter reported a five-year follow-up on 1,103 male patients with coronary disease, 548 of whom had a previous myocardial infarction (although criteria for diagnosis were not listed). The exercise program began with several months of mild strength-building activities, which included weight lifting. Specifics of this initial program are not provided. After about nine months, the men engaged in rhythmic endurance exercises such as running, hiking, swimming, cycling, rowing, and volleyball. Those who excelled in these activities and achieved a significant improvement in overall fitness then entered competitive team games. The participants in the general exercise program basically practiced on their own on a twice-daily schedule. There was obviously no medical supervision. Once a week, the men met as a group for instructions and practice. The most impressive results of the study are in the mortality rate data, which was 3.6 percent for the entire group over the five-year period in contrast to 12 percent of a comparable nonexercised group of Israelis with previous myocardial infarctions. Gottheiner described other objective effects of training, such as reductions of resting heart rate and of resting and exercise blood pressure levels. In addition, there was less S-T segment depression on electrocardiograms taken during and immediately postexercise. Unfortunately, the complete data on these observations are not given,

168

which makes the significance questionable. Hellerstein[1] noted the results of physical training on 656 middle-aged males, 203 of whom had angina pectoris and/or myocardial infarctions. An additional 51 men had resting or exercise stress test electrocardiograms compatible with silent coronary heart disease (utilizing the Minnesota code). Persons with valvular disease and uncompensated congestive failure were followed for an average of 2.7 years. They participated in at least a thrice-weekly exercise program and recreational activities. The latter included swimming, basketball, volleyball, and use of a punching bag. Detailed results were presented on the first 100 cardiac patients. The average weight loss was 2.5 kg. Sixty-five percent significantly improved their level of fitness, as measured by bicycle ergometric testing and oxygen consumption. Sixty-three percent showed improvement in their exercise electrocardiograms, mainly in terms of the initial slope and the junctional displacement of the S-T segment. The death rate for the exercise cardiac patients was 1.9 per 100 patient-years, which was less than half the expected rate.

Rechnitzer et al.[3] reported the results of physical training in men with previous documented myocardial infarctions. There were two aspects to the study. One consisted of a comparison of the incidence of nonfatal recurrences and cardiac deaths between 66 men in the exercise group and 71 controls who were matched according to age, year of infarction, and number of infarctions. All of the controls met the criteria for entry into the exercise program but did not enter for a variety of reasons (including job conflicts and personal physician disapproval). Over a seven-year follow-up period the results were as follows:

	No.	Nonfatal Recurrences	Cardiac Deaths
Exercise Group	77	1 (1.3%)	3 (3.9%)
Matched Control Group	111	31 (28%)	15 (11.8%)

There were several weaknesses of the above study, however, which might have had a bearing on the results. For one thing, the control groups were not "true" controls in the sense that they were randomly assigned to the inactive group. It is possible that certain members of the control group had severe angina pectoris and did not enter the exercise program for this reason. Another vulnerable area of the study concerns the documentation of nonfatal recurrence of myocardial infarction. In some instances, historical evidence supplied by the patient or his physician was utilized instead of much harder criteria such as enzyme and electrocardiographic changes. Still another deficit of the study was that the exercise and control groups were not matched for important risk factors such as cigarette smoking habits, hypertension, serum cholesterol levels, and family history.

Kennedy et al.[4] reported the Mayo Clinic experience with 8 men (ranging in age from forty-five to fifty-two years) who had stable angina pectoris. None of the men developed a myocardial infarction or died during the follow-up period. This has little significance, however, since the numbers are small, the follow-up was brief (one year), and a control group was not obtained. The study was of interest in that cardiac catheterization and coronary arteriography was performed prior to and at the completion of the one-year program. All patients had an increase in cardiac index after training (from a mean of 3.9 L/min/m² to 4.4 L/min/m²). Half of the patients showed a decrease in the magnitude of ischemic changes on follow-up exercise stress testing. Surprisingly, the left ventricular end-diastolic pressure increased in seven of the eight patients (from a mean of 16 mm Hg to 20 mm Hg). None of the individuals showed any increase in coronary collateral circulation post-training, nor were such increases found in two other series.[5, 6] Kattus et al.[7] noted enhanced collateral vessel development in three instances, however.

Perhaps the best-designed study of postinfarction physical training was that of Kentala,[8] who randomly assigned patients into control or exercise groups. Of those who were discharged from the hospital, 158 men met the diagnostic criteria for a documented myocardial infarction. The exercise group was comprised of 77 men, while the control group numbered 81 men. The groups were similar regarding age, smoking habits, preinfarction physical activities, severity of infarction, serum cholesterol levels, and lung vital capacities. Over a two-year follow-up period, there were no group differences as to coronary mortality or morbidity. However, only 10 of 77 (13%) in the training group had attended at least 70 percent of the thrice-weekly exercise sessions by the end of one year, while 11 of 81 controls (14%) had engaged in a regular physical training program on their own. Therefore, it is not too surprising that group differences were not detected. Those attending the exercise sessions on a regular basis showed significant weight loss, diminution of body fat, and decrease in serum triglyceride levels. In addition, they demonstrated greater improvement in physical work capacity on exercise testing ($p < .0025$), had more success in giving up cigarette smoking, and had faster disappearances in Q waves on the resting electrocardiogram.

In another randomized study of post-myocardial-infarction men and women (all born in 1913), 158 were allocated to the exercise group and 157 to the control group.[9] Over a four-year follow-up period, the group differences were minimal:

	Exercise Group (# of cases)	Control Group (# of cases)
Deaths	28	35
Nonfatal myocardial infarction	25	28

As in Kentala's study, the dropout rate was high, for after one year, only 39 percent of the exercise group were still training at the hospital (21% more trained at home or at work). Of those who adhered to the exercise program for at least one year, the mortality rate was half as high (5 of 67, or 7%) compared to the controls (20 of 142, or 14%). The dropouts tended to be sicker and smoked more than the high adherence subjects.

Bruce et al.[10] found that of 603 men and women in CAPRI (84.5% with clinical manifestations of coronary disease), over half dropped out after five to seven months of exercise participation. The dropouts and the active participants were fairly similar with regard to exercise test results and clinical diagnoses. The total mortality rates were reduced in the active group:

	Dropouts		Active	
	Men	Women	Men	Women
Total Mortality Rates (per 100 patient-years)	4.7	3.8	2.7	0

A wide variety of exercise programs have been utilized by the various investigators. Unfortunately, none are clearly and concisely outlined in the literature. In view of this, the three types of outpatient exercise programs utilized at Georgia Baptist Hospital are presented in detail.

HOME EXERCISE REGIMEN
(First Three Months Post-Coronary-Incident)

After completing the inpatient exercise and physical therapy program (Chapter 8), most patients will be ready for a home walking program. The purpose of this is to very gradually increase their exercise tolerance for the most strenuous group activity program which begins three months postinfarction. The walking should be done on level ground and in good weather. Other guidelines (Chapter 6) should be followed as well. In inclement weather, the patient may drive to an area shopping center and walk up and down the mall area. The specifics of the home regimen are seen in Table 8-III.

HOME EXERCISE REGIMEN
(Beginning Two Months Post-Coronary-Incident)

Certain patients are unable to participate in the physician-supervised exercise program beginning two to three months postinfarction, mainly because of logistical problems. For those who wish to advance to a higher level of endurance training, the program adapted from John L. Boyer, M.D. (San Diego, California) is recommended (Table 9-I).[11] Before starting the program, the individual is taught to check his own pulse rate. He is advised to not advance to the next stage (as from week one or two to week three or four) unless the immediate postexercise pulse rate is less than 120 beats per minute.

Prior to and at the completion of the twelve-week program, the patient should be tested on the treadmill to see whether he has achieved a significant improvement in oxygen uptake. If he has not done so, he is strongly urged to make arrangements to enter the physician-supervised exercise program, either at the parent center (GBH-AMC) or a satellite center (area YMCA or

TABLE 9-I
CARDIAC REHABILITATION HOME EXERCISE PROGRAM
GEORGIA BAPTIST HOSPITAL—ATLANTA MEDICAL CENTER

Week	Activity
1–2	Measure 1 mile distance with car. Walk to point and back (total of 2 miles) in 40 minutes. Pulse at end should be less than 115 per minute.
3–4	Measure 1.5 mile distance. Walk to point and back (3.0 miles) in 60 minutes.
5–6	Measure 2 miles distance. Walk to point and back (4.0 miles) in 72 minutes.
7–9	Measure 2 miles distance. Walk to point and back (4.0 miles) in 60 minutes. (15 minute mile pace)
10–12	Measure 2 miles distance. Walk to point and back (4.0 miles) in 56 minutes. (14 minute mile pace, just below a slow jog)

community recreation center). We do not advise a postcoronary patient to begin a jogging or vigorous swimming program on his own.

PHYSICIAN-SUPERVISED EXERCISE REGIMEN
(Beginning Two Months Post-Coronary-Incident)

This program was originally devised for a pilot project at the Mayo Clinic by Doctor Cantwell and several Mayo physicians. The program was tailored specifically for the postcoronary patient and can be modified according to the available laboratory facilities. In addition to the Mayo Clinic Study, which is in its tenth year, this exercise regimen is now being used in multiple rehabilitation centers in the United States and abroad. The fundamentals of the program are as follows:

1. Patients must be at least six weeks post-myocardial-infarction. They must be less than sixty-five years of age. Concomitant disease such as uncompensated congestive heart failure, severe hypertension (diastolic blood pressure greater than 120 mm Hg), cardiac rhythm disturbances (such as frequent PVCs, paroxysms of tachycardia), vascular disease, and chronic lung disease prohibit inclusion into the program.

2. A minimum of three exercise sessions, each forty-five minutes in duration, are conducted weekly at a YMCA,

local high school, or community recreation center. A physician is always in attendance. Resuscitation equipment, including a portable electrocardiograph machine, direct current defibrillator and emergency drug kit (Fig. 9-1), are on hand. The forty-five minute sessions are divided into three fifteen-minute periods. The first consists of calisthenics, the second of walk-jog activity, and the third of noncompetitive group activity such as volleyball, basketball, and swimming. A five-minute warm-up period and similar cool-down period is part of each session.

3. Patients are given an exercise prescription (Fig. 9-2) at the beginning of each week, indicating the calisthenic and walk-jog activity for that week. The prescription is based on three factors: (a) direct participant observation by the physician in attendance, who frequently exercises with the

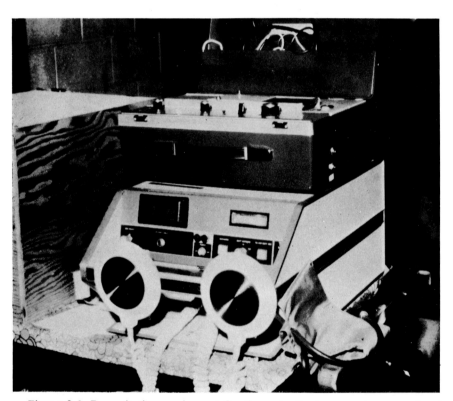

Figure 9-1. Resuscitation equipment for the outpatient gymnasium exercise program.

patients; (b) preliminary and follow-up data, based on treadmill performance and oxygen consumption; and (c) the patient's subjective response to the given level of exercise (in terms of musculoskeletal side effects and respiratory effort). It is updated approximately every two weeks.

The calisthenics are conducted in five different positions and are designed to exercise the major muscle groups. Initially, the number of repetitions is low to avoid undue muscular strain and discouragement to the participant. After the initial six months, the number of repetitions are increased to the point where the individual is averaging 70 percent of his maximum pulse rate during the actual exercises. This requires radiotelemetry recording during the calisthenic period or a manual check of the pulse rate midway during each calisthenic position. The number of repetitions for a given week (for the first six months of exercise) are listed in the chart following the illustration of each exercise, as seen in Figures 9-3 through 9-19.

EXERCISE PRESCRIPTION
GEORGIA BAPTIST HOSPITAL—ATLANTA MEDICAL CENTER
CARDIAC REHABILITATION—GEORGIA REGIONAL
MEDICAL PROGRAM

NAME: _____   DATE: _____

CALISTHENICS	REPETITIONS	CALISTHENICS	REPETITIONS
Arm and shoulder	_____	Bent leg raise	_____
Toe touch	_____	Straight leg raise	_____
Knee raise	_____	Double leg raise	_____
Lateral raise	_____	Sit-ups	_____
Arm circling	_____	Leg cross-over	_____
Small jumps	_____		
		Leg raise	_____
Trunk twist	_____		
Reverse push-ups	_____	Chest and leg raise	_____
Reach and touch	_____	Knee push-ups	_____

(Standing / Sitting; Supine / Side / Prone)

WALK-JOG		GROUP ACTIVITIES	
Walk slowly _____ laps		Volleyball	_____
Walk briskly _____ laps		Basketball	_____
Jog _____ laps		Bowling	_____
		Swimming	_____

SIGNED: _____ M.D.

Figure 9-2. Exercise card for walk-jog, calisthenic, and group activities.

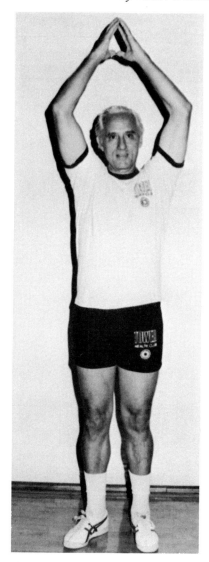

Figure 9-3. *Arm and shoulder loosen-ing.* With the subject in the standing position, the arms are raised over-head, bringing the palms together. The arms are then lowered to the side, completing the sequence.

Week	Repetitions per session	Week	Repetitions per session
1	6	13	18
2	6	14	18
3	8	15	18
4	8	16	18
5	10	17	18
6	10	18	18
7	12	19	20
8	12	20	20
9	14	21	20
10	14	22	22
11	16	23	22
12	16	24	22

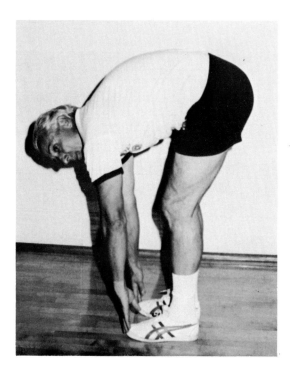

Figure 9-4. *Toe touching.** Keeping the knees slightly bent, the subject flexes at the waist and touches the right fingertips to the left toes. He assumes an erect position, then flexes again, touching the left fingertips to the right toes to complete the sequence.

---

* Omit if history of back injury.

Week	Repetitions per session	Week	Repetitions per session
1	6	13	16
2	6	14	16
3	6	15	16
4	6	16	18
5	8	17	18
6	8	18	18
7	10	19	20
8	10	20	20
9	12	21	20
10	12	22	22
11	14	23	22
12	14	24	22

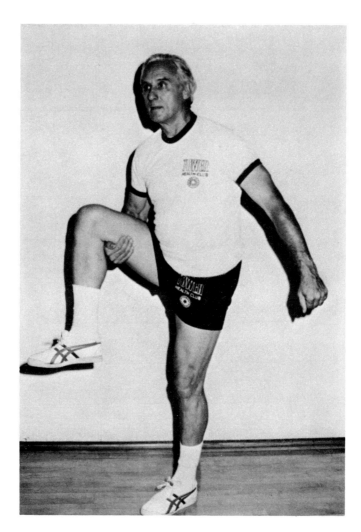

Figure 9-5. *Knee raising.* The subject grasps the right knee with his hand and raises it as high as he can. To complete the cycle, he repeats the above with the left knee.

Week	Repetitions per session	Week	Repetitions per session
1	6	13	16
2	6	14	16
3	8	15	16
4	8	16	18
5	8	17	18
6	8	18	18
7	10	19	20
8	10	20	20
9	12	21	20
10	12	22	22
11	14	23	22
12	14	24	22

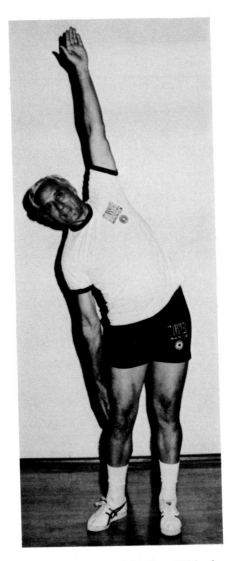

Figure 9-6. *Lateral bending.* With the arms elevated in a horizontal position, the subject bends laterally to the left, returns to an upright position, then bends laterally to the right.

Week	Repetitions per session	Week	Repetitions per session
1	6	13	12
2	6	14	14
3	6	15	14
4	8	16	14
5	8	17	16
6	8	18	16
7	8	19	18
8	10	20	18
9	10	21	20
10	10	22	20
11	12	23	22
12	12	24	22

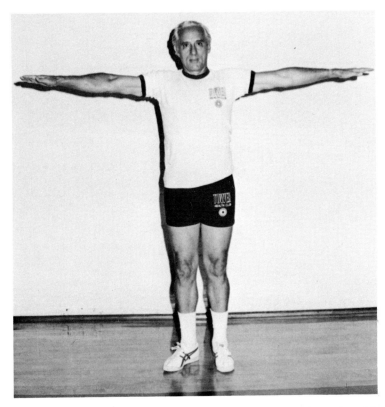

Figure 9-7. *Arm circling.* The arms are elevated in a horizontal position and are rotated, first clockwise for a given number of repetitions, then counterclockwise for the same number of times.

Week	Repetitions per session	Week	Repetitions per session
1	6	13	14
2	6	14	16
3	8	15	16
4	8	16	16
5	8	17	18
6	10	18	18
7	10	19	20
8	10	20	20
9	12	21	20
10	12	22	22
11	12	23	22
12	14	24	22

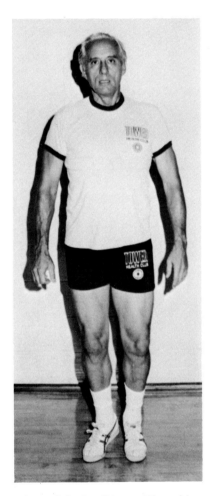

Figure 9-8. *Small jumps.* The subject jumps vertically about six inches off the ground, landing on the anterior aspect of the feet.

Week	Repetitions per session	Week	Repetitions per session
1	8	13	16
2	8	14	18
3	10	15	18
4	10	16	18
5	12	17	18
6	12	18	20
7	14	19	20
8	14	20	20
9	14	21	20
10	16	22	22
11	16	23	22
12	16	24	22

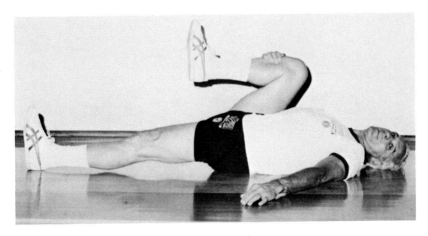

Figure 9-9. *Alternate bent leg raising.* While lying supine, the subject grasps the left knee and flexes the thigh. To complete the cycle, he repeats this maneuver with the right knee.

Week	Repetitions per session	Week	Repetitions per session
1	6	13	14
2	6	14	14
3	6	15	14
4	8	16	16
5	8	17	16
6	8	18	18
7	10	19	18
8	10	20	20
9	10	21	20
10	12	22	22
11	12	23	22
12	12	24	22

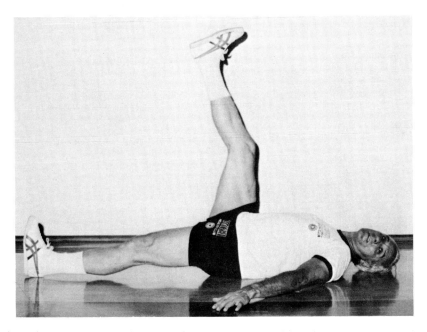

Figure 9-10. *Alternate straight leg raising.* While lying supine, the subject elevates the left leg to an eighty to ninety degree angle with the floor, keeping the knee straight. To complete the sequence, he repeats the above with the right leg.

Week	Repetitions per session	Week	Repetitions per session
1	6	13	14
2	6	14	14
3	6	15	14
4	8	16	16
5	8	17	16
6	8	18	16
7	10	19	18
8	10	20	18
9	10	21	20
10	12	22	20
11	12	23	22
12	12	24	22

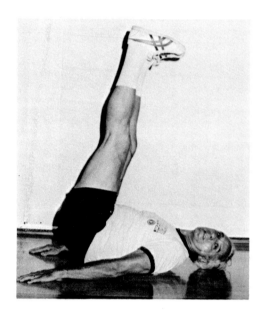

Figure 9-11. *Double leg raising and lowering.*
While lying supine, the subject elevates both
legs to an eighty to ninety degree angle with
the floor, keeping the knees straight.

Week	Repetitions per session	Week	Repetitions per session
1	6	13	14
2	6	14	14
3	6	15	14
4	8	16	16
5	8	17	16
6	8	18	16
7	10	19	18
8	10	20	18
9	10	21	20
10	12	22	20
11	12	23	22
12	12	24	22

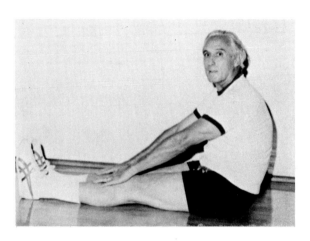

Figure 9-12. *Rocking situps.* While lying supine with arms extended, the subject rocks to a sitting position and touches both hands to the slightly flexed knees.

Week	Repetitions per session	Week	Repetitions per session
1	4	13	12
2	4	14	12
3	4	15	12
4	6	16	14
5	6	17	14
6	6	18	16
7	8	19	16
8	8	20	18
9	8	21	18
10	10	22	20
11	10	23	20
12	10	24	22

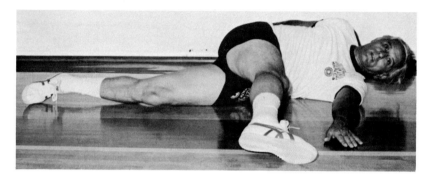

Figure 9-13. *Leg crossover.* While lying supine, the subject raises the right leg and touches the floor to his left with his toes. He then returns to the starting position. To complete one cycle, he raises his left leg and touches the floor to his right.

Week	Repetitions per session	Week	Repetitions per session
1	6	13	14
2	6	14	14
3	6	15	16
4	8	16	16
5	8	17	16
6	8	18	18
7	10	19	18
8	10	20	20
9	10	21	20
10	12	22	20
11	12	23	22
12	12	24	22

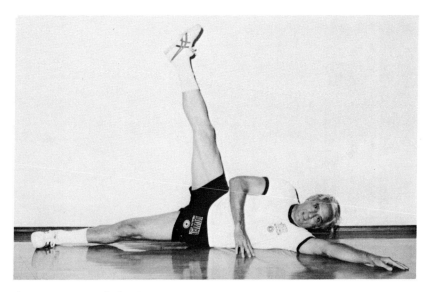

Figure 9-14. *Side leg raises.* While lying on the left side, the subject raises his right leg as high as he can for the recommended number of repetitions. He then switches to the right side and raises the left leg the same number of times.

Week	Repetitions per session	Week	Repetitions per session
1	6	13	14
2	6	14	14
3	6	15	14
4	8	16	16
5	8	17	16
6	8	18	18
7	10	19	18
8	10	20	18
9	10	21	20
10	12	22	20
11	12	23	22
12	12	24	22

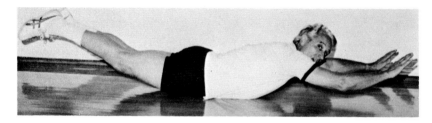

Figure 9-15. *Chest and leg raising.* Assuming a prone position, the subject places the arms overhead and raises both the upper part of the body and the legs as far off of the ground as possible.

Week	Repetitions per session	Week	Repetitions per session
1	6	13	14
2	6	14	14
3	6	15	14
4	8	16	16
5	8	17	16
6	8	18	16
7	10	19	18
8	10	20	18
9	10	21	20
10	12	22	20
11	12	23	22
12	12	24	22

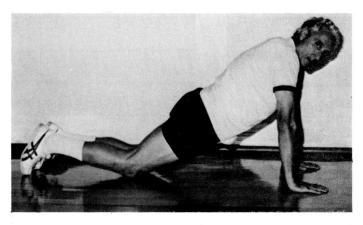

Figure 9-16. *Knee pushups.* The subject positions himself on his hands and knees and touches his chest to the floor.

Week	Repetitions per session	Week	Repetitions per session
1	4	13	14
2	4	14	14
3	6	15	14
4	6	16	16
5	8	17	16
6	8	18	16
7	8	19	18
8	8	20	18
9	12	21	20
10	12	22	20
11	12	23	20
12	12	24	22

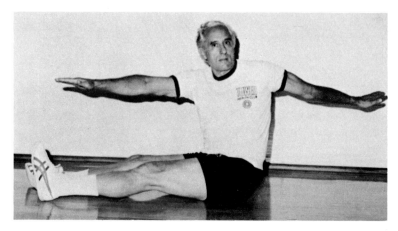

Figure 9-17. *Trunk twisting.* The subject sits with legs straight and with arms raised to a horizontal position. He twists his trunk to the left, returns to the original position, and completes one sequence by turning the trunk to the right.

Week	Repetitions per session	Week	Repetitions per session
1	6	13	14
2	6	14	14
3	6	15	14
4	8	16	16
5	8	17	16
6	8	18	16
7	10	19	18
8	10	20	18
9	10	21	20
10	12	22	20
11	12	23	22
12	12	24	22

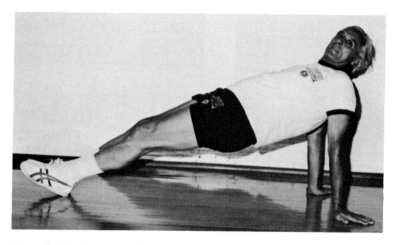

Figure 9-18. *Reverse pushups.* The subject assumes a sitting position with legs straight and hands on the floor behind his back. He pushes his body off of the floor and then returns to the original starting position.

Week	Repetitions per session	Week	Repetitions per session
1	4	13	12
2	4	14	14
3	6	15	14
4	6	16	16
5	6	17	16
6	8	18	16
7	8	19	18
8	8	20	18
9	10	21	20
10	10	22	20
11	12	23	22
12	12	24	22

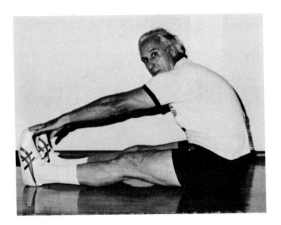

Figure 9-19. *Reach and touch.* The subject assumes a sitting position with legs slightly flexed and arms at the sides. He touches his toes with his fingertips and returns to the starting position.

Week	Repetitions per session	Week	Repetitions per session
1	6	13	14
2	6	14	14
3	6	15	14
4	8	16	16
5	8	17	16
6	8	18	18
7	10	19	18
8	10	20	20
9	10	21	20
10	12	22	20
11	12	23	22
12	12	24	22

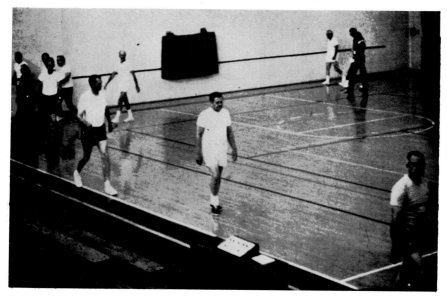

Figure 9-20. Post-myocardial-infarction patients engaging in supervised walk-jog activities.

The walk-jog activity (Fig. 9-20) for a given week is described in Table 9-II. The overall goal is to work up to a one-mile jog after twelve months, during which time the pulse is maintained at 70 percent of predicted maximum heart rate. A miniature heart-monitoring instrument (Fig. 9-21)* may be used initially to determine the level of exercise required to maintain this heart rate. The instrument is a battery-driven device which may be carried in a pocket or attached to the clothing. A pair of lightweight electrodes are applied to the chest, and a small earphone (hearing-aid type) is placed in the ear and plugged into the battery device. The device is set at the desired exercise heart rate and is switched on when exercise begins. The earphone relates the patient's own heartbeat until the target heart rate is approached, at which time the earphone remains silent as long as the pulse rate remains within a few beats of the desired rate. A warning tone is sounded when the heart rate

---

* MEDRAD, 4084 Mt. Royal Boulevard, Allison Park, Pa. 15101.

TABLE 9-II

CORONARY GROUP WALK AND JOG CHART
PRIOR TO CALISTHENICS

	(Perform minimum of 3 times per week)
Week 1 to 4	Walk slowly 100 yards, walk briskly 100 yards, alternately for $\frac{1}{4}$ mile.
Week 5 to 8	Walk slowly 100 yards, walk briskly 100 yards, alternately for $\frac{1}{2}$ mile.
Week 9 to 12	Walk slowly 100 yards, walk briskly 100 yards, jog 100 yards, alternately for $\frac{1}{2}$ mile.
Week 13 to 15	Walk briskly 200 yards, jog 200 yards, alternately for $\frac{3}{4}$ mile.
Week 16 to 24	Jog 400 yards, walk 200 yards, alternately for 1 mile.
Week 25 to 51	Jog 1 mile, maintain pulse rate at 70% maximal, adding 100 yards per month.
Week 52 and over	Jog 2 miles, maintaining pulse rate at 70% maximal.

exceeds the present rate. Patients can usually be instructed in checking their own pulse rate during interrupted jogging sessions and can thereby adjust their jogging pace with a satisfactory degree of accuracy.

If the patient misses three consecutive weeks of the program, he must undergo a repeat treadmill test and begin at the first week level of walking and flexibility exercise. If he knows in advance that he will be away for a week or two he may arrange to take his exercise prescription card with him and do the walking and calisthenic portions on his own. He is not permitted to jog.

The group activity portion is the most enjoyable to the patient but is potentially the most dangerous if noncompetitive rules are not adhered to. Volleyball has been highly successful and requires no special skill for enjoyment. Basketball routines such as free throws, lay-ups, passing, and full-court dribbling are also well accepted and necessitate almost constant motion. Swimming is a little harder to supervise but is an excellent form of exercise and provides a good change of pace periodically. Eight different exercise routines (Figs. 9-22–9-29) of pool exercises are performed under close supervision. Experienced bowlers may take advantage of the four bowling lanes and automatic pinsetters in the basement of the exercise facility (Fig. 9-30). The blood pressure and pulse rate are determined after the patient

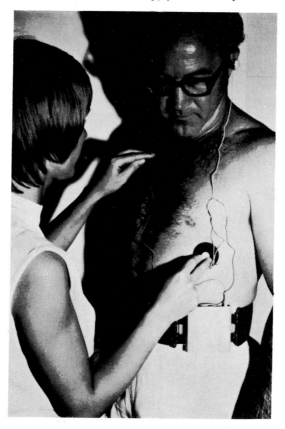

Figure 9-21. A subject demonstrates the use of a heart-monitoring instrument. The battery-driven device is seen attached to the subject's belt; lightweight electrode connections are applied to the chest wall. A small earphone is plugged into the device.

bowls a few frames to make sure that he is tolerating the somewhat isometric activity well. For the patient with some experience in tennis or paddleball, a modified version of wall-tennis is available (Fig. 9-31). When the weather permits, patients may exercise on the outdoor track (Fig. 9-32). Resuscitation equipment is set up nearby. Additional group activities such as badminton, ping pong, bicycle riding, darts, and golf practice can be added to the regimen. Coronary-prone patients are permitted to participate in half-court basketball games at a controlled pace. The dropout rate can be minimized by providing such a wide variety of group activities. Such activities are scheduled on a rotation basis, thereby preventing overcrowding of the volleyball court and exposing individuals to some new activities which most will find enjoyable. The physician in attendance exercises with the patients and is often the first to detect early signs of fatigue. He is always readily available to answer questions concerning any symptoms.

The progress of the exercising coronary patient can be followed in several ways. If a treadmill and equipment for oxygen consumption determination is available, this is used to determine the initial level of fitness and to record changes at three-month intervals. Using the Georgia Baptist treadmill test, an expired air sample is collected with a Douglas bag during the final minute of exercise. The resulting symptom-limited peak oxygen uptake is recorded in milliliters per kilogram per minute. In general, values below 25 are considered low, those

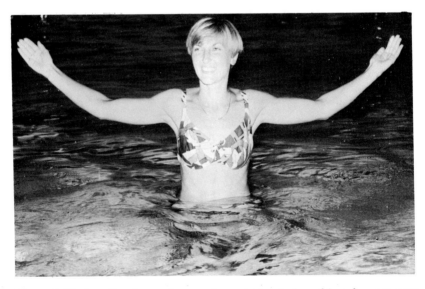

Figure 9-22. Standing in water up to the waist level, the subject does ten arm circles in a clockwise rotation and ten in a counterclockwise rotation.

between 30 and 40, average, and those above 40, high. The average initial value in Hellerstein's study[12] was 23.2 ml/kg/min. This rose to an average of 28.9 ml/kg/min. on follow-up testing. Clausen et al.[13] noted a similar increase in maximal oxygen uptake in nine patients with coronary disease who exercised regularly over a four– to six-week period. If one does not have the equipment to precisely measure oxygen uptake, it can be estimated from the treadmill test time, using normograms for the Bruce or Balke protocol (see Chapter 5).

Periodic screening for cardiac dysrhythmias or S-T segment

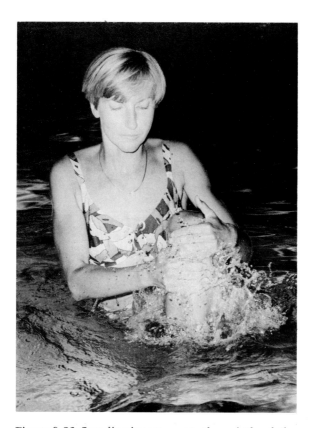

Figure 9-23. Standing in water up to the waist level, the subject alternately raises the knees for a total of fifteen repetitions.

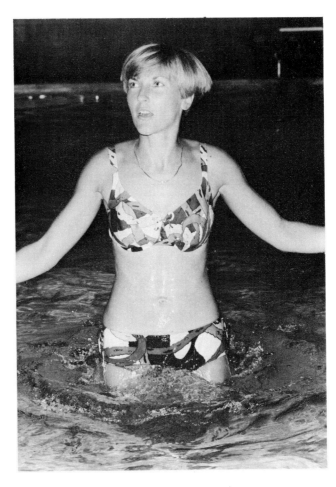

Figure 9-24. Standing in water up to the hip level, the subject performs twenty-two small jumps.

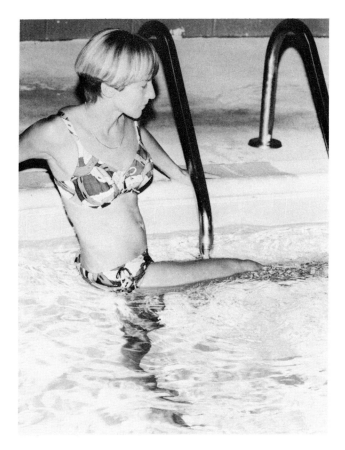

Figure 9-25. With the back against the wall, waist-deep in water, the subject first crosses the right leg (touching the wall to the left) and then crosses the left leg (touching the wall to the right) for a total of fifteen repetitions.

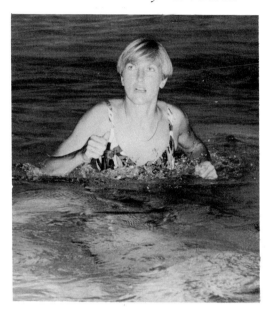

Figure 9-26. Waist-deep in water, the subject jogs back and forth across the pool for a total of four widths.

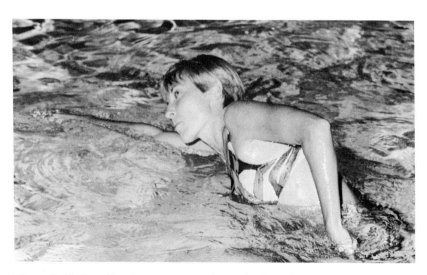

Figure 9-27. Standing in water up to the neck, the subject practices the crawl stroke, making fifteen strokes with each arm.

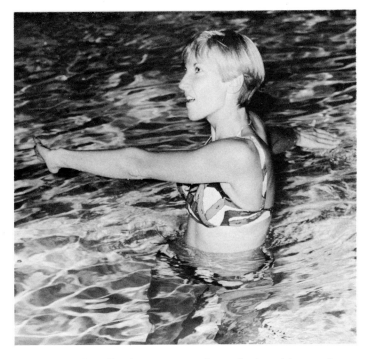

Figure 9-28. Standing in water up to the neck, the subject performs fifteen trunk twists.

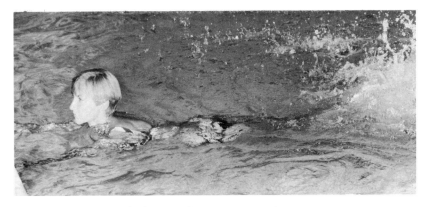

Figure 9-29. While holding onto the edge of the pool, the subject performs twenty-five flutter kicks.

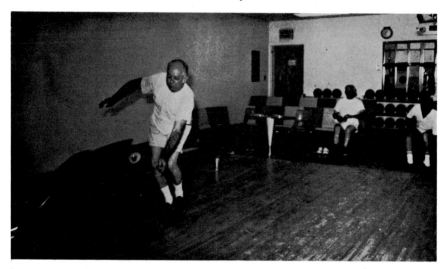

Figure 9-30. Postinfarction patients utilizing the gymnasium bowling lanes.

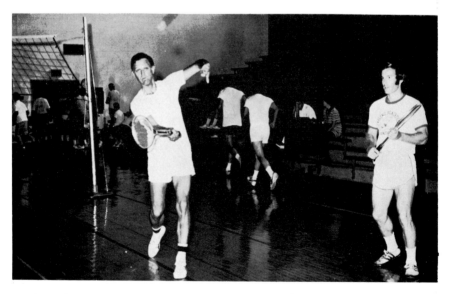

Figure 9-31. Patients engaging in wall tennis (using regulation tennis racquets and a rubber paddleball).

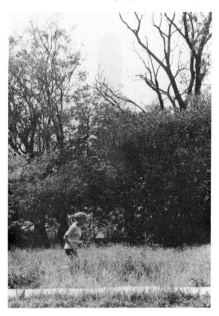

Figure 9-32. Subject jogging on a wood-chip outdoor track, across the street from the hospital gymnasium.

depression during exercise is recommended. This can be done either by the radiotelemetry monitoring or by utilizing the paddle electrodes on the defibrillator. One of our best volleyball players was found to have significant S-T segment depression by the former method (Fig. 9-33). Another man was found to have asymptomatic bouts of ventricular tachycardia during walk-jog activity (Fig. 9-34).

Charts are posted on the gym bulletin board listing the sequential results of treadmill testing, body composition analysis, and blood lipid levels. The patients enjoy comparing their progress with others in the group and have shown no embarrassment from such a listing.

It is unrealistic to think that all coronary patients can be reconditioned by physical training. Some patients have irreversible myocardial damage secondary to diffuse coronary atherosclerosis. If there is no improvement in treadmill performance,

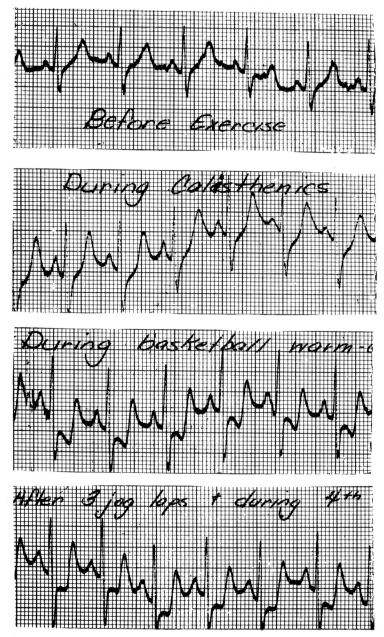

Figure 9-33. Telemetry monitoring during various activities; S-T changes are evident during basketball drills and walk-jog activities.

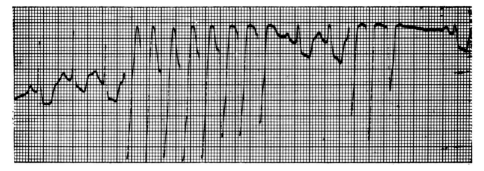

Figure 9-34. Asymptomatic episode of ventricular tachycardia in a fifty-seven-year-old man immediately after jogging 400 yards.

after six months of physical training, such individuals probably could be removed from the exercise program, as they tend to retard the progress of other group members and increase the risk of a cardiac catastrophe during the exercise sessions. Their removal from the program should be done with considerable tactfulness, and they should be encouraged to follow a daily walking program, mainly for subjective benefits.

A progress letter is sent to the referring physician at three-month intervals. Problems or situations arising in the interim that merit his attention are handled over the telephone. When the patient completes six months in the program, he receives a "graduation" letter, outlining his progress in lay terms and suggesting that he enroll in one of the satellite facilities (YMCA, community centers, etc.) which is physician-approved. In order to qualify for such approval, the center must have a portable defibrillator, an emergency drug kit, and allied health personnel (such as a physician's assistant or coronary care nurse) who are skilled in cardiac resuscitation.

To recapitulate, physical training is a promising new weapon in our armamentarium against coronary heart disease. The program described herein can be modified so that it can be used in a major medical center complete with sophisticated (and expensive) testing devices or in a relatively small community hospital equipped with only an interested physician and patient. To further illustrate the chameleonlike nature of this program, let us consider the following two cases.

Case 1

A forty-two-year-old man made an uneventful recovery from a myocardial infarction and five months later consulted his internist about physical activity. He was referred to the nearby university medical center, where he underwent a complete physical examination, which included having the following laboratory tests: electrocardiogram, chest x-ray, serum cholesterol and triglycerides, two-hour postprandial blood sugar, vital capacity, MMPI, and skinfold measurements. On initial treadmill testing he progressed only to the third level, stopping because of generalized fatigue. His maximal oxygen uptake was low, being 19 ml/kg/min. He was enrolled in the previously described exercise program and progressed according to schedule for the first eight weeks, experiencing no adverse musculoskeletal side effects. Repeat testing revealed that he was able to complete the fourth level of treadmill elevation. The oxygen uptake was now 24 ml/kg/min. As he began the ninth week of exercise, a cardiopacer was used to regulate his jogging pace at that necessary to maintain a pulse rate of 135 beats/minute. This pace was well tolerated by the patient. Radiotelemetry revealed no S-T segment depression or arrhythmias.

Case 2

A forty-nine-year-old man had been admitted to a small community hospital (eighty beds) for evaluation of severe angina pectoris. His physical examination was unremarkable, and there were no abnormalities in serum lipids or in glucose tolerance. He was advised to stop cigarette smoking and was on a combination of isosorbide dinitrate and propranolol. Despite maximum doses of the latter, he continued to require an average of fifteen nitroglycerine tablets daily and was unable to hold a job. Coronary arteriograms revealed a 75 percent narrowing of the distal left anterior descending coronary artery and a 60 percent occlusion of the right coronary artery. The patient chose to enroll in a physical training program at the local YMCA rather than to undergo coronary artery bypass grafting. The YMCA group was small, numbering only four men, and was supervised by a physical director and a physician. Initially, he was given a treadmill test (which was positive). Although quite apprehensive during the early exercise sessions, he had no difficulty in following the weekly exercise prescription. At three-month intervals, he had follow-up exercise testing which remained positive, although the S-T segment depression was reduced from 2 to 1 mm. With a little practice the patient was able to measure his radial pulse rate during interrupted jogging and adjusted his pace to maintain an average pulse rate of 135 beats/minute. He was able to return to work but still required approximately five nitroglycerine tablets per day.

REFERENCES

1. Hellerstein, H.K.: The effects of physical activity: Patients and normal coronary-prone subjects. *Minn Med, 52:*1335-1341, 1969.
2. Gottheiner, V.: Long range strenuous sports training for cardiac reconditioning and rehabilitation. *Am J Cardiol, 22:*426-435, 1968.
3. Rechnitzer, P.A., Pickard, H.A., Paivio, A.U., et al.: Long-term follow-up study of survival and recurrence rates following myocardial infarction in exercising and control subjects. *Circulation, 45:*853-857, 1972.
4. Kennedy, C.C., Spiekerman, R.E., Lindsey, M.I., et al.: Evaluation of a one-year graduated exercise program for men with angina pectoris by physiologic studies and coronary arteriography (Abstr). *Am J Cardiol, 31:*141, 1973.
5. Frick, M.H.: The effect of physical training in manifest ischemic heart disease. *Circulation, 40:*433-435, 1969.
6. Ferguson, R.J., Choquette, G., Chaniotis, L., et al.: Coronary arteriography and treadmill exercise capacity before and after 13 months physical training (Abstr). *Med Sci Sports, 5:*67-68, 1973.
7. Kattus, A.A., Jr., Hanafee, W.N., Longmire, W.P., Jr., et al.: Diagnosis, medical and surgical management of coronary insufficiency. *Ann Int Med, 69:*114-136, 1968.
8. Kentala, E.: Physical fitness and feasibility of physical rehabilitation after myocardial infarctions in men of working age. *Ann Clin Res 4: Suppl 9:*1-84, 1972.

9. Wilhelmsen, L., Sanne, H., Elmfeldt, D., et al.: A controlled trial of physical training after myocardial infarction. *Prevent Med, 4:*491-508, 1975.
10. Bruce, E.H., Frederick, R., Bruce, R.A., et al.: Comparison of active participants and dropouts in CAPRI cardiopulmonary rehabilitation programs. *Am J Cardiol, 37:*53-60, 1976.
11. Boyer, J.L.: Adult fitness starter program for individuals considered to be at high risk for coronary heart disease. *J SC Med Assoc, 65: Suppl 1.*99, 1969.
12. Hellerstein, H.K.: Exercise therapy in coronary disease. *Bull NY Acad Med, 44:*1028-1047, 1968.
13. Clausen, J.P., Larse, N.O.A., and Trap-Jensen, J.: Physical training in the management of coronary artery disease. *Circulation 40:*143-154, 1969.

Chapter 10

DANGERS OF EXERCISE

A S PHYSICIANS TURN MORE to exercise testing and training in the management of patients with coronary heart disease, we hear more of morbidity and mortality, perhaps related to and associated with exercise. These incidents, of course, are startling and of concern; however, the absolute incidence of such events remains quite low. Most current data on exercise testing (1971)[1] reported 2.4/10,000 serious events and 1.0/10,000 deaths immediately associated. With regard to exercise training programs for post-myocardial-infarction patients, Haskell[2] reported in 1975 only 3.3 percent mortality per year for current programs in the United States, or one death per 268,922 man-hours of participation.

Nevertheless, the potential dangers of exercise in "cardiac" patients cannot be overemphasized, and as we utilize dynamic exercise more and more in testing and training, physicians must be constantly aware of these dangers.

Complications of exercise can be subdivided into two groups, i.e. *cardiac* and *noncardiac*.

CARDIAC COMPLICATIONS

Regarding cardiac complications, the major factors to be concerned with are sudden death, myocardial infarction, and arrhythmias. Fox and Haskell[3] have reported that certain changes in physical activity may be instrumental in patients with myocardial infarction. On occasions, the news media report the occurrence of sudden unexpected death in a subject while jogging; not infrequently, we hear authenticated verbal reports of such complications. These deaths are most likely due to myocardial infarction, arrhythmias, or cerebral vascular accidents.

With regard to myocardial infarction, we have seen a typical example[4] in a forty-four-year-old insurance salesman who was hospitalized at the University Hospital of San Diego County complaining of severe chest pain which had developed while he was jogging in a "Run for your Life" exercise class. He had previously been well, although he had not actively exercised in over twenty years. He had smoked two packs of cigarettes per day, had been moderately overweight all his adult life, and recently had consumed alcoholic beverages in moderate to heavy amounts. His father died at forty-two years of age from an acute myocardial infarction. Prior to entering the exercise program, the patient obtained the recommended blood pressure, heart rate, and cholesterol levels from his private physician. An electrocardiogram was not taken. In the exercise program, he had been started in Plan B of Bowerman and Harris,[5] which is a program for individuals in average physical condition. After three weeks he had not lost his initial muscle soreness. On the day of admission, while attempting to jog one and a half miles, he was unable to keep up with the others in his group. Finally, he alternated walking and jogging, fifty steps each, and then jogged almost one mile, after which he noted severe substernal chest pain associated with dyspnea and diaphoresis.

On physical examination he was moderately obese but normotensive. Results of cardiopulmonary examination were normal, and no other pertinent physical findings were noted. Initial laboratory data included a normal x-ray film of the chest and normal cholesterol and blood glucose levels. Serial electrocardiograms showed changes of an acute inferior wall myocardial infarction (Fig. 10-1). Results of enzyme determinations supported this diagnosis. The hospital course was uneventful, and the patient was discharged at the end of the third week.

An example of an apparent dysrhythmia has been seen in a fifty-one-year-old man who had entered a running program

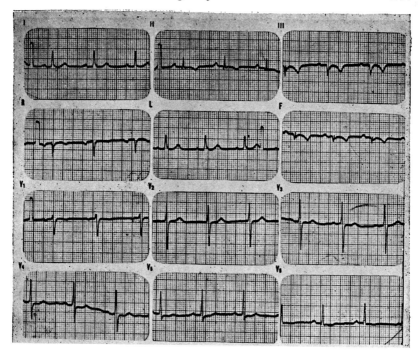

Figure 10-1. Twelve-lead electrocardiogram of a forty-four-year-old male who had an acute inferior myocardial infarction while jogging. The abnormal Q waves and ST-T segments are seen in leads II, III, and F.

following a physical examination which showed no abnormalities. He had noted malaise and fatigue two days before admission and chest pain on the right side posteriorly that persisted throughout the day of admission. Despite the latter, he played volleyball for forty-five minutes and ran one lap (440 yards). On completion of the latter, he suddenly collapsed, and a physician running behind him found him to be cyanotic, unresponsive, pulseless, and with fixed dilated pupils. He was successfully resuscitated in three minutes and hospitalized thirty minutes later. Family history was significant in that his father had died suddenly at forty-eight years of age. A brother had an initial myocardial infarction at the age of thirty-two and died from another at the age of thirty-eight. Another brother died at the age of fifty-eight of a "heart attack," and a third brother was hospitalized for several myocardial infarctions in his early fifties.

Results of physical examination on arrival at the hospital showed a blood pressure of 180/100 mm Hg. Other than a grade 1/6 early systolic murmur at the apex, findings from the cardiovascular examination were unremarkable. The white blood cell count was 6,400/cu mm with a normal differential count. The hemoglobin level was 14.1 gm/100 cc. The initial serum lactic dehydrogenase value was fourteen units on admission and, a week later, two units. The level of serum glutamic oxaloacetic transaminase drawn three days after admission was normal.

The aforementioned cases serve to suggest that complete screening of patients is of importance. Although it is appreciated that screening may not have detected the presence of coronary atherosclerotic disease in either of the cases reported, it is also probable that if high risk individuals were detected, such complications might be avoided.

In recent years, experimental data has confirmed the harmful effects of "overexercise." Arcos et al.[6] studied mitochondrial changes in young female rats during the time course of repeated exercise by swimming. With moderate exercise, there was a large increase in mitochondrial mass and few scattered foci of degenerative changes. With advanced stages of exercise (for 361 to 490 hours of swimming), the animals showed evidence of physical exhaustion and were unable to maintain the same rate of exercise. The distribution and extent of focal degenerative myocardial changes were much more pronounced. These findings suggest that the increase of mitochondrial mass is a compensatory response to exercise, and this increase brings about focal regions of hypoxia during overexercise which are responsible for the degenerative changes. Vatner[7] has studied the effects of exercise on the experimentally induced failing heart in dogs. He found that the failing heart responded differently to the stress of exercise in that inotropic responses are markedly attenuated and are not sufficiently powerful to augment stroke excursion. Therefore, experimental data supports the potentially harmful effects of excessive exercise.

In humans, the potential dangers of exercise should be emphasized both in the unsupervised "jogger" and in the supervised "cardiac" exerciser. Jogging deaths have been reported for many years, and based on the general statistics of Kuller,[8] coronary heart disease accounts for about 75 percent of deaths in unconditioned joggers.

Opie and Shephard[9, 10] have reported that sudden death can occur in sportsmen, and in 1975, Dayton[11] reported 3 cases of sudden death in long-distance runners. One patient, a thirty-eight-year-old marathon runner (fully tested for physical fitness one year before his death) developed chest pain while running and died several hours later. Postmortem exam reported evidence of ischemic heart disease with a number of small infarctions. Another man of nineteen and one half years "dropped dead" while running in a marathon. Postmortem exam revealed coronary atheroma. No mention is made of infarction, nor is there mention of a premortem evaluation or exercise test. A third subject died suddenly after a six– to eight-mile run. No mention is made of a previous evaluation or exercise test. Postmortem exam revealed marked myocardial fibrosis but no recent thrombosis.

Our personal experience has afforded a report of 2 physicians who died while running.[12] One was a young orthopedic resident-in-training who had a long history of regular running but no exercise test recorded. He died while running outside in very cold weather and was found with fist "clutched" over his precordium as if he were having chest pain or were attempting self-resuscitation using precordial thump. His heart and coronary arteries were normal at postmortem. The other, a fifty-two-year-old anesthesiologist, was a regular tennis player but not a runner and had never had an exercise test evaluation. He substituted running one day when tennis courts were not available and died in the locker room minutes after running a mile. His autopsy revealed severe, diffuse coronary athero-sclerotic disease with areas of myocardial fibrosis and recent infarction.

The aforementioned cases confirm the danger of extreme exercise in subjects, be they trained or untrained. Only 1 of the 5 had physical evaluations with exercise testing, the latter which may well have revealed abnormalities to warn those subjects of existing disease. As others[11] have related, competitive activities may well be more likely to precipitate sudden death than exercise training.

Another area of danger in exercise is that of the exercise test evaluation, usually more often seen with the treadmill. In 1976, Lintgen[13] reported death from acute infarction following a submaximal exercise test with a normal result in a fifty-six-year-old man. Death in his hospital room occurred thirty minutes after the test. Autopsy revealed hemorrhage into an intimal atherosclerotic plaque with superimposed intraluminal clot. It is likely that the cause of death existed prior to exercise testing; however, the hemodynamic stress was certainly associated and likely instrumental in the precipitation of his terminal event.

Even in lieu of such reports, exercise testing is considered quite safe but should be done only with direct medical supervision. The data of Rochmis and Blackburn[1] (though not current) certainly support this. It is our feeling that current data would show an even less frequent incidence of morbidity and mortality with exercise testing.

Exercise training programs for postinfarction patients, as suggested by Haskell,[2] do experience associated morbidity and mortality; however, the incidence is no greater (and probably less) than that usually expected with these patients. Individual reports from several programs are available with regard to postinfarction patients experiencing ventricular fibrillation during medically supervised exercise. Mead et al.[14] reported 15 cases of exercise-associated ventricular fibrillation occurring in the Seattle program since 1968. All were successfully resuscitated with no sequelae. They suggest that treating patients exhibiting exercise-induced premature ventricular contractions with antiarrhythmic drugs, proper attention to serum potassium levels, strict adherence to training heart rates, and proper warm-up will likely aid in prevention of future similar events in an exercise program.

In our experience at Georgia Baptist Medical Center in supervised gym cardiac exercise, there have been 5 cases of ventricular fibrillation associated with walk-jog exercise.[15] All of these patients were successfully defibrillated in the gym. All underwent coronary angiography, and 4 of the 5 had myocardial revascularization. All those operated upon have returned to an active exercise program; the other patient refused surgery and has not been permitted to return to active exercise.

As explained in other sections, it is truly felt that a detailed search for coronary risk factors should be undertaken prior to commencement of an exercise program.[16] Symptoms of chest discomfort, current medications, cigarette and alcohol consumption, previous exercise history, familial tendency toward coronary disease, and history of hypertension and diabetes mellitus should all be discussed. The physical examination should place emphasis on blood pressure, heart rate, cardiac murmurs, weight, and evidence of atherogenesis (such as xanthomas). Other screening laboratory work, such as exercise testing and blood studies are suggested and will be discussed in Chapter 11. During training, patients should be repeatedly warned not to exercise if they have recently noted ill health or experienced chest discomfort.

NONCARDIAC COMPLICATIONS

The noncardiac complications of exercise tend to debilitate the exercise enthusiast and cause dropouts from exercise programs. Such problems—usually involving the musculoskeletal system—are not infrequently seen. Harris and Bowerman[5] reported 7 subjects who developed acute gout in a group of 265 subjects who were involved in an exercise program. Other reported complications include development of petechiae,[17] jogger's heel,[18] exacerbations of osteoarthritis,[19] and severe, persistent muscular soreness which accounted for 34 of the 98 dropouts reported by Harris and Bowerman.[5] In addition, Doctor Cantwell has observed Achilles tendonitis and a march fracture directly related to jogging.

In a post-myocardial-infarction gym exercise program (described in detail in Chapter 9), we have seen a number of minor but notable problems. These include ecchymoses, sprained

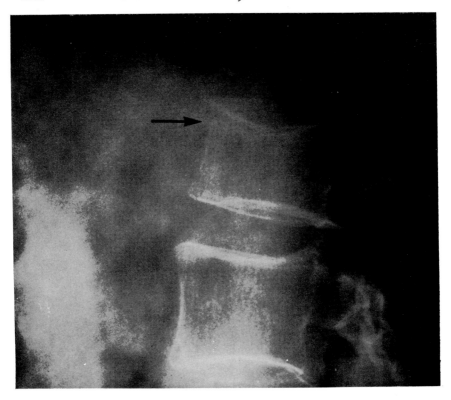

Figure 10-2. X-ray films of lumbosacral spine showing compression fracture as noted by arrow.

fingers (secondary to volleyball), muscular strains, aggravation of pseudogout, aggravation of previous knee injuries (cartilage or ligaments), and an occasional minor laceration. The most debilitating noncardiac complication occurring in our program has been that of a sixty-one-year-old man who fell in the "seated position" while playing volleyball. He suffered a compression fracture of the lumbar spine; x-ray changes are seen in Figure 10-2. He was treated conservatively and has subsequently returned to the program.

Noncardiac dangers of exercise continue to be reported and vary with extremes of minor soft tissue and musculoskeletal injury to more severe blunt and penetrating wounds. There is one recent (not well documented report) of a young lady who fell into an excavation site while running across a construction project. Her thorax and abdomen were penetrated by a steel spearlike portion of the incomplete foundation in the excavation. She miraculously survived and underwent several surgical procedures to have the foreign object removed. No information is available as to whether or not she has resumed her exercise. A well documented, less severe, but "socially important" danger was reported in the winter of 1977.[20] This involved a fifty-three-year-old physician who suffered penile frostbite while jogging outside in a reported air temperature of $-8°C$ with a severe wind chill factor. The subject utilized "self therapy" in a straddled, standing position and created a cradle for rapid rewarming by covering the penile tip with one cupped palm. The response to treatment was rapid and complete without consequence, except for the patient's wife returning home from a local shopping trip to observe him during the treatment procedure.

It is clear, therefore, that exercise programs for patients with coronary heart disease are, at times, interrupted by cardiac and noncardiac complications. These complications may delay the patient's progress in training but do not necessarily cause termination of his participation in the program. Further comments on the prevention of such complications and ways to make physical training more practical and efficient are forthcoming.

In summary, we cannot emphasize enough the importance of properly prescribed exercise, both for normal subjects and those with coronary disease, even if it involves imposing an element of fear. As will be discussed later, we feel that exercise testing is mandatory for anyone beginning a new exercise program and in most should be repeated at intervals. The potential dangers of exercise (both cardiac and noncardiac) are realistic. The more severe cardiac complications may range from death to irreversible myocardial damage, while the noncardiac complications may impose long-term interruption to exercise programs and often permanent soft tissue or musculoskeletal damage.

REFERENCES

1. Rochmis, P., and Blackburn, H.: Exercise tests: A survey of procedures, safety, and litigation experience in approximately 170,000 tests. *JAMA, 217:*1061-1066, 1971.
2. Haskell, W.: Cardiovascular complications during medically supervised exercise training of cardiacs. *Circulation, Suppl 11* to *51* and *52:*118, 1975.
3. Fox, S.M., III, and Haskell, W.L.: Physical activity and the prevention of coronary heart disease. *Bull NY Acad Med, 44.*950-965, 1968.
4. Cantwell, J.D., and Fletcher, G.F.: Cardiac complications while jogging. *JAMA, 210:*130-131, 1969.
5. Harris, W.E., Bowerman, W., McFadden, R.B., et al.: Jogging, An adult exercise program. *JAMA, 201:*759-761, 1967.
6. Arcos, J.C., Sohal, R.S., Sun, S.C., Argus, M.F., and Burch, G.E.: Changes in ultrastructure and respiratory control in mitochondria of rat heart hypertrophied by exercise. *Exp Mol Pathol, 8.*49-65, 1968.
7. Vatner, S.F.: Response of the failing heart to severe exercise. *Clin Res, 24, 3:*422 A (Abstr), 1975.
8. Kuller, L.: Sudden death in arteriosclerotic heart disease. *Am J Cardiol, 24.*617, 1969.
9. Opie, L.H.: Sudden death and sport. *Lancet, 1:*263-266, 1975.
10. Shephard, R.J.: Sudden death: a significant hazard of exercise? *Br J Sports Med, 8:*101-110, 1974.
11. Dayton, S.: Long-distance running and sudden death (Letter). *N Engl J Med, 293.*941-942, 1975.
12. Cantwell, J.D., and Fletcher, G.F.: Physician deaths while jogging. *Physician and Sports Medicine, March.*94-98, 1978.
13. Lintgen, A.B.: Deaths from myocardial infarction after exercise test with normal result. *JAMA, 235.*837-839, 1976.
14. Mead, W.F., Pyfer, H.R., Trombold, J.C., and Frederick, R.C.: Successful resuscitation of two near simultaneous cases of cardiac arrest with a review of fifteen cases occurring during supervised exercise. *Circulation, 53:*187-189, 1976.
15. Fletcher, G.F., and Cantwell, J.D.: Ventricular fibrillation in a medically supervised cardiac exercise program: clinical, angiographic and surgical correlation. *JAMA, 238(No. 24):* 2627, 1977.
16. Parmley, L.F.: Proceedings of the National Conference on exercise in the prevention, in the evaluation, in the treatment of heart disease. *J SC Med Assoc, 65.*i, 1969.
17. Cohen, H.L.: Jogger's petechiae. *N Engl J Med, 279:*109, 1968.
18. Siegel, I.M.: Jogger's heel. *JAMA, 206.*2899, 1968.
19. Hunder, G.G.: Harmful effect of jogging. *Ann Intern Med, 71.*664-665, 1969.
20. Hershkowitz, M.: Penile frostbite, an unforeseen hazard of jogging (Letter). *N Engl J Med, 296, 3:*178, Jan. 20, 1977.

Chapter 11

AN OUTPATIENT GYM EXERCISE PROGRAM FOR PATIENTS WITH RECENT MYOCARDIAL INFARCTION

AN UPDATE

A NUMBER OF CLINICAL STUDIES[1, 2, 3, 4, 5, 6, 7] from several countries emphasize the benefit of organized physical activity programs in patients with coronary heart disease and recent myocardial infarction. Although many of the known subjects with recent myocardial infarction are not incorporated into such programs, such management is becoming more popular among physicians as the feasibility and safety of these programs becomes more apparent and more patients become motivated.

Several studies have recently been reported regarding the results of exercise training programs for subjects with coronary heart disease. One of the most revealing was reported by Bruce et al.[8] from Seattle regarding their medically supervised program of physical training involving thirty to sixty minutes of graded levels of walk-jog and calisthenic activities three mornings per week. In this program, 230 men and 21 women remained active for twenty-two and twenty months respectively; 352 (58.4%) dropped out after an average of 8.6 months for men and 5.7 months for women. Results showed elapsed time to morbidity tended to be longer in active persons than in dropouts. Over one half of active men but only one third of dropouts were working. Among men, the respective total mortality rates were 2.7 and 4.7/100 person-years for active participants and dropouts; among women, the rates were 0 and 3.7 respectively. Twenty-four episodes of cardiac arrest occurred in 13 men with 3 deaths outside the training program, whereas in 11 instances of exertional arrests in supervised training, all defibrillations were successful. Therefore, the results of this follow-up study seem to support both the benefits and safety of medically supervised exercise training in post-infarction patients.

In another smaller group of 8 men with angina pectoris studied with both invasive and noninvasive techniques before and after training, Kennedy et al.[9] reported a decrease in oxygen consumption for a given repetitive workload and conversion of pretraining positive (for ischemia) exercise electrocardiograms to normal in 2 subjects. With training, all subjects had a decrease in angina, an increase in self-esteem, and a more positive attitude towards work and disability. However, there was no change in coronary lesions, in collaterals *or on arteriography.* In addition, left ventricular performance and hemodynamic response of the ventricle to supine leg exercise was unchanged.

In a well-controlled study by Wilhelmsen et al.[10] in Sweden, 158 post-myocardial-infarction patients were trained for one year, while 157 clinically comparable subjects served as controls. The training consisted of running, cycling, and calisthenics three times weekly, while other treatment for both groups was essentially the same. During four years of follow-up 28 patients died in the training group and 35 in the control group (Fig. 11-1). The numbers of nonfatal reinfarctions were 25 and 28, respectively. However, no differences in mortality between the trained group and the control group were statistically significant. Haskell[11] has recently summarized the results of data analysis regarding physical activity programs after myocardial infarction. He feels that the unique contribution of increased physical activity to reducing the severity and frequency of reinfarction has not been adequately established, but when combined with other behavior designed to reduce risk factors, the preliminary results are favorable. For those benefits to be obtained without undue risk, exercise for the post-myocardial-infarction patient needs to be individually prescribed and periodically reevaluated.

Therefore, data both in the United States and abroad continue to be reported regarding the likely benefits and safety

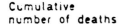

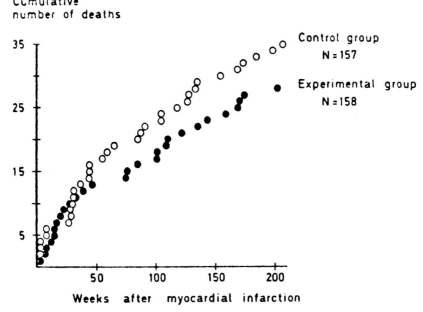

Figure 11-1. Total mortality after discharge from the hospital and during four years follow-up after myocardial infarction. From Wilhelmsen et al., A controlled trial of physical training after myocardial infarction. Effects on risk factors, nonfatal reinfarction, and death, *Preventive Medicine, 4*:491-508, 1975.

of exercise for the postinfarction patient. It is generally felt that such benefits are more abundant when an all-encompassing program of risk factor modification is utilized. Such programs should include dietary modifications and body weight control, cessation of cigarette smoking, and control of blood pressure as well as medically supervised and prescribed exercise.

The purpose of this chapter is to present the method of evaluation and training used and results of an outpatient exercise program for patients with recent myocardial infarction who were trained in the gymnasium of a large metropolitan community hospital. The method and training technique have also been used for patients in the post-myocardial-revascularization state and for some coronary-prone patients who have a high risk factor index.

GYMNASIUM EXERCISE PROGRAM

Patients were evaluated for the exercise phase of the cardiac rehabilitation program after receipt of a written clinical summary of hospitalization and referral from their individual private physicians. They were at least eight to ten weeks post-myocardial-infarction. No one was admitted to the program if he had persistent complicating dysrhythmias, heart failure, evidence of ventricular dysfunction, or a complicating systemic illness such as uncontrolled diabetes mellitus or obstructive lung disease. Angina pectoris was not considered a disqualifying complication. Some patients were receiving antianginal medications such as nitrates and beta blocking agents that could affect exercise performance. Candidates for the program were evaluated by the team of physicians, physician's assistants, and nurses in charge of the rehabilitation program. At this time, a brief history was taken and physical examination (including careful cardiac palpation and auscultation) was performed. Emphasis was placed on a coronary risk factor profile to include history of hypertension, smoking, and family history of coronary disease. The mechanics and purpose of the exercise program and testing were explained to the patient and his family. The subjects were submitted to a baseline resting electrocardiogram which was reviewed by the physician, followed by a submaximal treadmill exercise test (as a measure of exercise capacity) with oxygen consumption studies at rest and with exercise. Patients on medications continued these during their testing periods. The method of exercise testing involving a motor-driven treadmill has been described elsewhere. Additional evaluation included body weight, skinfold measurements and abdominal, chest and thigh circumferences. The mechanics and purpose of the exercise program were explained to the patient and his family.

The patient was then scheduled for the second part of his evaluation for the exercise program, to be done one day later. At this time, the bench test, (a simple step test) was performed. This was done in order to have a simple exercise evaluation that can be done in any physician's office to compare with the more elaborate treadmill test.

However, evaluation of 35 patients with both treadmill and bench testing revealed that the latter did not show an increase in bench steps or an increase in heart rate with training. To the contrary, on the treadmill, the subjects showed significant increases in oxygen consumption, test time, and maximal heart rate. In addition, of the 4 patients who had positive S-T segment changes of ischemia on treadmill testing, none were positive with the bench test. It was, therefore, concluded that bench step testing used alone is an unreliable gauge of testing exercise capacity after myocardial infarction,[12] and this method of testing has henceforth been discontinued in this program.

Spirometry for evaluation of pulmonary function and blood studies for lipid profile (including serum cholesterol and triglyceride determination) were also performed. SMA-12 determinations were done to include glucose and uric acid levels. All blood studies were done in the fasting state—twelve hours after the last meal. At this visit (eight to twelve weeks after myocardial infarction), the patient was informed of his official acceptance into the program (unless the evaluation revealed some of the aforementioned complications that required further evaluation by the private physician) and any further questions regarding the program were answered by the staff for him or his family. At the final part of the second evaluation, the subject was given a tour of the hospital gymnasium facility.

The gymnasium utilized in the program is a 19,500-square-foot building which houses a full-size basketball court which is also utilized as a volleyball court. The view of the hospital facilities in Figure 11-2 shows the gym and its relation to the hospital. There are spectator stands adjacent to the volleyball court with a seating capacity of 500 persons. A thirty-by-thirty-foot swimming pool, ping pong area (two tables), a four-lane bowling alley, and areas for shuffleboard and indoor horseshoes are also utilized. The exercise sequence for the subjects involves classes on Monday, Wednesday, Friday (forty-five minutes per class). Four classes meet each day. Each session is divided into a fifteen-minute period each of walk-jog sequence, calisthenics and team sports—usually volleyball; the specifics of each of these periods are described elsewhere, as is the walk-jog sequence.

The sequence serves only as a guideline and is modified individually according to the subject's treadmill exercise test performance. The level of exercise in each of these categories is prescribed by individual prescription for each patient by the program director or his associate based on the initial work load attained in testing heart rate, blood pressure, and S-T segment response. Prescriptions are altered and increased according to the subject's exercise heart rate, longevity in the program, and degree of conditioning. At each session, the nurse or technologist checks and records the patient's resting blood pressure by cuff sphygmomanometer. At this time, the physician, nurse, recreational therapist, or technologist has the opportunity to converse briefly with the patient in order to detect any obvious acute emotional or physical change; specific note is made of symptoms of chest discomfort, dizziness, faintness, or palpitation, and the daily exercise may be decreased accordingly. The patient himself then checks and records his own heart rate by radial or carotid palpation before and after each fifteen-minute exercise period (Fig. 11-3).

In addition to medical personnel trained in cardiopulmonary resuscitation, the gym is equipped with closed circuit television monitoring from the swimming pool, ping pong area, and volleyball court with a central receiving set in the gym office. Cardiopulmonary resuscitation equipment (including airway, defibrillator, electrocardiogram machine, and ambu bag) as well as cardiac drugs are located on an emergency cart. Both a litter and a wheel chair are available in the gym for patient transportation to the hospital emergency room, which is only a five-minute walk from the gym and employs a direct telephone extension.

INSTANT ELECTROCARDIOGRAPHY

Instant electrocardiogram rhythm strips are available through recorded signals via defibrillator paddles as seen in Figure 11-4.

Ten patients with suspected arrhythmias have been evaluated

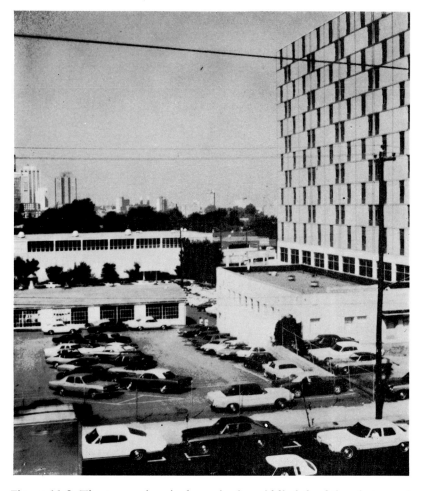

Figure 11-2. The gymnasium is shown in the middle-left of the photograph (several large shrubs in front) as it relates to the hospital facility (tallest building on the right). The metropolitan skyline of Atlanta is seen in the background.

with instant electrocardiography; tracings were obtained three times weekly for three to six months. Four patients developed S-T segment depression equal to or greater than 2 mm immediately after walk-jog activities, and 1 of the 4 had ventricular ectopy. Three other subjects had asymptomatic bouts of ventricular tachycardia. Two of the latter subsequently

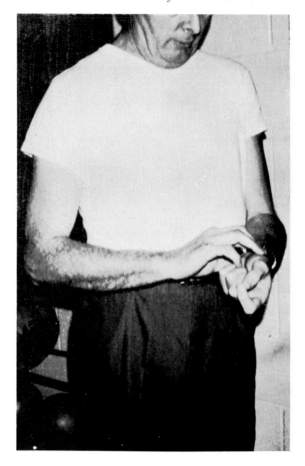

Figure 11-3. Patient is shown checking heart rate after
an exercise sequence by palpation of the radial pulse.

developed ventricular fibrillation during moderate physical
activity, and 1 ultimately died suddenly while engaged in
week-end yard work. It was concluded that instant ECG is a
simple method of screening arrhythmia-prone participants in a
supervised exercise program. It is felt that such persons should
be considered candidates for antiarrhythmic treatment and be
limited to rather light physical activity such as mild flexibility
exercises, noncompetitive sports, and slow walking.[13]
    All patients admitted to the program understand that they are

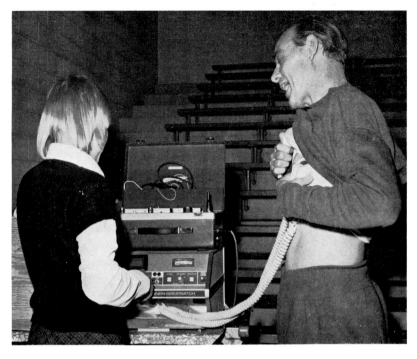

Figure 11-4. Nurse coordinator is shown recording "instant" electrocardiographic rhythm strip on patient prior to walk-jog sequence. The signal is transmitted through the defibrillator paddles to the graphic recorder.

to have repeat testing (identical to that on entering the program) at three-month intervals for at least nine months. The subjects are also given instruction in coronary risk factor modification, and as their study results return, if indicated, they are given private or group instruction on dietary modification for the purpose of alleviating coronary risk factors such as smoking, abnormal lipid patterns and control of hypertension. Educational conferences are also held weekly for the patients and their families by physicians, nurses, dietitians, social workers, and chaplains.

At the six-month point in the program, the subjects are given the privilege of continuing in the hospital program or are given an exercise prescription by which to continue their individual program at home or at some other facility. After the nine-month testing, patients are submitted to the exercise test only every six months as a method of follow-up evaluation. At the end of exercise, the patient's private physician receives a written progress report.

DATA FROM OUTPATIENT EXERCISE PROGRAM

From January, 1971 through April, 1974, 230 patients were enrolled in the program after having qualified through evaluation and testing. Ninety-eight patients had completed six months of training with an overall average of 70 percent attendance. Of these 98, 91 were male and 7 were female; all were white. The age ranged from 35 to 70 years, with a mean of 50.6 years. Forty-one subjects had anterior myocardial infarction by electrocardiogram, 50 had inferior infarction, and seven had subendocardial infarction. Thirteen additional patients dropped out of the program prior to three months but cooperated in returning for follow-up studies.

Data were calculated on the 98 patients who completed six or more months of the training program as well as on the 13 who dropped out. All exercise testing data were recorded for the same heart rate end point. There was an increase in mean exercise oxygen consumption in ml/kg/min from 15.6 (initial) to 18.4 at three-month testing ($p \leq 0.01$) and subsequently from 18.4 (three months) to 19.2 at six-month testing. There was also an increase in mean treadmill test time from 11.5 minutes (initial) to 16.7 minutes at three months ($p \leq 0.01$) and from 16.7 at three months to 19.5 minutes at six-month testing ($p \leq 0.01$). The exercise quotient (systolic blood pressure in millimeters of mercury × heart rate in beats per minute divided by treadmill test time in minutes) decreased from a mean of 2289.1 (initially) to 1361.2 at three months ($p \leq 0.01$) and subsequently from 1361.2 at three months to 1191.1 at six months ($p \leq 0.05$). These data on oxygen consumption, exercise quotient, and treadmill test time are seen in Figure 11-5.

The mean resting systolic blood pressure decreased from 129.0 mm Hg (initially) to 119.9 at three months ($p \leq 0.01$) but

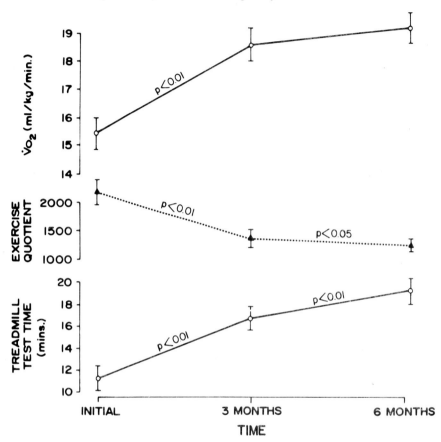

Figure 11-5. Graph showing changes in mean oxygen consumption, exercise quotient, and treadmill test time in trained subjects from the initial to the three– and six-month testing. From G.F. Fletcher and J.D. Cantwell, Outpatient gym exercise and risk factor modification for patients with recent myocardial infarction: Methodology and results in a community program, *Journal of the Louisiana State Medical Society, 127:*52-57, 1975.

rose slightly from 119.9 at three months to 123.2 at six months. The mean peak exercise systolic blood pressure decreased from 156.9 mm Hg initially to 147.9 at three-month testing ($p \leq 0.05$) and subsequently increased slightly from 147.9 (three months) to 154.8 at six months. The mean systolic blood pressure immediately postexercise decreased from 149.5 mm Hg (initially) to 145.2 at three months ($p \leq 0.05$) but increased from 145.2 at three months to 149.3 at six months ($p \leq 0.05$). The mean diastolic blood pressure at rest decreased from 85.6 mm Hg (initially) to 81.7 at three months ($p \leq 0.05$) and from that point to 81.5 at six months. The exercise diastolic pressure decreased from 84.4 mm Hg (initially) to 79.1 at three months ($p \leq 0.05$) but remained the same at six months. The mean diastolic blood pressure immediately postexercise increased from 79.6 mm Hg (initially) to 83.3 at three months ($p \leq 0.05$) but remained essentially the same from three months to six months. The pressure three minutes postexercise remained the same in follow-up testing—both in systole and diastole.

The mean resting heart rate in beats per minute decreased from 78.6 (initially) to 74.8 at three months ($p \leq 0.05$) and then to 74.3 at six months. Exercise and postexercise testing heart rate did not change significantly during the six-month training period.

With regard to other studies, there was essentially no change in the mean body weight, serum cholesterol, and uric acid. However, the mean serum triglycerides decreased from 214.4 mgm/dl initially to 181.23 mg/dl at three-month testing and subsequently to 169.0 mg/dl at six months (Fig. 11-6). There was a significant change in triglyceride levels from initial to three months ($p \leq 0.05$) and from initial to six months ($p \leq 0.01$).

Of 81 cigarette smokers, 68 percent (55 of 81) stopped from initial to six-month testing. There were no deaths and no recurrent infarctions, and 95 percent (93 of 98) of the group are gainfully employed.

Of 13 patients who dropped out of the program within the first three weeks, treadmill test times increased significantly on retesting three months after the baseline study (mean of 11.3 minutes to 15.8 minutes—$p \leq 0.05$). However, the oxygen consumption did not change significantly, nor were there significant changes in triglyceride, cholesterol, and exercise pressure rate product. In addition, only 54 percent were gainfully employed. Reasons for dropping out included work conflicts in 7, unrelated medical problems in 3 and lack of interest in 3.

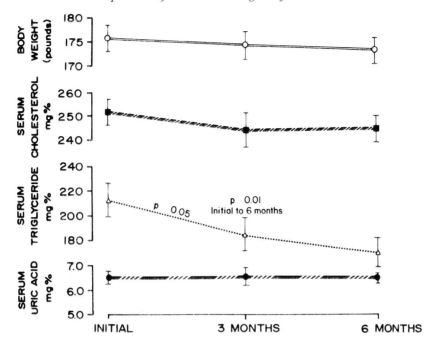

Figure 11-6. Graph showing changes in the mean body weight, serum cholesterol, triglycerides, and uric acid in the trained subjects from the initial to the three– and six-month testing. From G.F. Fletcher and J.D. Cantwell, Outpatient gym exercise and risk factor modification for patients with recent myocardial infarction: Methodology and results in a community program. *Journal of the Louisiana State Medical Society, 127:*52-57, 1975.

One of the most notable and significant results of this follow-up study is the improvement in oxygen consumption. These data reflect that the most impressive training effect seems to be in the first three months. A similar trend is seen with the treadmill test time and exercise quotient. These latter data show a significant change both at three and six months, with the greatest change in mean values occurring in the first three-month period of training. The value, perhaps, of the effectiveness of training being seen as early as three months is that some patients may need only this three-month period of supervised training in order to obtain the desired level of long-term and safe exercise prescription. Therefore, earlier "graduation" from the program to an unsupervised home or community program would be both feasible and safe for selected patients. A more rapid turnover of such patients would make facilities more available for others as these programs become popular.

It is felt that with the addition of the aforementioned multiple coronary risk factor modification techniques to the gym training program, a more effective result in secondary prevention will be obtained in the postinfarction patients. Whether or not this will significantly affect the ultimate morbidity and mortality of patients with recent myocardial infarction remains to be seen when a group of comparable control patients are followed along with the patients in training for a period of several years. Regardless, exercise training for myocardial infarction patients appears to be safe and beneficial as manifested by increased oxygen consumption and treadmill test time and decreased heart rate—blood pressure product as indices of improved exercise capacity and is associated with beneficial changes in triglyceride levels and smoking habits.[14]

DIETARY INTERVENTIONS IN EXERCISE TRAINING

In order to further assess the effect of multifactoral risk intervention in the outpatient gym exercise program, a subset of 60 postinfarction patients were evaluated with regard to the effect of dietary control and exercise training on daily food intake and serum lipids.[15]

From a total of 60 volunteers, patients were randomized by standard random number technique into two groups. Group I (no diet control, n = 30, mean 49.2 years, 179.24 ± 4.7 lb.) underwent exercise training without dietary control. Group II (diet control, n = 30, mean 51.1 years, mean 171.2 ± 3.2 lb.) combined exercise training with dietary control by individual counseling with a therapeutic dietitian.

Sources of dietary composition and related nutritional information were recorded initially and at twelve weeks by a registered dietitian from documentation of food type and source by personal interview. These data were obtained following randomization using a three-day dietary record, recall interview, and standard reference tables. No dietary alterations were suggested in Group I. An individualized diet was prescribed for patients in Group II. The diet prescription was based on lipid phenotyping and individual caloric requirements. Six patients followed a combination fat– and caloric-controlled diet, and four patients followed a regular fat-controlled diet with no caloric restriction. Two patients had a type IIb lipid pattern indicative of elevations both in serum cholesterol and triglycerides. Eighteen patients were phenotyped as type IV. (The type IIb diet strictly limits dietary cholesterol, while in type IV diets, the cholesterol intake is only moderately restricted. Both types limit carbohydrate intake.) Caloric requirements were determined by the degree of physical activity and the patients' need to either reduce or maintain an ideal body weight. Fasting (twelve-hour) blood samples were obtained prior to exercise participation initially and at the end of the study. Total cholesterol and triglycerides were determined by standard methods. None of the subjects studied were taking lipid-reducing medications. Body weight was obtained during similar conditions at the beginning and end of the experimental period. An uncorrelated t test was used to determine significant differences between group means.

Both groups showed reductions ($p \leq 0.01$) in mean total daily kilocalories consumed (2867 ± 82 versus 2088 ± 77 and 2848 ± 15 versus 1285 ± 68, respectively); however, no significant change occurred in total body weight. The dietary control group consumed relatively more kilocalories as protein than the group without dietary control (285 of 1,285 versus 389 of 2,088, respectively) and less ($p \leq 0.05$) as fat (443 of 1285 versus 804 of 2,089, respectively). Both groups had lower ($p \leq 0.01$) mean daily dietary cholesterol after 12 weeks (811 ± 44 versus 232 ± 17 mg) versus (325 ± 18 versus 309 ± 23 mg, respectively). A reduction in serum cholesterol ($p \leq 0.05$) was seen in the dietary control group (270 ± 8 versus 243 ± 7 mg/dl) but not in the group without dietary control (260 ± 6 versus $261 = 7$ mg/dl) (Fig. 11-7). The dietary control group had a lower mean triglyceride

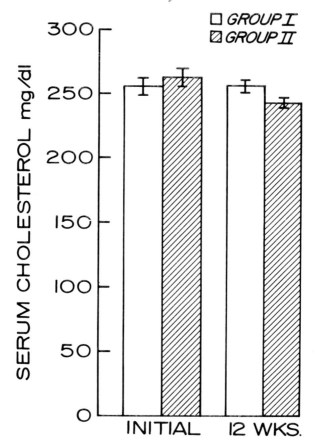

Figure 11-7. Bar graph showing levels of serum cholesterol in mg/dl initially and after twelve weeks of exercise training. Group I had no dietary control; group II had dietary control. From Watt et al., Effect of dietary control and exercise training on daily food intake and serum lipids in post-myocardial infarction patients, *American Journal of Clinical Nutrition, 29.*900-904, 1976.

level ($p \leq 0.05$) (229 ± 24 versus 155 ± 18 mg/dl), but no differences were seen in the group without dietary control (189 ± 15 versus 180 ± 13 mg/dl) (Fig. 11-8). It was concluded that significant reductions in caloric intake and daily dietary

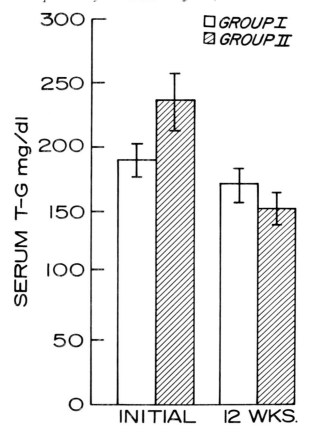

Figure 11-8. Bar graph showing serum triglycerides (T-G) in mg/dl initially and after twelve weeks of exercise training. Group I had no dietary control; group II had dietary control. From Watt et al., Effect of dietary control and exercise training on daily food intake and serum lipids on post-myocardial infarction patients, *American Journal of Clinical Nutrition, 29*:900-904, 1976.

cholesterol complement the effects of exercise training in post-myocardial-infarction patients by increasing substrate protein and fat consumption ratio and by reducing serum cholesterol and triglycerides. These effects are not seen with exercise training alone.

AMBULATORY ELECTROCARDIOGRAPHIC MONITORING

Other more recent techniques of patient monitoring have been utilized in the evaluation of the patients in the exercise program. In order to evaluate cardiac rate and rhythm in 20 patients, continuous ambulatory electrocardiographic monitoring was performed during an exercise training class and the subsequent twenty-four hours, which included activities at work and home. Sixty-five percent (13) of the 20 patients had abnormal findings on recordings. Of the 20 patients studied, 40 percent (8) had arrhythmias detected by ambulatory recording that had not been detected by resting or exercise electrocardiograms (Fig. 11-9). Three patients with ventricular ectopia (multiform premature ventricular beats, couplets, and bigeminy) had exercise activities temporarily curtailed and therapy with antiarrhythmic drugs begun, with subsequent resolution or improvement. Two other patients (with recorded heart rates of 160 beats per minute) were instructed to carefully monitor their heart rate in order to not exceed the target maximum. It was concluded that twenty-four-hour continuous electrocardiographic monitoring is beneficial in evaluating patients in cardiac exercise programs and frequently influences the management of such patients.[16]

OXYGEN CONSUMPTION STUDIES

Preliminary data in the gym program has been collected to assess the oxygen cost (VO_2-ml/kg/min) and hemodynamic response of various exercises used in training. Eleven male post-myocardial-infarction patients (PMIP) were studied by means of a modified Max Planck respirometer technique. Heart rate (HR) and systolic blood pressure product response (RPP) were also obtained. All patients were considered exercise trained (ET), having been in the program at least twelve weeks. Exercise activities (EA) included thirteen standard calisthenics (C) of fifteen repetitions (reps) each, walk-jogging (WJ) of five minutes at five to seven miles per hour, volleyball (VB)—a twenty-minute

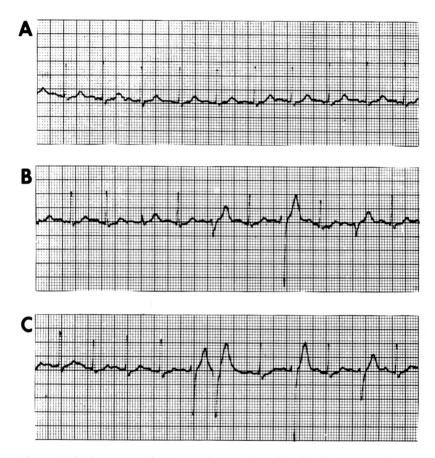

Figure 11-9. Home recordings. (A) Sinus tachycardia of 106 beats per minute just prior to coitus. (B) Subsequent sinus tachycardia of 118 beats per minute with a period of ventricular bigeminy. (C) Ensuing sinus tachycardia of 118 beats per minute with ventricular bigeminy and couplets. (Both B and C were recorded during coitus.) From G.F. Fletcher and J.D. Cantwell, Continuous ambulatory electrocardiographic monitoring: Use in cardiac exercise programs, *Chest, 71:*27-32, 1977.

game, swimming (SW) for a nontimed forty yard freestyle sequence, and a combination of three exercise dance (Pelican, Evil Ways, and Nite Owl) routines (ED). The results were as follows:

	VO_2	METS	RPP
C	9.87 ± 0.5	2.8	$10,260 \pm 37$
WJ	$23.15 \pm 2.2*$	6.6	$19,402 \pm 195$
VB	$11.68 \pm 0.5*$	3.3	$11,125 \pm 57$
SW	$30.10 \pm 2.2*$	8.6	$21,000 \pm 129$
ED	21.07 ± 3.4	6.02	$17,300 \pm 187$

In efforts to introduce variety in prescriptive exercise while maintaining the efficacy and safety of such activities, these data suggest that energy demands, with the exception of SW, do not appear to be overly severe for the uncomplicated patient. Contrary to speculation, ED was slightly less demanding than WJ, while VB demanded less ($p < 0.01$) VO_2 ml/gk/min than all other activities studied. The higher VO_2 ($p < 0.01$) seen in SW versus WJ and ED support our contention that this activity should be used with caution. Increased RPP seen in SW, WJ, and ED encourage careful monitoring of HR and BP as PMIP progress in these activities.

EVALUATION OF COITAL ACTIVITIES

In order to evaluate the effects of exercise training on coital habits in the post-myocardial-infarction and the postrevascularization state, questionnaires were mailed to 130 patients enrolled in the gymnasium exercise program. Of 87 (67%) responding, 68 were post-myocardial-infarction and 19 had undergone myocardial revascularization. The postinfarction group significantly decreased their coital frequency after infarction by 28 percent; the revascularization group, however, decreased by only 10 percent. The myocardial infarction group waited 9.4 weeks after infarction to resume sexual intercourse, while the revascularization group waited only a mean of 5.7 weeks. These data suggest that physically trained post-myocar-

---

$*p < 0.01$

dial-infarction patients decrease frequency of coitus significantly more than physically trained patients with myocardial
revascularization. The overall decrease, however, is notably less
than reported in nontrained post-myocardial-infarction patients and therefore supports the possible "bedroom benefit" of
medically supervised exercise both in postinfarction and
postrevascularization patients.

GENERAL DATA

General overall data regarding the program at Georgia
Baptist Medical Center over a six-year period (1970-1976)
revealed that approximately 500 patients have been involved in
the program; approximately 133 are active at any one time. The
patients are referred from 140 different primary physicians.
The dropout rate has been 65%; however, many of these have
continued their exercise at other nonsupervised facilities in the
area, such as YMCAs, other gyms, or "on their own" in
neighborhood areas. To date, 14 patients have had recurrent
infarctions while in the exercise program; none of these
occurred with exercise nor were they related in time to the
exercise. Seventy-one patients had angina pectoris or developed
same while in the program. Of these, 23 have eventually had
coronary angiographic studies, and 10 have had revascularization. At this point, a total of 22 patients in the program are
postrevascularization.

ELECTRICAL INSTABILITY

In the six-year period, 5 subjects experienced ventricular
fibrillation exercising in the gymnasium. All were successfully
resuscitated. Four were post-infarction and 4 had a history of
angina pectoris. Two had previously recorded ventricular
ectopy; 1 was on treatment. All subsequently had coronary
angiography; 4 of 5 had 75 percent obstruction of at least two
major coronary arteries, while 1 had a high grade proximal left

anterior descending lesion. Four subsequently had successful myocardial revascularization (3 prior to hospital discharge), and, except for the patient who refused surgery, all have returned to an active exercise prescription. It was concluded that multivessel, operative coronary disease is common in patients experiencing ventricular fibrillation and that ventricular fibrillation may occur unpredictably (two to forty-eight months) in duration of exercise exposure.[17]

NATIONAL EXERCISE AND HEART DISEASE PROJECT

Irregardless of the apparent benefit and safety of exercise programs for post-myocardial-infarction patients, there is still a lack of controlled data to support this. In order to study all aspects of the question, the National Exercise and Heart Disease Project (NEHDP)[18] was initiated in 1972 as a multicenter study involving Emory University School of Medicine with Georgia Baptist Medical Center, Case Western Reserve University, University of Alabama, George Washington University and Lankenaw Hospital. After a prerandomization period of exercise, 651 post-myocardial-infarction patients were randomized into either an organized medically supervised exercise class (323) or to free activities at home (328). The study will continue for five to seven years to study primarily the effect of exercise on mortality and morbidity involving recurrent myocardial infarction, angina pectoris, or complications of infarction. Early results are available for the first phase of the study only.

Characteristics of the study population revealed that the patients were predominantly married, white, middle class, educated, with good incomes, and with average age of fifty-two years. More than half entered the study within one year of experiencing the myocardial infarction. Most patients (83%) had only one myocardial infarction, the qualifying one.

The exercise test taken at the end of the prerandomization exercise period as the final evaluation before entry to the study revealed that the candidates could perform quite well—78 percent of them went to stage seven or further.

More than 81 percent were already back at work; therefore, only 103 patients were available to study the rehabilitation effects of the exercise program, in respect to return to work. The percent already working did not seem to depend upon the "months elapsed" since the myocardial infarction.

The initial psychological evaluations indicated that a fair proportion of the patients had scores above the upper limits of normality, indicating potential room for improvement from the exercise program or other influences.

The follow-up rates are good but not excellent. At least 84 percent have been followed for one year. The follow-up for the exercise group is better (88%) than for the control group (79%).

Changes observed during the prerandomization exercise period (PREP) were clearly noticeable; measures of systolic blood pressure and heart rate suggest that the PREP had some conditioning effect.

Changes were also noted in various psychological scores. Most of these are of questionable clinical significance even though "statistically significant" at the customary .05 level.

No serious events occurred during the PREP sessions, no deaths, and no recurrent myocardial infarctions. There were two deaths after first evaluation before scheduled entry into the study. One of these died of unknown causes before entering the PREP. The other died of a myocardial infarction two weeks after successfully completing PREP. He had not come in for the second evaluation but was continuing PREP-like exercising at the clinic. He died at the racetrack one day after his last (nontraining) exercise session. One nonfatal myocardial infarction occurred during the trial period. This patient had completed the PREP, had been through the second evaluation, and was awaiting the randomization step. He had been continuing in PREP-like sessions and experienced the myocardial infarction on a nonexercising day. He did not complain of pain in the previous exercise session and withdrew from candidacy for the study.[19]

The final phase of the study is in progress, and results will be available in two to three years.

REFERENCES

1. Naughton, J., Shanbour, K., Armstrong, R., et al.: Cardiovascular responses to exercise following myocardial infarction. *Arch Intern Med, 117:*541-545, 1966.
2. Frick, M.H., and Katila, M.: Hemodynamic consequences of physical training after myocardial infarction. *Circulation, 37:*192-202, 1968.
3. Gottheiner, V.: Long range strenuous sports training for cardiac reconditioning and rehabilitation. *Am J Cardiol, 22:*426-435, 1968.
4. Hellerstein, H.K.: The effects of physical activity: Patients and normal coronary-prone subjects. *Minn Med, 52:*1335-1341, 1969.
5. Rechnitzer, P.A., Pickard, H.A., Paivio, A.U., et al.: Long-term follow-up study of survival and recurrence rates following myocardial infarction in exercising and control subjects. *Circulation, 45:*853-857, 1972.
6. Boyer, J.L.: Physical activity program following myocardial infarction. *Hosp Med, 8:*95-112, 1972.
7. Morgan, C.M.: Supervised training after myocardial infarction (Abstr). *Br Heart J, 34:*203, 1972.
8. Bruce, E.H., Frederick, R., Bruce, R.A., and Fisher, L.D.: Comparison of active participants and dropouts in Capri Cardiopulmonary Rehabilitation Programs. *Am J Cardiol, 37:*53-60, 1976.
9. Kennedy, C.C., Spiekerman, R.E., Lindsay, M.I., Jr., Mankin, H.T., Frye, R.L., and McCallister, B.D.: One-year graduated exercise program for men with angina pectoris. Evaluation by physiologic studies and coronary arteriography. *Mayo Clin Proc, 51:*231-236, 1976.
10. Wilhelmsen, L., Sanne, H., Elmfeldt, D., Grimby, G., Tibblin, G., and Wedel, H.: A controlled trial of physical training after myocardial infarction. Effects on risk factors, nonfatal reinfarction, and death. *Prev Med, 4:*491-508, 1975.
11. Haskell, W.L.: Physical activity after myocardial infarction. *Am J Cardiol, 33:*776-782, 1974.
12. Fletcher, G.F., Watt, E.W., and Cantwell, J.D.: Bench step testing of exercise capacity: Unreliable gauge after recent myocardial infarction. *Arch Phys Med Rehabil, 55:*553-556, 1974.
13. Cantwell, J.D., and Fletcher, G.F.: Instant electrocardiogram: Use in cardiac exercise programs. *American College of Cardiology, 50:*962-966, November, 1974.
14. Fletcher, G.F., and Cantwell, J.D.: Outpatient gym exercise and risk factor modification for patients with recent myocardial infarction: Methodology and results in a community program. *J La State Med Soc, 127:*52-57, 1975.
15. Watt, E.W., Wiley, J., and Fletcher, G.F.: Effect of dietary control and exercise training on daily food intake and serum lipids in post-myocardial infarction patients. *Am J Clin Nutr, 29:*900-904, 1976.

16. Fletcher, G.F., and Cantwell, J.D.: Continuous ambulatory electrocardiographic monitoring: Use in cardiac exercise programs. *Chest, 71:*27-32, 1977.
17. Fletcher, G.F., and Cantwell, J.D.: Ventricular fibrillation in a medically supervised cardiac exercise program: Clinical, angiographic and surgical correlation. *JAMA, 238:*2627-2629, 1977.
18. Naughton, J., Taylor, J., Gorman, P., and Rios, J.: National Exercise and Heart Disease Project. *Med Ann D C, 43:*5-6, 1974.
19. Shaw, L.W.: The character and present status of the National Exercise and Heart Disease Project. Lecture given to the Conference on Cardiovascular Disease Epidemiology, Council of Epidemiology of the American Heart Association, San Diego, California, March 1-6, 1977.

Chapter 12

SURVEY OF CURRENT "CARDIAC" EXERCISE PROGRAMS IN THE UNITED STATES

A S THE PROBLEM OF CORONARY atherosclerotic heart disease prevails in the Western world and as facilities for the care of these patients become widely spread and readily available, the need for preventive and rehabilitative services for post-myocardial-infarction patients also increases. In addition, with the more recent and frequent utilization of myocardial revascularization procedures (predominantly aortocoronary vein bypass), the need emerges for the rehabilitation of this group of patients. Most exercise training programs for post-myocardial-infarction subjects are beginning to incorporate (in near equal numbers) those patients with coronary artery disease who have had revascularization surgery. In many instances, these subjects are more needful of rehabilitation-exercise activities than are many post-myocardial-infarction patients who often have considerably more residual myocardial disease.

The purpose of this chapter is to itemize and basically describe, as completely and as currently as possible, the various outpatient supervised exercise training programs for post-myocardial-infarction and post-myocardial-revascularization patients that exist and are active in the United States today. Most of the data included has been obtained from existing written data and from data gathered by telephone discussions and written questionnaires. We are most appreciative to William Haskell, Ph.D., of Stanford University, who provided us with an important "nucleus" of this program directory, and to Nanette Wenger, M.D., of Emory University School of Medicine and the Rehabilitation Committee of the American Heart Association, who was instrumental in helping us complete the list.

Arizona

Tucson 81711

Cardiac Rehabilitation Center
350 North Wilmot Road
DIRECTOR: L.J. Buckels, M.D.
PHONE: (602) 296-3211, ex. 2712
TYPE: Hospital—St. Joseph's
SUPERVISION:
Medical—M.D., cardiologist, and
exercise physiologist
Other—

California

Anaheim 92801

Martin Luther Hospital
1825 West Ronneya Drive
DIRECTOR: Richard L. Wellner, M.D.
PHONE: (714) 772-1200
TYPE: Hospital
SUPERVISION:
Medical—Richard L. Wellner, M.D.
Other—Ilean Lungren, R.N.
Pamela Weiss, R.N.

Arcadia 91006

Arcadia Methodist Hospital CT Center
300 West Huntington Drive
DIRECTOR: Julian Love, M.D.
PHONE: (213) 445-4441, ex. 357/358
TYPE: Hospital
SUPERVISION:
Medical—Julian Love, M.D.
Other—Lois Middleton, R.N.
Barb Sedgwick, R.N.

Bakersfield 93301

Mercy Hospital CT Center
2215 Truxtun Avenue
DIRECTORS: Richard C. Dickmann, M.D.
Charles W. Holeman, M.D.
Lewis Sandige, M.D.
PHONE: (805) 327-3371, ex. 394
TYPE: Hospital
SUPERVISION:
Medical—Richard C. Dickmann, M.D.
Charles W. Holeman, M.D.
Lewis Sandige, M.D.

California
  Other—Dalee Girod, R.N.
         Barbara Meeks, R.N.
Corona 91720
  Circle City Hospital
  Cardiopulmonary Stress Test and Work Evaluation Unit
  730 Old Magnolia
  DIRECTOR: Norman H. Mellor, M.D.
  PHONE: (714) 735-1211
  TYPE: Hospital
  SUPERVISION:
  Medical—N.H. Mellor, M.D. and
           Bittal Maheshwar, M.D.
  Other—Two technicians and one physical therapist
Davis 95616
  Adult Fitness Program
  Department of Physical Education
  University of California
  DIRECTOR: Rudolph H. Dressendorfer, Ph.D.
  PHONE: 752-0511
  TYPE: University and community service
  SUPERVISION:
  Medical—Physician-supervised stress testing
  Other—Exercise leaders and voluntary physicians
Downey 90242
  Cardiac Rehabilitation Program
  7601 East Imperial Highway
  DIRECTORS: Doctor John Camp
             Doctor Ron Selvester
  PHONE: (213) 922-7221
  TYPE: Hospital, private and public
  SUPERVISION:
  Medical—M.D. Director
  Other—Full-time physical therapists
Downey 90241
  Downey Community Hospital CT Center
  11500 South Brockshire Avenue
  DIRECTORS: John D. Alexander, M.D.
             John R. Judge, M.D.
             Joseph M. Oyster, M.D.
             Alvin Frey, M.D.
             Henry M. McLaughlin, M.D.
  PHONE: (213) 869-3061
  TYPE: Hospital

California

SUPERVISION:

Medical—Gary E. Marsh, M.D.
Harry I. Riegel, Jr., M.D.
Sheldon S. Zinberg, M.D.
and others

Other—Katherine Hoyt, R.N.
Joanne Alison, R.N.

Fullerton   92635

Fullerton CT Center

401 West Bastanchury Road

DIRECTOR: Donald D. Mahoney, M.D.

PHONE: (714) 870-9577

TYPE: Private

SUPERVISION:

Medical—Donald D. Mahoney, M.D.

Other—Irlys Harris, R.N.
Jacquie Dorr, R.N.

Glendale   91204

Cardiac Treatment Center

Memorial Hospital of Glendale,

1420 South Central Avenue

DIRECTOR: J. Dooley, M.D.

PHONE: (213) 246-6711, ex. 303

TYPE: Hospital

SUPERVISION:

Medical—Physician-monitored (telemetry) exercise

Other—

Glendale   91204

Memorial Hospital of Glendale CT Center

1420 South Central Avenue

DIRECTORS: Santo Polito, M.D.
James Dooley, M.D.

PHONE: (213) 246-6711

TYPE: Hospital

SUPERVISION:

Medical—Santo Polito, M.D.
James Dooley, M.D.

Other—Evelyn Sutherland, R.N.
Delores Dayan, R.N.

Glendora   91740

Foothill Presbyterian Hospital CT Center

250 South Grand Avenue

DIRECTORS: Robert Armstrong, M.D.
Byron Song, M.D.

California

PHONE: (213) 963-8411, ex. 242
TYPE: Hospital
SUPERVISION:
Medical—Robert Armstrong, M.D.
  Byron Song, M.D.
Other—Donna Fickey, R.N.
  Annette Whistler, R.N.

Harbor City 90701
Bay Harbor Hospital CT Center
1437 West Lomita Boulevard
DIRECTOR: Roberto Unguez, M.D.
PHONE: (213) 325-1221, ex. 220
TYPE: Hospital
SUPERVISION:
Medical—Roberto Unguez, M.D.
Other—Carol Taylor, R.N.
  Steve Martino, R.N.

Hawaiian Gardens 90716
Cerritos Gardens General Hospital CT Center
21530 South Pioneer Boulevard
DIRECTOR: Doctor Murray Mentor
PHONE: (213) 860-0401
TYPE: Hospital
SUPERVISION:
Medical—Doctor Murray Mentor
Other—Barbara Morck, R.N.

Hawthorne 90250
Hawthorne Community Hospital CT Center
11711 Garevillea Avenue
DIRECTORS: G. Broder, M.D.
  W. Miller, M.D.
PHONE: (213) 973-1711, ex. 359/360
TYPE: Hospital
SUPERVISION:
Medical—G. Broder, M.D.
  W. Miller, M.D.
Other—Janet Meyer, R.N.
  Rhonda Stevens, R.N.

La Jolla 92037
Cardiac Treatment Center
Scripps Memorial Hospital
9888 Genesee Avenue
DIRECTORS: Ames Early, Executive Director
  Fredric C. Shean, M.D.,

California
Chairman, Cardiopulmonary Committee
PHONE: (714) 453-3400
TYPE: Hospital
SUPERVISION:
  Medical—Panel of stress testing physicians
  Other—Two CPR-trained nurses
Lancaster 93534
  Antelope Valley Hospital CT Center
  1500 West Avenue "J"
  DIRECTOR: Henry Shibata, M.D.
  PHONE: (805) 948-4577, ex. 408/406
  TYPE: Hospital
  SUPERVISION:
    Medical—Henry Shibata, M.D.
    Other—Pam Williams, R.N.
          Judy Pooley, R.N.
Los Angeles 90017
  Good Samaritan Hospital CT Center
  616 South Witmer Street
  DIRECTOR: Eugene J. Ellis, M.D.
  PHONE: (213) 488-8371
  TYPE: Hospital
  SUPERVISION:
    Medical—Eugene J. Ellis, M.D.
    Other—Helen Gwozda, R.N.
Marina del Rey 90291
  Marina Mercy Hospital CT Center
  4650 Lincoln Boulevard
  DIRECTOR: David N. Edlebaum, M.D.
  PHONE: (213) 823-8911, ex. 281/282
  TYPE: Hospital
  SUPERVISION:
    Medical—David N. Edlebaum, M.D.
    Other—Majorie Rogers, R.N.
          Jeannie Bercier, R.N.
Mission Viejo 92675
  Cardiac Treatment Center
  27852 Puerta Real, Suite 118
  DIRECTOR: Carl R. Tassistro, M.D.
  PHONE: (714) 495-4400, ex. 365
  TYPE: Hospital
  SUPERVISION:
    Medical—General internist
    Other—R.N. in attendance at all time

California
Mission Viejo 92675
Mission Community Hospital CT Center
27802 Puerto Real Highway
DIRECTOR: Carl R. Tassistro, M.D.
PHONE: (714) 831-2300, ex. 365
TYPE: Hospital
SUPERVISION:
Medical—Carl R. Tassistro, M.D.
Other—Carol Catalono, R.N.
Montebello 90640
Beverly Hospital CT Center
309 West Beverly Boulevard
DIRECTOR: Masao Ishihama, M.D.
PHONE: (213) 726-1222, ex. 295/296
TYPE: Hospital
SUPERVISION:
Medical—Masao Ishihama, M.D.
Other—Valia Silvius, R.N.
Jean Sais, R.N.
Newport Beach 92660
Hoag Memorial Hospital
301 Newport Boulevard
DIRECTOR: James C. Shelburne, M.D.
PHONE: (714) 645-8600
TYPE: Hospital
SUPERVISION:
Medical—James C. Shelburne, M.D.
Other—Carol Covington, R.N.
North Hollywood 91607
Riverside Hospital CT Center
12629 Riverside Drive
DIRECTOR:
PHONE: (213) 980-9200
TYPE: Hospital
SUPERVISION:
Medical—Robert W. Oblath, M.D.
Richard L. Cockey, M.D.
Donald Danzig, M.D.
Harry Kahan, M.D.
Charles King, M.D.
Joan Marie King, M.D.
Edward Shulkin, M.D.
Sam H. Stone, M.D.
Jerome Hamburger, M.D.

California
    Other—Barbara Pinnell, R.N.
Orange 92668
    Orange CT Center
    1201 West LaVeta, Suite 101
    DIRECTOR:
    PHONE: (717) 997-1222
    TYPE: Private
    SUPERVISION:
    Medical—B.E. Ball, M.D.
            C.H. Sears, M.D.
            and others
    Other—Judy Brownfield, R.N.
Palm Desert 92260
    Eisenhower Medical Center CT Center
    39000 Bob Hope Drive
    DIRECTORS: Richard N. Roger, M.D.
               Charles W. Shaffer, M.D.
    PHONE: (714) 346-3911
    TYPE: Hosptial
    SUPERVISION:
    Medical—Richard N. Roger, M.D.
            Charles W. Shaffer, M.D.
    Other—Sue Hejdak, R.N.
Palo Alto 94303
    Y. M. Cardiac Therapy
    3412 Ross Road
    DIRECTOR: Gary Fry, M.D.
    PHONE: (415) 494-1300
    TYPE: YMCA
    SUPERVISION:
    Medical—Physician, CCU nurse
    Other—Physical educator
San Diego 92103
    Alvarado Hospital Cardiac Rehabilitation Program
    6655 Alvarado Road
    DIRECTOR: John L. Boyer, M.D.
    PHONE: (714) 287-3270
    TYPE: Private community hospital
    SUPERVISION:
    Medical—In-hospital cardiology staff
    Other—Nonphysician program director and exercise leaders
San Diego 92103
    Mercy Hospital and Medical Center CT Center
    4077 Fifth Avenue

California

DIRECTOR: John Mazur, M.D.
PHONE: (714) 294-8111
TYPE: Hospital
SUPERVISION:
  Medical—John Mazur, M.D.
  Other—Nancy Perry, R.N.
        Glenda Bell, R.N.

San Diego 92182
San Diego State University—Adult Fitness Program
San Diego State University
DIRECTOR: Fred W. Kasch, Ph.D.
PHONE: (714) 286-5560
TYPE: University
SUPERVISION:
  Medical—John L. Boyer, M.D.
  Other—Fred W. Kasch, Ph.D.

San Francisco 94115
Garden Sullivan—YMCA Cardiac Rehab
2340 Clay Street, Annex 200
DIRECTOR: William T. Armstrong, M.D.
PHONE: (415) 563-3950
TYPE: In-hospital, Rehab gym, and YMCA
SUPERVISION:
  Medical—Yes
  Other—

San Pedro 90732
San Pedro and Peninsula Hospital CT Center
1300 West Seventh Street
DIRECTOR: Milford G. Wyman, M.D.
PHONE: (213) 832-3311
TYPE: Hospital
SUPERVISION:
  Medical—Milford G. Wyman, M.D.
  Other—Alena Goralik, R.N.

Santa Barbara 93111
Goleta Valley Hospital CT Center
351 South Patterson Avenue
DIRECTOR: J.H.K. Vogel, M.D.
PHONE: (805) 967-3411, ex. 230
TYPE: Hospital
SUPERVISION:
  Medical—J.H.K. Vogel, M.D.
  Other—Caroline Conner, R.N.

California

Santa Monica   90400

St. John's Hospital and Health Center

1328 22nd Avenue

DIRECTOR: Steven C. Berens, M.D.

PHONE: (213) 829-5511

TYPE: Hospital

SUPERVISION:

Medical—Steven C. Berens, M.D.

Other—Pat McCoy, R.N.

Santa Monica   90404

Santa Monica Hospital Medical Center

1225 Fifteenth Street

DIRECTORS: Arnold Nedelman, M.D.

Burt Rosenthal, M.D.

PHONE: (213) 451-1511

TYPE: Hospital

SUPERVISION:

Medical—Arnold Nedelman, M.D.

Burt Rosenthal, M.D.

Other—Kathleen Hunt, R.N.

Ann Ronders, R.N.

Torrance   90503

Little Company of Mary Hospital CT Center

4101 Torrance Boulevard, Suite 300

DIRECTOR: Robert Astone, M.D.

PHONE: (213) 540-7152, ex. 440

TYPE: Hospital

SUPERVISION:

Medical—Robert Astone, M.D.

Other—Anita Erickson, R.N.

Leah Diehl, R.N.

Whittier   90605

Whittier Hospital CT Center

15151 Janine Drive

DIRECTORS: Morton Futterman, M.D.

Alan Dauer, M.D.

PHONE: (213) 945-3561

TYPE: Hospital

SUPERVISION:

Medical—Morton Futterman, M.D.

Alan Dauer, M.D.

Other—Marilynn Boedicker, R.N.

Mary Johnson, R.N.

Jo Lyn Taylor, R.N.

Colorado

Aspen 81611
ACT (Aspen Cardiac Training Program)
100 Main
DIRECTOR: Bruno Balke, M.D.
PHONE: (303) 925-5440
TYPE: Private but connected with Internal Medicine Associates, Aspen Clinic
SUPERVISION:
 Medical—Yes
 Other—

Grand Junction 81501
Hilltop House Cardiac Reconditioning Program
515 Patterson Road
DIRECTOR: G. Paul Smith, M.D.
PHONE: (303) 242-2801
TYPE: Public nonprofit rehabilitation center
SUPERVISION:
 Medical—Internist
 Other—R.N. and R.P.T.

District of Columbia

Washington 20006
Washington Cardiovascular Evaluation Center
Suite 815, 916 19th Street NW
DIRECTOR: James R. Snyder, M.D.
PHONE: (202) 223-6664
TYPE: Private
SUPERVISION:
 Medical—Cardiologist
 Other—

Connecticut

New Britain
New Britain General Hospital/New Britain
YMCA Cardiac Rehabilitation
DIRECTOR: Charles N. Leach, Jr., M.D.
             Director of Cardiology, New Britain General Hospital
PHONE: (203) 224-5274
TYPE: Four-stage program utilizing hospital and YMCA Medical School affiliated supervision
SUPERVISION:
 Medical—Doctor Leach screens patients for admission and makes
             administrative decisions; attends YMCA jogging program
 Other—Phase I and Phase II: physical therapists
             Phase III: cardiovascular nurse
             Phase IV: cardiovascular nurse and YMCA physical director

Delaware

Wilmington 19810
Wilmington CT Center
104 Hagley Building, Concord Plaza
3411 Silverside Road
DIRECTORS: Mark G. Cohen, M.D.
Abid Mohiuddin, M.D.
Paul C. Pennock, M.D.
Kenneth M. Corrin, Jr., M.D.
Alfred E. Bacon, Jr., M.S.
Henry A. Claggett, Jr., M.D.
PHONE: (302) 478-7930
TYPE: Private
SUPERVISION:
Medical—Mark G. Cohen, M.D.
Abid Mohiuddin, M.D.
Paul C. Pennock, M.D.
Kenneth M. Corrin, Jr., M.D.
Alfred E. Bacon, Jr., M.S.
Henry A. Claggett, Jr., M.D.
Other—Lynne Simpkins, R.N.
Doris Vola, R.N.

Florida

Miami 33133
Mercy Cardiac and Pulmonary
Rehabilitation Center (AMSCO-Rehab)
3661 South Miami Avenue, Room 2
DIRECTOR: Edward W. St. Mary, M.D.
PHONE: (305) 854-0982
TYPE: Private-soon to be hospital-based, Mercy Hospital
SUPERVISION:
Medical—Edward W. St. Mary, M.D.
Other—Monitored exercise supervised by R.N.
Orlando 32803
Cardiac Rehabilitation Unit
601 East Rollins Street
DIRECTOR: Zeb Burton, M.D.
PHONE: (305) 896-6611
TYPE: Hospital
SUPERVISION:
Medical—Zeb Burton, M.D.
Other—Barbara Schuett, R.N.
Roxanne Reilly, R.N.
Pat Feree, R.N.

Florida

Pensacola 32503
 Heart and Lung CT Center
 1717 Northeast Street, Suite 502
 DIRECTOR: Charles Reily, M.D.
 PHONE: (904) 434-4666
 TYPE: Hospital
 SUPERVISION:
  Medical—Charles Reily, M.D.
  Other—Diane Register, R.N.

Georgia

Atlanta 30312
 Georgia Baptist Cardiac Rehabilitation Program
 300 Boulevard NE
 DIRECTORS: Gerald Fletcher, M.D.
       John Cantwell, M.D.
 PHONE: (404) 659-4211
 TYPE: Hospital
 SUPERVISION:
  Medical—Yes
  Other—R.N., P.T., recreational therapist

Atlanta 30303
 Grady Memorial Hospital
 80 Butler Street SE
 DIRECTOR: Nanette K. Wenger, M.D.
 PHONE: (404) 659-1212
 TYPE: Hospital
 SUPERVISION:
  Medical—Yes
  Other—R.N. and P.T.

Atlanta 30309
 Jewish Community Center
 1745 Peachtree Street NE
 DIRECTOR: Joel Felner, M.D.
 PHONE: (404) 875-7881
 TYPE: Community Center
 SUPERVISION:
  Medical—Yes
  Other—R.N.

Atlanta 30342
 Northside Cardiac Rehabilitation Program
 1000 Johnson Ferry Road
 DIRECTOR: Barry Silverman, M.D.
 PHONE: (404) 256-8803
 TYPE: Community Center

Georgia
SUPERVISION:
Medical—Yes
Other—R.N.

Hawaii
Honolulu 96814
Cardiac Rehabilitation Program
Central YMCA, 401 Atkinson Drive
DIRECTOR: Jack H. Scaff, Jr., M.D.
PHONE: (808) 941-3344, ex. 116
TYPE: YMCA
SUPERVISION:
Medical—Two M.D.s (one per class)
Other—Three R.N.s, one EKG technician

Illinois
Danville 61832
St. Elizabeth Hospital
600 Sager Street
DIRECTOR: Doctor Mushtag
PHONE: (217) 442-6300
TYPE: Hospital
SUPERVISION:
Medical—Doctor Mushtag
Other—Marie Hires, R.N.
Galesburg 61401
Galesburg Cottage Hospital CT Center
695 North Kellogg Street
DIRECTORS: Morton Willcutts, M.D.
　　　　　 Fred Stansbury, M.D.
　　　　　 Madan Gupta, M.D.
　　　　　 and others
PHONE: (309) 343-8131, ex. 439
TYPE: Hospital
SUPERVISION:
Medical—Morton Willcutts, M.D.
　　　　　 Fred Stansbury, M.D.
　　　　　 Madan Gupta, M.D.
　　　　　 and others
Other—Mitzie Tarleton, R.N.
Rockford 61101
Cardiac Rehabilitation Exercise Program
Rockford Memorial Hospital
DIRECTOR: Joseph Valaitis, M.D.
PHONE: (815) 968-6861

Illinois

TYPE: Hospital—YMCA being developed

SUPERVISION:

Medical—Cardiologist

Other—CCU-trained R.N. and physical therapist

Rock Island 61201

Franciscan Medical Center Cardiac Treatment Center

2701 17th Street

DIRECTOR: A.W. Wise, M.D.

PHONE: (309) 793-1000, ex. 2000/2001

TYPE: Hospital

SUPERVISION:

Medical—A.W. Wise, M.D.

Other—Russ Scott, R.N.

Phyllis Martin, R.N.

Springfield 62702

Cardiac Rehabilitation

800 East Carpenter

DIRECTOR: Doctor Carvalho

PHONE: (217) 544-6464

TYPE: YMCA

SUPERVISION:

Medical—

Other—

Wheaton 60187

Marianjoy Rehab Hospital CT Center

P.O. Box 795

DIRECTORS: R.N. Pesch, M.D.

Neil Agruss, M.D.

PHONE: (312) 653-7600, ex. 367

TYPE: Hospital

SUPERVISION:

Medical—R.N. Pesch, M.D.

Neil Agruss, M.D.

Other—Carol Klipp, R.N.

Indiana

Anderson 46015

Fitness and Rehabilitation

28 West 12th Street P.O. Box 231

DIRECTOR: Rudolf R. Jirka, M.D.

PHONE: (317) 644-7796

TYPE: YMCA

SUPERVISION:

Medical—

Other—Physiologist

Indiana

Indianapolis 46218
Vital Cardio Rehabilitation
5508 East 16th Street, Suite 3
DIRECTORS: Robert E. Edmands, M.D.
Richard E. Linback, M.D.
PHONE: (317) 353-9307
TYPE: Private
SUPERVISION:
Medical—Two physicians
Other—Four nurses

Michigan City 46360
Memorial Hospital CT Center
Fifth and Pine Streets
DIRECTOR: W. Haze, M.D.
PHONE: (219) 879-0202
TYPE: Hospital
SUPERVISION:
Medical—W. Haze, M.D.
Other—Diane Jensen, R.N.
Barbara Logan, R.N.

South Bend 46622
Cardiac Treatment Center of South Bend, Inc.
919 East Jefferson Boulevard, Suite 104
Jefferson Medical Arts Building
DIRECTOR: Donald T. Olson, M.D.
PHONE: (219) 233-1300
TYPE: Private
SUPERVISION:
Medical—Donald T. Olson, M.D.
Other—Andrea Byrns, R.N.

Kansas

Kansas City 66112
Cardiac Treatment Center
8929 Parallel Parkway
DIRECTOR: Murray D. Corbin, M.D.
PHONE: (913) 334-2500
TYPE: Hospital
SUPERVISION:
Medical—
Other—Judith Franiuk, R.N.

Kansas City 66101
Providence-St. Margaret Hospital CT Center
759 Vermont Avenue

Kansas
DIRECTORS: Murray D. Corbin, M.D.
Ray A. Schwegler, M.D.
PHONE: (913) 621-0700, ex. 311
TYPE: Hospital
SUPERVISION:
Medical—Murray D. Corbin, M.D.
Ray A. Schwegler, M.D.
Other—Judith Franiuk, R.N.
Margie Schroeder, R.N.

Kentucky
Lexington 40508
310 South Limestone
DIRECTOR: Stuart Lowenthal, L.P.T.
PHONE: (606) 252-6612
TYPE: Outpatient
SUPERVISION:
Medical—R.A. McAllister, Jr., M.D.
Other—H.R. Groden, P.T.
Whitney Atcheter, P.T.

Maryland
Columbia 21044
Howard County General Hospital CT Center
Little Patuxent Parkway and Cedar Lane
DIRECTOR: Jerome Hantman, M.D.
PHONE: (301) 730-5000, ex. 338/339
TYPE: Hospital
SUPERVISION:
Medical—Jerome Hantman, M.D.
Other—Anne Orthner, R.N.
Cumberland 21502
Cardiac Treatment Center
Memorial Hospital, Memorial Avenue
DIRECTOR: Peter B. Halmos, M.D.
PHONE: (301) 777-4086 or 4087
TYPE: Hospital
SUPERVISION:
Medical—Two cardiologist advisors
One internist advisor
Other—Cardiac nurse-therapist—direct medical supervision
Cumberland 21502
Memorial Hospital CT Center
Memorial Avenue

Maryland

DIRECTORS: Peter Halmos, M.D.
R.J. Barrera, M.D.
PHONE: (301) 777-4086
TYPE: Hospital
SUPERVISION:
Medical—Peter Halmos, M.D.
R.J. Barrera, M.D.
Other—Jeanne Schaidt, R.N.
Barbara Tice, R.N.
Rachel Hoyer, R.N.

Fallston 21047
Fallston General Hospital CT Center
200 Milton Avenue
DIRECTORS: Kermit Bonovich, M.D.
V.S. Nair, M.D.
PHONE: (301) 877-3700
TYPE: Hospital
SUPERVISION:
Medical—Kermit Bonovich, M.D.
V.S. Nair, M.D.
Other—Connie Francis, R.N.
Peggy Sawyer, R.N.
Janice Nickolsi, R.N.

Massachusetts

Jamaica Plain 02130
Faulkner Hospital CT Center
1153 Centre Street
DIRECTORS: A. Ramirez, M.S.
Laurence Ellis, M.D.
PHONE: (617) 522-5800
TYPE: Hospital
SUPERVISION:
Medical—A. Ramirez, M.S.
Laurence Ellis, M.D.
Other—Patricia Blackmer, R.N.
Julie Kehler, R.N.

Michigan

Battle Creek 49016
Community Hospital CT Center
183 West Street
DIRECTOR: Robert Brown, M.D.
PHONE: (616) 963-5521, ex. 623
TYPE: Hospital

Michigan

SUPERVISION:
  Medical—Robert Brown, M.D.
  Other—Myrtle Evans, R.N.
         Debbie Richie, R.N.
         Jean Vaughan, R.N.

Flint 48502
  St. Joseph's Hospital CT Center
  302 Kensington Avenue
  DIRECTOR: John Brady, M.D.
  PHONE: (313) 238-2601
  TYPE: Hospital
  SUPERVISION:
  Medical—John Brady, M.D.
  Other—Linda Newbury, R.N.
         Carolyn Coon, R.N.

Midland 48640
  Midland Hospital CT Center
  4005 Orchard Drive
  DIRECTOR: Doctor Harold Kwast
  PHONE: (517) 631-7700
  TYPE: Hospital
  SUPERVISION:
  Medical—Doctor Harold Kwast
  Other—Jo David, R.N.

Minnesota

Duluth 55805
  St. Mary's Hospital Postcoronary Rehabilitation Program
  407 East Third Street
  DIRECTOR: Richard Goese, M.D.
  PHONE: (218) 727-4551
  TYPE: Hospital
  SUPERVISION:
  Medical—Under cardiology supervision
  Other—Physical therapy participates

Minneapolis 55454
  St. Mary's Hospital Cardiac Rehabilitation Program
  DIRECTOR: Herbert A. Schoening, M.D.
  PHONE: (612) 332-8111
  TYPE: Hospital
  SUPERVISION:
  Medical—Each patient must have a referring M.D.
  Other—Hospital cardiologist available in emergencies. Cardiac resusci-
         tation team within 50 yards on adjacent coronary care unit.
         Occupational therapist supervises exercises.

Minnesota
St. Paul 55101
Cardiac Rehabilitation—St. Paul Ramsey Hospital and Medical Center
640 Jackson Street
DIRECTOR: John M. McBride
PHONE: (612) 221-3462
TYPE: University-affiliated city-county hospital and medical center
SUPERVISION:
Medical—Director part of section of Cardiology
Other—Physical medicine and rehabilitation

Missouri
Joplin 64801
Freeman Hospital CT Center
1102 West 32nd Street
DIRECTOR: W. Kohler, M.D.
PHONE: (417) 623-2801
TYPE: Hospital
SUPERVISION:
Medical—W. Kohler, M.D.
Other—Doris Surbrugg, R.N.
Christine Hoag, R.N.
Kansas City 64106
Kansas City Cardiac Exercise Rehabilitation Program
404 East 10th Street
DIRECTORS: Ben McCallister, M.D.
Ralph Hall, M.D.
PHONE: (816) 842-6649
TYPE: YMCA
SUPERVISION:
Medical—Medically supervised
Other—R.N.s and technicians

New Jersey
Hackensack 07601
YM-YWHA Cardiac Exercise Program
211 Essex Street
DIRECTOR: Consultant of the program—Irving M. Levitas, M.D.
PHONE: (201) 489-5900
TYPE: YM-YWHA
SUPERVISION:
Medical—
Other—Physical Educator
Summit 07901
Summit Medical Group
120 Summit Avenue

New Jersey

DIRECTORS: T.V. Inglesby, M.D.
R.G. Sachs, M.D.
K.F. Murphy, M.D.

PHONE: (201) 273-4300

TYPE: Private

SUPERVISION:

Medical—T.V. Inglesby, M.D.
R.G. Sachs, M.D.
K.F. Murphy, M.D.

Other—Rosemary Simmons, R.N.
Debbie Freund, R.N.

Trenton 08629

Cardiac Rehabilitation Center
601 Hamilton Avenue

DIRECTOR: Doctor John A. Kinczel

PHONE: (609) 396-7676

TYPE: Hospital

SUPERVISION:

Medical—Five cardiologists oversee patients in the program
Other—One full-time nurse therapist and one part-time nurse therapist

Trenton 08629

St. Francis Medical Center CT Center
601 Hamilton Avenue

DIRECTORS: Doctor Jaferi
A.J. Migliori, M.D.
J. Lucarella, M.D.
M.I. Khan, M.D.

PHONE: (609) 396-7676, ex. 415/439

TYPE: Hospital

SUPERVISION:

Medical—Doctor Jaferi
A.J. Migliori, M.D.
J. Lucarella, M.D.
M.I. Khan, M.D.

Other—Nancy Peoples, R.N.
Linda Schwinn, R.N.

New Mexico

Albuquerque 87108

Lovelace-Bataan Cardiopulmonary Prevention,
Detection and Rehabilitation Program
5200 Gibson Boulevard SE

MEDICAL DIRECTOR: Frank Jones, M.D.

PROGRAM DIRECTOR: Ralph LaForge, M.Sc.

PHONE: (505) 842-7088

New Mexico
    TYPE: Hospital (outpatient); also alcoholic rehabilitation
    SUPERVISION:
    Medical—
    Other—Ralph LaForge; exercise physiologist and nursing personnel
New York
  Bronx 10467
    Montefiore Hospital Exercise Testing and Training Program
    111 East 210 Street
    DIRECTOR: Lenore R. Zohman, M.D.
    PHONE: (212) 920-5046
    TYPE: Hospital-based exercise testing.
        Five satellite exercise training gymnasium group programs.
    SUPERVISION:
    Medical—All testing by physicians plus nurse, clinician, or physiologist
    Other—Training supervised by physical educators knowledgeable in
        cardiac class leadership and CPR (including defibrillation)
  Brooklyn 11228
    Bay Ridge CT Center
    666 92nd Street
    DIRECTORS: Joseph Florio, M.D.
    F. Garofalo, M.D.
    C. Govindarag, M.D.
    Thomas LaBarbara, M.D.
    PHONE: (212) 833-3388
    TYPE: Private
    SUPERVISION:
    Medical—Joseph Florio, M.D.
            F. Garofalo, M.D.
            C. Govindarag, M.D.
            Thomas LaBarbara, M.D.
    Other—Elaine Sarfati, R.N.
            Maureen Fiorilla, R.N.
  Brooklyn 11215
    The Methodist Hospital Cardiopulmonary Reconditioning Program
    506 Sixth Avenue
    DIRECTOR: Doctor Vojin N. Smodlaka
    PHONE: (212) 780-3266
    TYPE: Hospital
    SUPERVISION:
    Medical—Cardiologist
    Other—Physiologist
  Buffalo 14215
    Buffalo VA Hospital Cardiac Rehab Program
    3495 Bailey Avenue

New York

DIRECTORS: David C. Dean, M.D.

K.H. Lee, M.D.

PHONE: (716) 834-9200

TYPE: Hospital

SUPERVISION:

Medical—

Other—Monitored by trained physical therapist with oscilloscope

Buffalo 14209

Millard Fillmore Hospital Cardiac Reconditioning Program

3 Gates Circle

DIRECTORS: Italo Besseghini, M.D.

David Conti, M.D. (Coordinator)

PHONE: (716) 845-4615

TYPE: Hospital

SUPERVISION:

Medical—Cardiologist

Other—Cardiac nurse, exercise leader, secretary

Cedar Hurst 11516

South Shore Medical Group P.C.

366 Pearsal Avenue

DIRECTOR: Doctor Ruskin

PHONE: (516) 239-7744

TYPE: Private

SUPERVISION:

Medical—Doctor Ruskin

Other—Betty Bloom, R.N.

East Meadow 11756

Central Nassau CT Center

1900 Hempstead Turnpike

DIRECTORS: Erwin Friedman, M.D.

Stephen Richmond, M.D.

Robert J. Rabinowitz, M.D.

PHONE: (516) 794-9797

TYPE: Private

SUPERVISION:

Medical—Erwin Friedman, M.D.

Stephen Richmond, M.D.

Robert J. Rabinowitz, M.D.

Other—Virginia Kinions, R.N.

Susan Pawlenko, R.N.

June Egge, R.N.

East Meadow 11554

Nassau County Medical Center

2201 Hempstead Turnpike

New York
DIRECTOR: Doctor David R. Adamovich
PHONE: (516) 542-3581
TYPE: Hospital
SUPERVISION:
  Medical—Doctor Adamovich (exercise physiologist)
              Doctor Lugell (cardiologist)
  Other—
New York 10022
  Manhattan CT Center
  211 East 51st Street
  DIRECTOR: Michael Wolk, M.D.
  PHONE: (212) 371-6281
  TYPE: Private
  SUPERVISION:
    Medical—Michael Wolk, M.D.
              Leslie Kuhn, M.D.
              O. Alan Rose, M.D.
              Isadore Rosenfeld, M.D.
    Other—Pat O'Keefe, R.N.
              Eileen Raftery, R.N.
              Chris Tekverk, R.N.
North Tarrytown 10591
  Cardiopulmonary Rehabilitation Center, Phelps Memorial Hospital
  North Broadway
  DIRECTOR: Arnold Salop, M.D.
  PHONE: (914) 631-5100
  TYPE: Hospital
  SUPERVISION:
    Medical—Yes
    Other—
Oceanside 11572
  Cardiac Work Evaluation Unit
  S. Nassau Communities Hospital
  DIRECTOR: H.D. Ruskin, M.D.
  PHONE: (516) 378-2884
  TYPE: Hospital-based
  SUPERVISION:
    Medical—H.D. Ruskin, M.D.
              E. Braverman, M.D.
    Other—Social worker, clinical psychologist, vocational psychologist
Olean 14760
  St. Francis Hospital CT Center
  2221 West State Street
  DIRECTOR: D. Wormer, M.D.

New York

PHONE: (716) 372-5300

TYPE: Hospital

SUPERVISION:

Medical—D. Wormer, M.D.

Other—Laura Ludwick, R.N.

Dorothy Neilson, R.N.

Staten Island 10304

Staten Island Diagnostic and Rehab Center

11 Ralph Place

DIRECTOR: F. Suarez, M.D.

PHONE: (212) 727-4900

TYPE: Private

SUPERVISION:

Medical—F. Suarez, M.D.

Other—Mary Picciotto, R.N.

Mary Jo Thompson, R.N.

Eileen Shea, R.N.

West Islip 11795

Suffolk Cardiac and Pulmonary Associates

1111 Montauk Highway

DIRECTORS: M. Beyers, M.D.

V. William Caracci, M.D.

D.J. Kearney, M.D.

and others

PHONE: (516) 422-1000

TYPE: Private

SUPERVISION:

Medical—J.J. Lambert, M.D.

R.F. Levine, M.D.

D.J. Kearney, M.D.

and others

Other—Margaret Kramer, R.N.

Veronica Mulcahey, R.N.

Nevada

Las Vegas 89109

Cardiac Treatment Center

Sunrise Hospital

DIRECTOR: Michael P. Sawaya, M.D.

PHONE: (702) 732-8218

TYPE: Private

SUPERVISION:

Medical—

Other—Cardiac rehabilitation nurse therapist

Nevada
Las Vegas 89109
Sunrise Hospital CT Center
3186 Maryland Parkway
DIRECTORS: John Bowers, M.D.
Michael Sawaya, M.D.
PHONE: (702) 731-8218
TYPE: Hospital
SUPERVISION:
Medical—John Bowers, M.D.
Michael Sawaya, M.D.
Other—Linda Ames, R.N.
Valeria McGuire, R.N.
North Carolina
Winston-Salem 27109
Wake Forest Cardiac Rehabilitation
Wake Forest University
DIRECTOR: Paul M. Ribisl, Ph.D.
PHONE: (919) 761-5395
TYPE: University-based
SUPERVISION:
Medical—Henry S. Miller, Jr., M.D. (cardiologist)
Other—Exercise physiologists
Ohio
Cleveland 44109
Cleveland Metropolitan General Hospital Cardiac
Evaluation and Rehabilitation Program
3395 Scranton Road
DIRECTORS: C. Long, M.D.
L. Rokita, M.D.
PHONE: (216) 398-6000
TYPE: Hospital
SUPERVISION:
Medical—Yes
Other—
Cleveland 44122
Highland View Hospital Cardiac
Evaluation and Rehabilitation Program
3901 Ireland Drive
DIRECTOR: Charles Long, M.D.
PHONE: (216) 464-9600
TYPE: Hospital
SUPERVISION:
Medical—Yes
Other—

Ohio

Cleveland Heights 44118
Physical Fitness Testing and Evaluation Program
Jewish Community Center
DIRECTOR: F.H. Protkin, M.D.
PHONE: (216) 382-4000
TYPE: Community center
SUPERVISION:
  Medical—Internist-cardiologist
  Other—Physical educator

Dayton 45406
Cardiac Treatment Center
Good Samaritan Hospital
DIRECTOR: Sylvan Lee Weinberg, M.D.
PHONE: (513) 278-2612
TYPE: Hospital
SUPERVISION:
  Medical—M.D.s for stress test
  Other—R.N.s for rehabilitation visits

Dayton 45406
Good Samaritan Hospital CT Center
2222 Philadelphia Drive
DIRECTOR: Doctor Brecount
PHONE: (513) 278-2612
TYPE: Hospital
SUPERVISION:
  Medical—Doctor Brecount
  Other—Joanne Helms, R.N.
        Vickie Redrick, R.N.

Lima 45804
Cardiac Treatment Center
Linden and Mobel Streets
DIRECTOR: Alexander C. Reed, M.D.
PHONE: (419) 225-5967
TYPE: Hospital
SUPERVISION:
  Medical—Alexander C. Reed, M.D.
  Other—Joan K. Reynolds, R.N.
        Madge Stubbs, R.N.
        Joyce Money, R.N.

Portsmouth 45662
Mercy Hospital CT Center
12548 Kinneys Lane
DIRECTOR: Sol Asch, M.D.
PHONE: (614) 353-2131

Ohio
> TYPE: Hospital
> SUPERVISION:
>   Medical—Sol Asch, M.D.
>   Other—Becky Lampen, R.N.
> *Youngstown* 44501
>   Professional Cardiac Rehabilitation (Procare)
>   17 North Champion Street
>   DIRECTOR: L. Anthony Whitney
>   PHONE: (216) 743-8345
>   TYPE: Private
>   SUPERVISION:
>   Medical—Physician
>   Other—Two exercise technicians, R.N., Medical tech., and physical
>   therapist

Oklahoma
> *Tulsa* 74104
>   Cardiac Treatment Center
>   1923 South Utica
>   DIRECTORS: Lotfy Basta, M.D.
>   C.S. Lewis, M.D.
>   PHONE: (918) 744-2699
>   TYPE: Hospital
>   SUPERVISION:
>   Medical—M.D.
>   Other—R.N.
> *Tulsa* 74104
>   St. John's Hospital CT Center
>   1923 South Utica Avenue
>   DIRECTORS: C.S. Lewis, M.D.
>   R.W. Neal, M.D.
>   R.I. Lubin, M.D.
>   H.A. Ruprecht, M.D.
>   PHONE: (918) 744-2699
>   TYPE: Hospital
>   SUPERVISION:
>   Medical—C.S. Lewis, M.D.
>   R.W. Neal, M.D.
>   R.I. Lubin, M.D.
>   H.A. Ruprecht, M.D.
>   Other—Donna Shallenburger, R.N.

Oregon
> *Portland*
>   Capri
>   Seattle and Yakima, Washington, and Portland, Oregon

Oregon

DIRECTOR: Howard R. Pyfer, M.D.

PHONE: (206) 323-7550

TYPE: Nonprofit organization lease community facilities at Jewish community centers, universities and YMCA

SUPERVISION:

Medical—Physician 33-100%

Other—CCU nurse 100%

Portland 97201

YMCArdiac Therapy

2831 SW Barber Boulevard

DIRECTOR: M. Rene Malinow, M.D.

PHONE: (503) 223-9622, ex. 247

TYPE: YMCA

SUPERVISION:

Medical—Physician and R.N.

Other—YMCA physical director

Pennsylvania

Allentown 18103

Allentown Sacred Heart Hospital CT Center

1200 South Cedarcrest Boulevard

DIRECTOR: Stanley Zeeman, M.D.

PHONE: (215) 821-2121, ex. 3004

TYPE: Hospital

SUPERVISION:

Medical—Stanley Zeeman, M.D.

Other—Faye Baylor, R.N.

Cindy Kostolsky, R.N.

Berwick 18603

Berwick Hospital CT Center

701 East 16th Street

DIRECTOR: Doctor Gedwick

PHONE: (717) 752-4551

TYPE: Hospital

SUPERVISION:

Medical—Doctor Gedwick

Other—Sharon Slowick, R.N.

Sharleen Sorber, R.N.

Bethlehem 18018

Bethlehem CT Center

35 East Elizabeth Avenue

DIRECTOR: Doctor R.L. Shields

PHONE: (215) 694-0595

TYPE: Private

Pennsylvania

SUPERVISION:

Medical—Doctor R.L. Shields

Other—Charlene Dunn, R.N.

Camp Hill 17011

Holy Spirit Hospital CT Center

North 21st Street

DIRECTORS: Doctor Durbeck

Doctor Sullivan

Doctor Grandon

Doctor Bricknell

PHONE: (717) 761-0202, ex. 391/394

TYPE: Hospital

SUPERVISION:

Medical—Doctor Durbeck

Doctor Sullivan

Doctor Grandon

Doctor Bricknell

Other—Pat Carnes, R.N.

Linda Aloise, R.N.

Kathy Calhoun, R.N.

Darby 19023

Mercy Catholic Medical Center CT Center

Fitzgerald Mercy Division, CT Center

Lansdowne Avenue and Baily Road

DIRECTOR: O. Mueller, M.D.

PHONE: (215) 586-5020, ex. 2242

TYPE: Hospital

SUPERVISION:

Medical—O. Mueller, M.D.

Other—Mary Coll, R.N.

Clare Pierri, R.N.

DuBois 15801

Maple Avenue CT Center

Maple Avenue Hospital, Maple Avenue

DIRECTOR: Howard Fugate, M.D.

PHONE: (814) 371-3440, ex. 235

TYPE: Hospital

SUPERVISION:

Medical—Howard Fugate, M.D.

Other—Mary Ellen Verne, R.N.

East Stroudsburg 18301

Heart Evaluation Program

Human Performance Lab, E. Stroudsburg State College

MEDICAL DIRECTOR: Doctor Berman

Pennsylvania

ADMINISTRATIVE DIRECTOR: Doctor Weber
PHONE: (717) 424-3336
TYPE: Cooperative private and college
SUPERVISION:
Medical—Doctor Berman, Board Certified Cardiologist
Other—Doctor Weber, Certified Program Director (ACSM)

Easton 18042
Easton Cardiac Rehab Center
2024 Lehigh Street
DIRECTOR: AMSCO/REHAB Corporation
PHONE: (215) 252-0301
TYPE: Private
SUPERVISION:
Medical—Doctor Liberta (medical advisor)
Other—Tina Lobb, R.N.

Erie 16500
Doctors Osteopath Hospital CT Center
252 West 11th Street
DIRECTOR: W.A. Rowane, M.D.
PHONE: (814) 455-3961, ex. 204
TYPE: Hospital
SUPERVISION:
Medical—W.A. Rowane, M.D.
Other—Louise Koscelnik, R.N.

Erie 16502
Erie CT Center
225 West 25th Street, Medical Arts Building, Room 208
DIRECTORS: Gene Mercier, M.D.
Charles A. Joy, M.D.
PHONE: (814) 453-5485
TYPE: Private
SUPERVISION:
Medical—Gene Mercier, M.D.
Charles A. Joy, M.D.
Other—Marcia Lethaby, R.N.
Ethal Burch, R.N.

Erie 16512
Hamot Medical Center
104 East Second Street, Professional Building
DIRECTOR: William Underhill, M.D.
PHONE: (814) 455-6711, ex. 480
TYPE: Hospital
SUPERVISION:
Medical—William Underhill, M.D.

Pennsylvania

Other—Gayle Dobson, R.N.
Nancy Rose, R.N.
Carole Muye, R.N.
Sherry Horl, R.N.

Hazleton 18201
Cardiac Rehabilitation Pacemaker Evaluation Clinic
Suite 1109, Northeastern National Bank Building
DIRECTORS: Doctor Peter Saras
Doctor Herman Auerbach
Doctor Leo Corazza
PHONE: (717) 455-9070
TYPE: Private clinic
SUPERVISION:
Medical—Three internists
Other—CCU nurses:
Kathleen Bertuola, R.N.
Pat Colangelo, R.N.

Lancaster 17603
St. Joseph Hospital Cardiac Rehab Program
250 College Avenue
DIRECTOR: Ronald M. Logan, M.D.
PHONE: (717) 299-8091
TYPE: In-hospital program
Gym program opens 7/77
SUPERVISION:
Medical—Cardiology staff:
R.M. Logan, M.D.
M.B. McKee, M.D.
Other—

Lancaster 17604
St. Joseph's Hospital CT Center
250 College Avenue
DIRECTORS: Kenneth Carroll, M.D.
Ronald Legum, M.D.
Michael McKee, M.D.
PHONE: (171) 291-8291
TYPE: Hospital
SUPERVISION:
Medical—Kenneth Carroll, M.D.
Ronald Legum, M.D.
Michael McKee, M.D.
Other—Mary Ann Rettig, R.N.
Sandy Myford, R.N.

Pennsylvania

Lewisburg 17837

Evangelical Community Hospital CT Center

One Hospital Drive

DIRECTORS: T. Savidge, M.D.

John Persing, M.D.

Donald Steckel, M.D.

PHONE: (171) 523-1241, ex. 258

TYPE: Hospital

SUPERVISION:

Medical—T. Savidge, M.D.

John Persing, M.D.

Donald Steckel, M.D.

Other—Corine Pausa, R.N.

Lena Renock, R.N.

Ginny Zimmerman, R.N.

Meadville 16335

Spencer Hospital Cardiac Treatment Center

1034 Grove Street

DIRECTOR: Hendrik DeKruif, M.D.

PHONE: (814) 724-6622

TYPE: Located in hospital—AMSCO Corporation

SUPERVISION:

Medical—Hendrik DeKruif, M.D.

Other—Zeline Euler, R.N.

Jayne Pickens, R.N.

Mechanicsburg 17055

Mechanicsburg CT Center

4950 Wilson Lane

DIRECTORS: Raymond Grandon, M.D.

Frank Jackson, M.D.

PHONE: (717) 697-8350

TYPE: Private

SUPERVISION:

Medical—Raymond Grandon, M.D.

Frank Jackson, M.D.

Other—Jackie Kreitzer, R.N.

Ruth Matthews, R.N.

Vivian Wisniewski, R.N.

Roxanne Stoner, R.N.

Philadelphia 19124

JFK Memorial Hospital CT Center

Cheltenham Avenue and Langdon Street

DIRECTORS: Gilbert Grossman, M.D.

Phillip Lisan, M.D.

Pennsylvania

PHONE: (215) 289-6000, ex. 266
TYPE: Hospital
SUPERVISION:
Medical—Gilbert Grossman, M.D.
        Phillip Lisan, M.D.
Other—Elizabeth Rhoades, R.N.
        Pamela Leos, R.N.

Philadelphia 19107
Jefferson University Hospital Rehabilitation Program
1025 Walnut Street
DIRECTOR: Doctor Frank Naso
PHONE: (215) 829-6571
TYPE: Hospital
SUPERVISION:
Medical—Yes
Other—

Philadelphia 19139
Pennsylvania Hospital Cardiac Rehabilitation Program
111 North 49th Street
DIRECTOR: Norman Makous, M.D.
PHONE: (215) 829-3456
TYPE: Hospital and private
SUPERVISION:
Medical—Physician and Nurse
Other—Physiotherapist

Pittsburgh 15232
Cardiac Rehabilitation Institute
532 South Aiken Avenue, Suite 108
DIRECTOR: Lawrence N. Adler, M.D.
PHONE: (412) 682-6201
TYPE: Private
SUPERVISION:
Medical—Thirteen M.D.s
Other—Four R.N.s

Scranton 18510
Scranton Cardiac Rehabilitation Center
748 Quincey Avenue
DIRECTOR: Sandy O. Furey, M.D.
PHONE: (717) 961-3090
TYPE: Private
SUPERVISION:
Medical—Sandy Furey, M.D.
Other—Marta Taglianite, R.N.

Pennsylvania

Sharon 17146
Sharon General Hospital Cardiac Treatment Center
740 East State Street
DIRECTOR: Joseph Bolotin, M.D.
PHONE: (412) 981-1700
TYPE: Hospital
SUPERVISION:
  Medical—Joseph Bolotin, M.D.
  Other—Helen Benes, R.N.
          Fran Giroski, R.N.
          Ruth Roth, R.N.
          Rose Palmer, R.N.

Wilkes-Barre 18705
Cardiac Rehab Center
8 Church Street
DIRECTOR: J.P. Brennan, M.D.
PHONE: (717) 822-1136
TYPE: Hospital
SUPERVISION:
  Medical—
  Other—Two full-time specially trained nurses with a minimum of four
        years ICU experience

Wilkes-Barre 18702
Mercy Cardiac Rehabilitation Center
8 Church Street
DIRECTOR: John Brennan, M.D.
PHONE: (717) 822-8101, ex. 365
TYPE: Hospital
SUPERVISION:
  Medical—John Brennan, M.D.
  Other—Geri Buczewski, R.N.
          Dena Nackley, R.N.

York 17403
York Cardiac Training Center
924 South Colonial Avenue
DIRECTOR: Benjamin A. Hoover II, M.D.
PHONE: (171) 854-4698
TYPE: Private (Division of AMSCO/REHAB)
SUPERVISION:
  Medical—Benjamin A. Hoover II, M.D.
  Other—Coronary Care trained R.N. monitors exercise program

Tennessee

Knoxville
Cardiac Rehabilitation Outpatient Program (CROP)

Tennessee
St. Mary's Medical Center, Oakhill Avenue, Knoxville 37917 and
Ft. Sanders Presbyterian Hospital, Clinch Avenue, Knoxville 37928
DIRECTOR: Joseph E. Acker, M.D.
PHONE: (615) 971-6641
TYPE: Hospital
SUPERVISION:
  Medical—Yes
  Other—CCU nurse
Knoxville 37917
  Oak Hill Avenue
  DIRECTOR: Joseph Acker, M.D.
  PHONE: (615) 971-6641
  TYPE: Outpatient
  SUPERVISION:
  Medical—Yes
  Other—Rose Wilson, R.N.

Texas
Houston 77030
  Cardiac Rehabilitation
  1333 Moursund
  DIRECTOR: David Cardus, M.D.
  PHONE: (713) 797-1440, ex. 345
  TYPE: Hospital
  SUPERVISION:
  Medical—Physician
  Other—Technician (trained)

Utah
Salt Lake City 84143
  LDS Hospital Cardiac Rehabilitation Program
  325 Eighth Avenue
  DIRECTOR: Frank G. Yanowitz, M.D.
  PHONE: (801) 350-1185
  TYPE: Hospital
  SUPERVISION:
  Medical—
  Other—

Virginia
Lynchburg 24503
  Virginia Baptist Hospital CT Center
  3300 Rivermont Avenue
  DIRECTOR: Charles H. Sackett, M.D.
  PHONE: (804) 384-4000
  TYPE: Hospital

Virginia
SUPERVISION:
Medical—Charles H. Sackett, M.D.
Other—Wanda Roadcap, R.N.
Richmond 23221
Virginia Heart Institute
205 North Hamilton Street
DIRECTOR: C.L. Baird, Jr., M.D.
PHONE: (804) 359-9265
TYPE: Private outpatient clinic
SUPERVISION:
Medical—Yes
Other—
Waynesboro 22980
Waynesboro Community Hospital CT Center
501 Oak Avenue
DIRECTOR: Thomas L. Gorsuch, M.D.
PHONE: (703) 943-3101, ex. 469
TYPE: Hospital
SUPERVISION:
Medical—Thomas L. Gorsuch, M.D.
Other—Wanda Roadcap, R.N.
Washington
Seattle 78122
914 East Jefferson Street
DIRECTOR: Howard Pyfer, M.D.
PHONE:
TYPE: Gymnasium
SUPERVISION:
Medical—Yes
Other—
Benton 98055
17105 156th Avenue SE
DIRECTOR: Manuel Cooper, M.D.
PHONE: (206) 271-1631
TYPE: Outpatient
SUPERVISION:
Medical—Yes
Other—
Wisconsin
La Crosse 54601
(1) Gunderson Clinic—La Crosse Lutheran Hospital Inpatient Rehabilitation Program
(2) La Crosse Cardiac Rehabilitation Program 1836 South Avenue
DIRECTOR: J.W. Edgett, Jr., M.D.

Wisconsin

PHONE: (608) 782-7300

TYPE:

    (1) Inpatient and immediately posthospital rehabilitation

    (2) Late aggressive phase cardiac rehabilitation

SUPERVISION:

  Medical—

    (1) Inpatient covered by primary physician

    (2) Forty volunteer physicians

  Other—

    (1) Nursing and Physical Therapy departments

    (2) Paramedical personnel, primarily graduate students; Department of Physical Education, University of Wisconsin-La Crosse, under direction of Philip K. Wilson, Ed.D.

COMMENTS

The preceding directory was compiled from answers to questionnaires mailed to various cardiac exercise programs currently active in the United States today. We are appreciative to the directors of these programs for their cooperation and feel that the program listing is as complete as possible under the circumstances that exist today with the rapid development and variety of such programs. As noted in the directory, there is some variation in presentation of many programs; however, each is presented in nearly the exact words of the questionnaire responses we received in order to avoid any degree of "editorialization."

There are a total of 142 programs listed in alphabetical order by states and cities within states. The distribution of these programs around the United States is displayed in Figure 12-1. Of the 142, 92 percent (131 of 142) are supervised by a physician; 101 of the total are hospital based. Thirty-six of the programs listed are in California.

Other data is listed, and it is felt that the program directors or other personnel would be cooperative in affording more information as requested by mail or telephone.

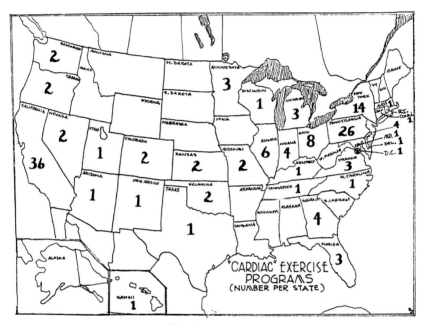

Figure 12-1. Map of the United States showing distribution of "cardiac" exercise programs. Numbers denote totals for each state.

Chapter 13

CARDIAC REHABILITATION
IN OTHER COUNTRIES

T HE PURPOSE OF this section is to review briefly the activities and results of programs of exercise training for patients with coronary heart disease that are presently underway in other countries. Much of the information included, especially from West Germany, originates from our personal observations and interviews. This discussion will include current data (much of which is unpublished) derived from these programs, and the illustrations will include photographs of testing and training activities.

It is felt that international interest in physical training is increasing and that the experiences of other countries have had in the past, and will have in the future, a considerable impact on our attitude toward exercise in the management of coronary heart disease. It is obvious that each population differs in baseline physical activities and in physical activity after myocardial infarction; also, the coronary risk factors (such as hypertension, smoking, and lipid abnormalities) vary from one country to another. Hopefully, this section will not only inform the reader but will also elicit critique regarding methods of testing and training utilized in these countries compared to those described in American programs.

HELSINKI, FINLAND

Kentala,[1] in the second Department of Medicine at Helsinki University, has recently summarized the results of exercise training in 298 consecutive male patients under sixty-five years

289

of age who were treated in the hospital with a diagnosis of acute myocardial infarction. The patients were divided in the hospital into a control group and a training group by their year of birth in order to make a controlled study in physical rehabilitation after myocardial infarction. Forty-five patients died in the hospital. Patients with other severe diseases were excluded from the follow-up study. Of the patients discharged from the hospital, 158 met the diagnostic criteria of acute myocardial infarction defined in this study and lived so close to the hospital that they could be accepted for a twelve-month follow-up study of supervised physical training. The training group was made up of 77 patients, with a mean age of fifty-three years. The physical working capacity of these men was measured by means of a bicycle ergometer test six to eight weeks after the infarction.

After this test, the members of the training group were given an opportunity to participate in supervised training exercises, at first twice and later three times per week. In these exercises, the patient's heart rate was kept for twenty minutes about ten beats below the level reached at the first maximal test The loads were increased when the working heart rate slowed. In order to ensure uniform basic treatment, all the patients in both the control group and the training group attended the outpatient department once a month for consultation with the doctor. In addition to the first exercise test, the patients underwent maximal exercise tests five and twelve months after the infarction. Clinical findings, anthropometric measurements, ECG, chest x-rays, serum lipid values, and the two-hour glucose tolerance test were recorded at these times.

There were only minor differences between the groups in the anamnestic data, anthropometric measurements, and clinical findings recorded in the hospital. A statistically significant difference was observed in the serum cholesterol value three weeks after the infarction; it was 238 mg/100 ml in the control and 256 mg/100 ml in the training group ($p < 0.05$). The vital capacity (in percent of the predicted value) was 100 in the control and 95 in the training group ($p < 0.05$).

Physical working capacity at the first measurement six to eight weeks after the infarction was 498 kpm/minute in the control and 470 kpm/minute in the training group (Fig. 13-1). The corresponding mean heart rates at maximal load were 129 and 128 beats/minute.

The initial physical working capacity was only approximately half of that of healthy men of the same age and occupation. The variation in physical working capacity was wide, ranging from under 150 kpm/minute to 1,050 kpm/minute.

Stepwise regression analysis was applied to find out the determinants of physical working capacity six to eight weeks after the infarction. Variables of the first myocardial infarction recorded during the hospital phase turned out to be of relatively small significance except variables related to cardiac failure. The patient's physical fitness prior to the infarction had an important influence on the subsequent physical working capacity.

The feasibility of participation in the regular examinations was good, i.e. almost all the patients attended. However, it was possible to implement an adequate, supervised physical training program for only a minority of the training group. Four patients died within five months of the infarction. Poor functional capacity precluded participation in the training program for a further 12 of the 77 patients in the training group. Of the remaining 61 patients, 29 participated adequately up to the first follow-up study five months after the infarction. Later, the number of patients with an adequate attendance rate diminished further to only 10 between the sixth and twelfth months. However, in addition to these patients, another 16 patients maintained physical activity of training level on their own accord.

The physical activity of the control group also increased. After a year, 11 control patients maintained physical activity of full training level.

This shows that physical reconditioning can be carried out completely on the patient's own initiative. To sum up, supervised physical training appeared to be indicated and feasible in only about one-fifth of an unselected infarction series. Patients with poor prognostic features need especially close supervision of the physical training, if this is applied.

One recurrence of infarction occurred during the training

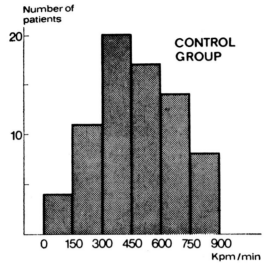

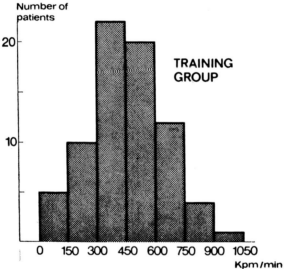

Figure 13-1. Bar graph showing the distribution of physical work capacity six to eight weeks after myocardial infarction in the control group and in the training group. From E. Kentala, Physical fitness and feasibility of physical rehabilitation after myocardial infarctions in men of working age, *Annals of Clinical Research, 4:Suppl 9:*1-84, 1972.

sessions. There was no difference between the control and training groups in morbidity and mortality (Fig. 13-2). Locomotor complications were few.

Because the intergroup difference in physical activity turned out to be small for the reasons mentioned above, it follows that no statistically significant difference in physical working capacity was established in the follow-up study between the original control and training groups. Both groups displayed a clear decrease in the heart rate/blood pressure product measured at the same submaximal load, while an increase was elicited at maximal workload.

Those individuals in whom supervised physical training was feasible, i.e. with an attendance rate of 70 percent or more, improved their physical working capacity markedly more ($p < 0.0025$) than the other members of the training group by the five-month test, although the mean initial capacities were practically the same.

On the basis of an interview made at the twelve-month follow-up, the whole patient series was regrouped into those with a training level physical activity and those without, regardless of whether they were initially in the control or training groups. The physical working capacity of the high activity subgroup increased significantly more than that of the others by the five-month follow-up examination ($p < 0.0001$) and started from better initial capacity ($p < 0.05$). This increase in the course of one year was 56 percent in the patients maintaining the high level of physical activity (Grade III) against 26 percent for the rest of the total series divided in this way.

The initial physical working capacity six to eight weeks after the infarction was the most important single variable in the training group in predicting the physical working capacity achieved by training in twelve months. Next in the stepwise regression analysis came the average training heart rate, participation rate, FEV 1.0, cardiac failure complicating the acute infarction, paradoxical cardiac pulsation, and heart volume.

The subjects participating adequately in supervised physical training showed the most distinct decrease in the skinfold

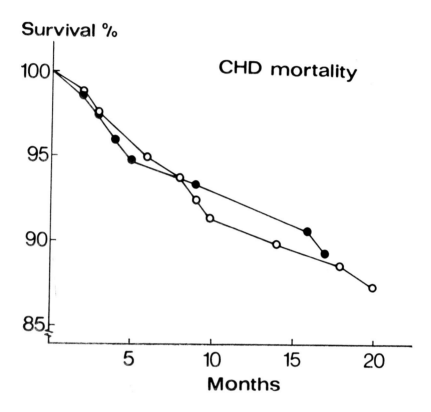

Figure 13-2A. Graph showing survival rates during the twenty-month follow-up in the control group and in the training group. From E. Kentala, Physical fitness and feasibility of physical rehabilitation after myocardial infarctions in men of working age, *Annals of Clinical Research, 4:Suppl 9:*1-84, 1972.

Incidence %

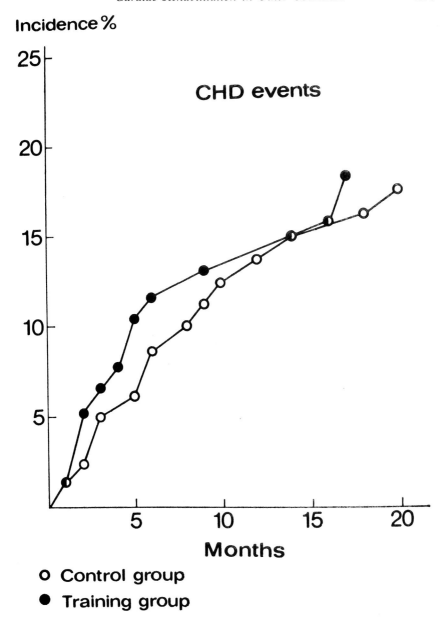

Figure 13-2B. Graph showing the incidence of coronary heart disease (CHD) events during the follow-up in the control group and in the training group. From E. Kentala, Physical fitness and feasibility of physical rehabilitation after myocardial infarctions in men of working age, *Annals of Clinical Research,* *4:Suppl 9:*1-84, 1972.

measurements and weight loss. These patients were also somewhat better able to give up smoking. Further, the patients with training level activity gave initially significantly ($p < 0.001$) more numerous Q-QS findings in accordance with Minnesota Code, but they disappeared considerably faster in the course of the twelve-month follow-up. No corresponding changes were noted in regard to ST-T alterations.

Return to work was not influenced by the supervised physical training. Sixty-eight percent of the patients in the total series who had been at work before the current infarction and who were alive twelve months after it returned to work. This percentage is only 26.5 in an unselected series from the Ischemic Heart Disease Register of Helsinki. It became evident that regular follow-up examinations by a doctor, measurement of physical working capacity, adequate medical therapy, and the sense of security given by continuous contact with a physician contribute at least as much to return to work as does supervised physical training. The number of sustained myocardial infarctions was the most important determinant of retirement in the multiple discriminating analysis. The patients who retired in conjunction with the current infarction were distinguished from the rest of the series in that they had been in the physically heaviest work; these jobs had been frequently too heavy for their actual work capacity. The myocardial infarction appeared to be overestimated in the evaluation of the working capacity of some patients, leading fairly readily to their retirement on pension. At other times, patients with ischemic heart disease may have to work for a long time in conditions that are beyond their functional capacity without vacation or pension even being considered.

The prognosis for the next one to two postinfarction years was most clearly associated with paradoxical cardiac pulsation noted during the treatment of acute infarction. If this finding was easily established on palpation of the chest, it implied a poor prognosis. Other predictors of poor prognosis were an increasing frequency of ventricular extrasystoles during the hospital stay, low arterial blood pressure, poor physical working capacity measured six to eight weeks after the infarction, and various signs of cardiac or respiratory failure. Whether the patient belonged to the control or training group was of no prognostic importance.

On the basis of the study by Kentala, some physicians in Helsinki now feel less enthusiastic about the benefits of programs of supervised physical activities for patients with recent myocardial infarction. They feel, however, that this could reflect the characteristics of their specific population sample and do not attempt to apply this rigidly to other populations.

The noted differences in skinfold measurements, weight loss, and ease of giving up cigarette smoking in the supervised trained group as opposed to the control group is certainly encouraging as regards alleviation of coronary risk factors. This may influence the future, especially in lieu of the high intake of saturated fats in the Finnish population, i.e. cheeses and milk, the latter reportedly in the range of one liter per person per day.

GOTEBORG, SWEDEN

At Sahlgrens Hospital, University of Goteborg, an outpatient facility has been utilized for exercising patients with recent myocardial infarction. The facility is part of the physical therapy department, and the exercise program is under the supervision of the physiotherapists. The program consists of sessions of walking and calisthenics three times weekly. Personal conversation with Doctor Lars Wilhelmsen reveals that the physician staff members have been pleased with their results in programmed exercise in patients with recent myocardial infarction. They feel that one of the most important aspects of this type of patient management has been the evolution of methods of patient and family education and the study of coronary risk factors.

One of the studies reported relating to the experience in Goteborg was with primary intervention of high risk factors related to myocardial infarction. In this, Wilhelmsen et al.[2] described a preventive trial aiming at treatment of the risk factors—hypertension, elevated serum cholesterol, smoking, and, to some degree, low physical activity. At the time of the study report, 305 subjects had been found with previously undiagnosed and untreated hypertension. Of these, 210 have been placed on drug therapy, and in most, blood pressure has become normal. Regarding hypercholesterolemia, diet information is provided by a doctor and a dietician. Clofibrate and nicotinic acid are also utilized accordingly to the type of lipid abnormality. A seasonal variation has been noted, with the mean serum cholesterol recorded of 233 mg% in December and 256 mg% in March.

With regard to smoking, of special interest has been the utilization of an antismoking clinic for those who smoked less than fifteen cigarettes per day. The introduction information meeting comprised around 40 participants followed by group sessions of 7 to 10 participants. Only rarely were they treated individually. All smokers received information about the positive consequences of not smoking and were advised on steps in a cessation program, although they were advised to stop completely. Some decreased their tobacco consumption by changing from cigarettes to cigars or pipes.

In addition, chewing gum containing nicotine has been used in the early cessation period. Of the 295 men who have entered the program, 93 (32%) have stopped smoking completely and 65 (22%) have reduced their smoking by less than 50 percent.

Little emphasis was placed on physical activity except for increasing activity in those with very low levels of activity. The specifics are not described.

Later in the same year, Gustufson et al.[3] reported a series of 229 post-myocardial-infarction patients studied up to two years following hospitalization with comparison to a random population sample of men of comparable age. Hyperlipoproteinemia, cholesterol, and triglycerides elevation were more common in myocardial infarction patients, especially in the younger group. There was a trend toward higher mortality among patients with hyperlipoproteinemia. Types IIA and B were very common in young patients. Serum cholesterol values were significantly higher in the youngest patients and serum triglyceride higher in the controls in age groups forty to forty-five, forty-six to fifty, and fifty-one to fifty-five years.

More recently, unpublished data by Wilhelmsen and Tibblin[4] (obtained by personal interviews) has been revealing regarding coronary risk factors. The study population was made up of 973 men (all age fifty) recruited from a general Swedish urban population. Of the 855 participants, 834 were free from coronary heart disease on entry and have been observed for nine years and four months. All except 2 of 55 deaths were autopsied. Twenty-five near-fatal and 19 fatal cases of coronary heart disease occurred.

By a multiple model, nine probable risk factors were analyzed. Serum cholesterol, smoking, systolic blood pressure, dyspnea, and conviction for drunkenness were significantly related to coronary heart disease, but not serum triglycerides, hematocrit, or social mobility (place of birth), while physical inactivity during work showed a slight tendency to relationship.

The predictive capability of the logistic function (with cholesterol, smoking, and systolic blood pressure) was tested in another randomly selected population sample of 5,146 men (ages fifty-one to fifty-five years) and found to be quite accurate. Thus, it was possible to isolate the highest decile group of men with a twenty-nine times higher risk of suffering coronary heart disease than the lowest decile.

Thus, efforts in Sweden (particularly in Goteborg) seem to be predominantly directed toward risk factor detection and modification. The structure of the city registry in Goteborg and the accessibility of data and cooperation of the registry with the physician investigators make such studies most realistic and rewarding. The studies being done at the time under the direction of Doctor Wilhelmsen are most impressive, and the methodology seems worthy of the stature of an international model for coronary risk factor detection, evaluation, and modification.

HOHENRIED, GERMANY

A most elaborate and extensive European cardiac exercise rehabilitation center is the Klinik Hohenried, Germany, located twenty kilometers south of Munich on the Starnberger Sea. The facility (seen in aerial view in Fig. 13-3) has approximately 600 beds with a four-bed coronary care unit; the total surrounding area encompasses almost twenty acres. The area was originally the land surrounding a large castle (seen in Fig. 13-4 as it relates to the rehabilitation center); the castle is now used as a recreation facility for the physicians and staff of the rehabilitation center. The center is a modern unit complex with a connecting closed corridor. There is a large gymnasium (Fig. 13-5) and an indoor pool with additional area for a sauna and various types of physical therapy. In the adjacent outdoor area, there is minigolf (Fig. 13-6) and lawn bowling (Fig. 13-7). The beach and sea nearby are utilized as a part of the daily recreational and training activities (Fig. 13-8).

The patient population is obtained by private referral—mainly from the sourthern part of Germany. The population is of middle-class derivation, and the rehabilitation program is supported by national health insurance. Referral of patients takes place from four to six months after myocardial infarction, and at any one time there are approximately 550 patients in the facility. Each patient remains at the Klinik for a period of six weeks in his own private room (Fig. 13-9) and is allowed visits by his family only on weekends. After initial bicycle ergometer stress testing (Fig. 13-10), the patient undergoes a progressive program of training and recreation. The activities include running, calisthenics (Fig. 13-11), minigolf, lawn bowling, and swimming (Fig. 13-12). In addition to the above, the patients are trained by bicycle ergometry twice weekly, at which time they have constant telemetry monitoring of their electrocardiogram (Fig. 13-13). After the six-week period, the patients are discharged and are monitored by consultation in the rehabilitation clinic and in their own homes.

In addition to the 550 post-myocardial-infarction patients, the Klinik usually has 75 to 100 coronary-prone patients in training. These patients spend four weeks at the Klinik and have a similar program to the post-myocardial-infarction patients; however, it is more strenuous and involves more use of isometric maneuvers such as weight lifting.

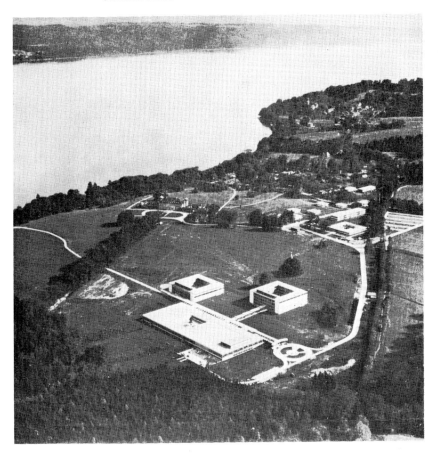

Figure 13-3. Aerial view of the Hohenried Klinik with the castle and Starnberger Sea in the background.

In 1972, Stocksmeier and Halhuber[5] reported preliminary results of the Hohenried longitudinal cross section study of patients with myocardial infarction. Patients under comprehensive care for myocardial infarction were observed for ten years, and information concerning recurrence of myocardial infarction and mortality, readjustment of mode of living, capacity to earn living, and diet utilization ratio were recorded and evaluated. In 92 workers and salaried employees suffering from myocardial infarction, an adjustment of diet lasting eleven

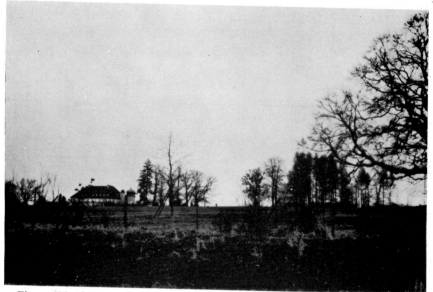

Figure 13-4. Castle about which Hohenried Klinik is built.

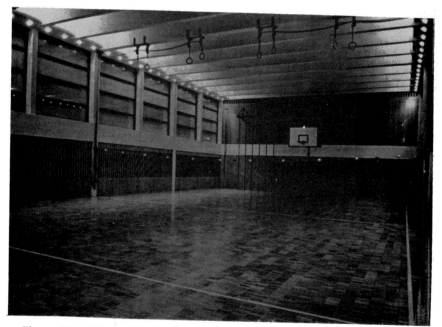

Figure 13-5. View of the gymnasium facility at Hohenried Klinik.

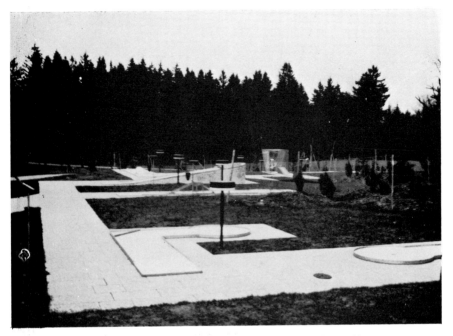

Figure 13-6. View of the minigolf course at Hohenried Klinik.

months could be achieved by intensive consultation in the rehabilitation clinic and in the household. The results showed a change in the ratio of polyunsaturated to saturated fatty acid of 0.3 to 1.2. During the six weeks in rehabilitation it was possible to reduce significantly the mean levels of body weight, blood pressure, and blood lipids of 273 myocardial infarction patients. The effect of the modification lasted at least nine months after discharge from the rehabilitation center. As about one third of the 490 myocardial infarction patients accepted in the meantime received follow-up treatment (early rehabilitation), the time between the occurrence of the myocardial infarction and return to work was of interest. It was found that with the follow-up treatment, there was an advance of about three months in beginning work. It was felt, however, that the only way to obtain sufficient information as to whether such an advance is beneficial or harmful to the patient is by prolonging the duration of the study.

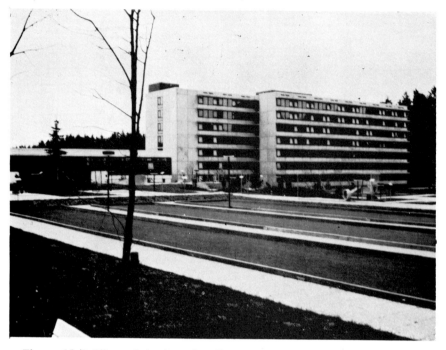

Figure 13-7. View of the lawn bowling lanes with Klinik buildings in the background.

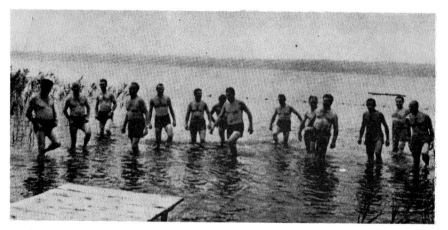

Figure 13-8. Bathers seen in shallow water of the sea during daily beach activities.

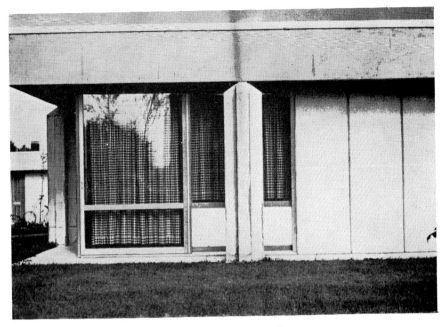

Figure 13-9. Outside view of individual living units.

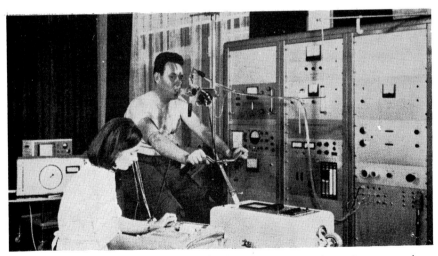

Figure 13-10. A patient undergoing ergometry stress testing prior to exercise training at Hohenried Klinik.

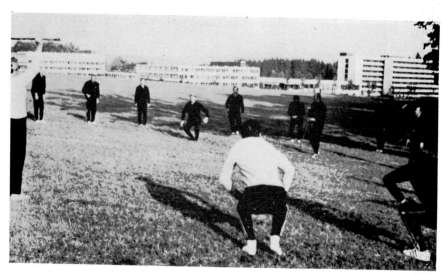

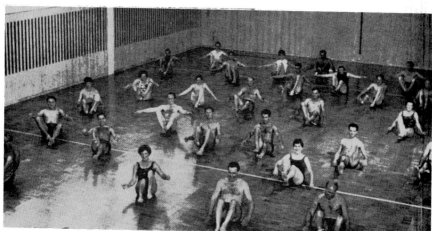

Figure 13-11. Views of calisthenics both outside (above) and inside the gymnasium (below).

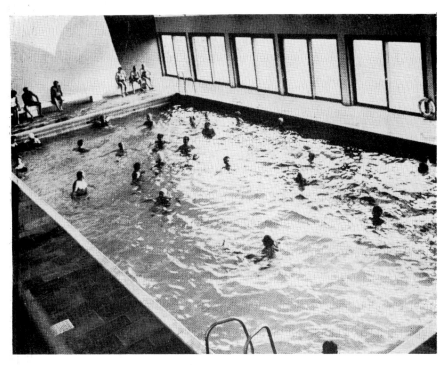

Figure 13-12. Patients in gym swimming pool during daily swimming activities.

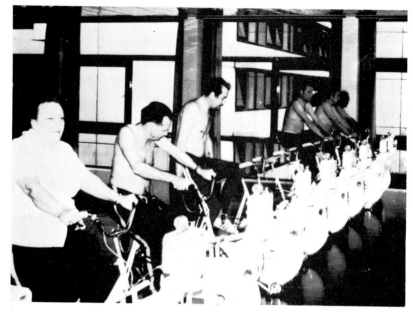

Figure 13-13. Patients undergoing follow-up exercise testing during telemetry ECG monitoring.

In summary, the Klinik Hohenried is the epitomy of an all-encompassing facility for cardiac rehabilitation. The 35 physicians and 50 nurses, along with physiotherapists and other personnel who supervise the program, form an adequate number of capable staff. The experience in evaluation of patient data is inconclusive at this point but suggests a benefit of more rapid return to work and a consistent fall in blood pressure and blood lipids up to a year thereafter. As with other programs, there is a need for a longer duration of study involving more patients before conclusive evidence can be available.

BAD KROZINGEN, GERMANY

In this area, at the Benedikt Kreutz Klinik, a more thorough diagnostic center has been established. This center is quite different from Hohenried. It is smaller (250 beds), limited to secondary coronary prevention, and more like a hospital environment because most of the activities are limited to the facility itself.

Many patients come directly to Bad Krozingen (Benedikt Kreutz Klinik) from the hospital where they were treated for the acute attack. At five weeks postinfarction, according to the general schedule, patients undergo low level exercise stress testing. At eight to nine weeks, the stress test is done in conjunction with right heart catheterization, looking for the response of the pulmonary capillary wedge pressure to the challenge of exercise. If the response is appropriate, the patient then undergoes progressive exercise training. Those patients who have abnormal hemodynamics, persistent angina pectoris, or who are less than forty years of age will be candidates for coronary arteriography, to be performed no sooner than nine to ten weeks postinfarction.

In addition to exercise testing, physical training, and invasive diagnostic studies, the center also provides psychosocial counseling and dietary instructions. The food served in the cafeteria is low in saturated animal fat and in salt content. Spouses are instructed in the patient's diet before discharge from the clinic. Impressive aspects of rehabilitation at Benedikt Kreutz are the vocational rehabilitation, occupational therapy (Fig. 13-14), and educational efforts. Patients may take courses in subjects ranging from language to electronics (Fig. 13-15) and select their own videotapes to be played on their private room television set. They may enroll in job-retraining sessions which include activities ranging from metal work to advanced executive training. Telemetry monitoring of heart rate and rhythm is frequently performed during such job-simulated work activities. The physical therapist once again plays a vital role in supervising the various physical activities.

CURRENT STATUS OF CARDIAC
REHABILITATION IN WEST GERMANY

The concept of cardiac rehabilitation in West Germany has its origin in the time of Bismark. During this period social

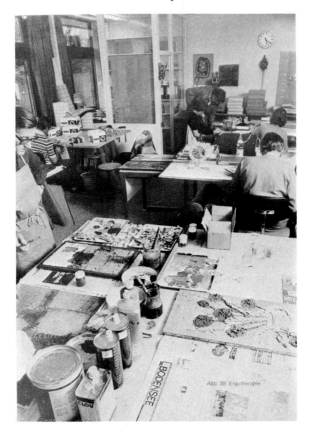

Figure 13-14. Occupational therapy activities at Benedikt Kreutz. Reprinted with permission of H. Roskamm, M.D. from *Rehabilitation fur Herz– und Kreislaufkranke.*

legislation reforms and attitudes developed that were conducive to rehabilitation in many spheres of life. Early in German history the concept of the Kur (pronounced *coor*) also evolved. The Kur were developed in various locations and were typified by the elaborate resort (Kur) at Baden-Baden. Here, the wealthy Germans took periodic (each year for several weeks) leaves from work for rest, relaxation, social diversion, and physical activity. Often the Kur was prescribed by a physician as part of patient management. The Kur at Baden-Baden in the Black Forest area

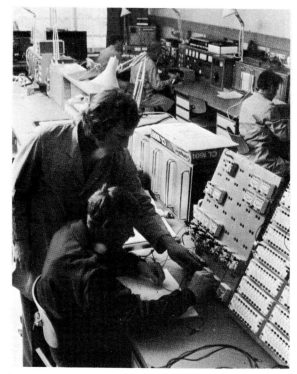

Figure 13-15. Electronic workshop activities at Benedikt Kreutz. Reprinted with permission of H. Roskamm, M.D. from *Rehabilitation fur Herz– und Kreislaufkranke.*

was one of the most elaborate. Here a subject combined "medicinal health" activities, such as hiking, exercises, sauna, massage, and aerobic games, with "social" activities, such as gambling, dancing, cocktail hours, and dinner parties. Other such centers were developed around the country and exist today; however, the gardens and activities at Baden-Baden are the most attractive and interesting.

In the last decade or so, a greater frequency of coronary atherosclerotic heart disease has been seen in both West Germany and the United States. In Germany, a high degree of disability is permitted by physicians largely because of an apparent problem with misdiagnosis and management of two different subsets of patients. The *first group* is made up of those individuals who present to a primary physician with upper respiratory symptoms and S-T segment changes on electrocardiogram and are "labeled" as having coronary disease without further diagnostic workup. These patients frequently attain levels of disability because of this misdiagnosis. The *other group* includes those with definite transmural myocardial infarction with no complications who are placed on disability status because of their diagnosis without consideration of their functional capacity.

Because of these patient problems and their impact on the German economy secondary to the high incidence of disability status in these patients, industry and insurance companies have turned to the use of cardiac rehabilitation centers with their specialists for proper diagnosis and treatment as well as rehabilitation.

The several types of classes of rehabilitation centers in West Germany are outlined below.

1. *The Sophisticated Kur*—as in Klinik Hohenried. These centers accept insurance-paid patients primarily for rehabilitation, recreational, and preventive reasons. Less diagnostic work is done, and the patients are frequently well subjects.

2. *The Private facility*—as in Waldkirch. Such clinics accept private-paid and insurance-paid patients with the diagnosis of coronary disease. The patients are admitted for work-up and rehabilitation. Although coronary angiography and surgery are not performed, careful evaluation and prescribing of oral therapy is done.

3. *The Diagnostic Center*—as the Klinik in Bad Krozingen. Patients with all degrees of coronary disease are referred to these centers for detailed noninvasive and invasive diagnostic evaluation. Medical therapy is incorporated as needed with all phases of rehabilitation. These type of centers seem to be the ultimate resource in Germany for the evaluation and management of the patient with coronary disease. Their approach is clearly displayed in

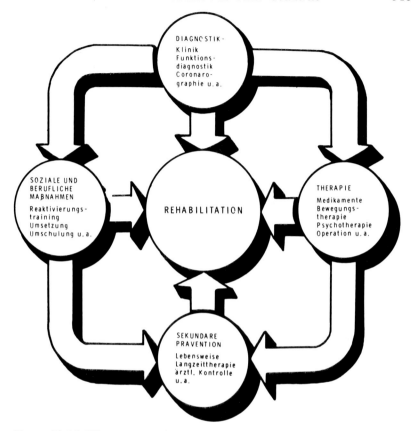

Figure 13-16. The concept of rehabilitation at Benedikt Kreutz. Reprinted with permission of H. Roskamm, M.D. from *Rehabilitation fur Herz– und Kreislaufkranke.*

Figure 13-16. Physicians and staff at the rehabilitation centers in West Germany seem to have a logical approach to the problems with which they are faced; however, efficacy and efficiency, especially of the Type 1 center, is doubtful. The success they have had with "insurance coverage" of the center activities is impressive and is a method for the United States to seriously consider. However, more careful administration and utilization of such funds would be mandatory in the United States for such a program to "survive" long-term.

Irregardless of the current evidence for success or failure of cardiac rehabilitation in Germany or the United States, the concept of avoiding unnecessary disability and returning patients to work with their coronary disease stabilized is realistic, practical, and beneficial to our society and our economy.

CURRENT DEVELOPMENTS IN OTHER COUNTRIES

In recent years, rehabilitative activities have been reported in countries as close as Canada or as distant as Israel, India, and Australia.

Kavanagh[6] from Toronto, *Canada*, reported that 7 of 8 post-myocardial-infarction patients completed the Boston Marathon. Four kilograms weight loss were reported in each, with associated degrees of "heat stress" and elevated blood area nitrogen, creatinine, and creatine phosphokinase. Kavanagh also relates that "such strenuous exercise should not be routine in such patients." Also from Canada, Ogirimah et al.[7] reported 12 postinfarction patients trained with jogging compared to 12 trained with swimming, volleyball, and bowling. The results revealed a significantly better training effect in the joggers.

In Belgium, Debacker et al.[8] have reported a statistically significant difference in training effect, especially the rate-pressure product, in 36 postinfarction patients who were exercised as opposed to a group of nonexercised controls.

The *Russians* have recently discussed the principles of stepwise therapy of the post-myocardial-infarction patient and the need of designing programs of interval training and evaluation of same as well as the necessity of investigation of the psychological aspects of rehabilitation.[9]

The *British*[10] have described beneficial effects of physical training in 23 trained patients compared to 15 controls, especially with regard to the lesser heart rate response to stress in the trained group. Another British study by Carson et al.[11] described rehabilitative exercise in 59 men two times weekly for three months. The results were especially supportive of the increased rate of return to work in the exercisers.

In *Sweden*,[12] a study of 34 trained post-myocardial-infarction patients (PMIP) versus 29 controls revealed a twentyfold increase in work capacity and less increase in lactate and free fatty acid for a given work load.

One study in *Singapore*[13] revealed a decreased heart rate, systolic blood pressure, and tension time index along with increased work capacity in 150 trained PMIP. Another study[14] there of 94 PMIP (1955-69) reported on the efficacy and safety in the training of PMIP, stating that it could be done without expensive equipment.

The *Swiss*[15] have related benefits of PMIP training in returning the patient to previous life activities with positive psychological, physical, social, and vocational rewards.

In *Geneva*, most recently, Doctor Antoine Bloch has presented well-controlled studies supporting the concept of early mobilization and discharge in the uncomplicated post-myocardial-infarction case. Doctor Bloch recently started an outpatient gym program which begins two months postinfarction. The classes are divided into two sections, one for those recently enrolled and the other for those who have been in the program for several months. Patients engage in activities with a medicine ball, skip rope, run through a slalom course, and jump over low hurdles. After a six– to eight-month period, the patients attend only once per week (versus three times weekly in the beginning) and are encouraged to be active on their own during other days. During Doctor Cantwell's recent visit to this program he observed a middle-aged former boxer (whose saphenous vein graphs had closed and whose left ventricular ejection fraction was less than 25%) who was the most active member of the class. This man has continued a hobby of long-distance cycling (against medical advice) and had just completed a 120-mile event, averaging over 30 miles per hour.

Kellerman,[16] in *Israel*, has reported that greater than 85 percent of a population of PMIP who did not return to work were able to do so after four months in an exercise training program. He feels that the future of rehabilitation must be adapted to the newer medical therapy and surgical interventions.

In *India*,[17] an uncontrolled study of 150 trained PMIP

revealed beneficial changes in heart rate, systolic blood pressure, and tension time index and an increase in work capacity. The authors emphasized the improved behavioral, social, and sexual adjustment in these patients. A two year follow-up has revealed a low morbidity and mortality.

In *New Zealand*, Nye et al.[18] reported on 130 PMIP, one-half committed to an exercise club and one-half being control. They recorded no excessive mortality in the exercise group and good adherence.

In *Denmark*,[19] there was a small PMIP study of 12 trained subjects and 15 subjects who were submitted to free activities. The trained group developed a decreased heart rate and systolic blood pressure to a given workload; however, there was no change in cardiac output between the groups.

In *Australia*, Samios and Watson[20] reported that rehabilitation and prevention in coronary disease established a psychological benefit and an improved work aptitude.

In *Czechoslovakia*, Ressel et al.[21] reported results of a small study in 23 PMIP—12 trained and 11 untrained. The trained group had a decreased heart rate response for a given workload and increased work capacity compared to the controls. In addition, their invasive evaluations revealed no adverse changes in hemodynamics, i.e. pulmonary artery and diastolic pressure.

In *Italy*, Doctor Vincenzo Rulli (Rome) and Doctor Bruno Cary (Milan), among others, have been actively engaged in inpatient and outpatient cardiac rehabilitation efforts.

Therefore, recent published data on a worldwide scale supports, in general, the beneficial effect and safety of exercise in the PMIP. Although adequate controlled studies are still not complete, the "trend of benefit" seems apparent.

REFERENCES

1. Kentala, E.: Physical fitness and feasibility of physical rehabilitation after myocardial infarctions in men of working age. *Ann Clin Res, 4: Suppl 9:*1-84, 1972.
2. Wilhelmsen, L., Tibblin, G., and Werko, L.: A primary preventive study in Gothenburg, Sweden. *Prev Med, 1:*153-160, 1972.
3. Gustufson, A., Elmfeldt, D., Wilhelmsen, L., et al.: Serum lipids and lipo-proteins in men after myocardial infarction compared with representative population sample. *Circulation, 46:*709-716, 1972.
4. Wilhelmsen, L., and Tibblin, G.: Personal interviews, April, 1973.
5. Stocksmeier, V.U. and Halhuber, M.J.: Die Hohenrieder Langschitt-Studie an Herzingarlg-patienten. *Munch Med Wochenschr, 114:*1349, 1972.
6. Kavanagh, T., Shephard, R.H., and Pandit, V.: Marathon running after myocardial infarction. *JAMA, 229:*1602-1605, 1974.
7. Ogirimah, A.M., Cunningham, D.A., Rechnitzer, P.A., and Yuhasz, M.S.: Comparison of effects of two types of exercise programs on work capacity and electrocardiogram of patients with previous myocardial infarction. *J Sports Med Phys Fitness, 14:*1-7, 1974.
8. Debacker, G.D., Deporter, A.M., Willems, P., and Varewijck, E.: The influence of rehabilitation on the physical performance after myocardial infarction. *Acta Cardiol*, XXIX:427-440, 1974.
9. Shkhvatsabaya, L.K., and Aronov, D.M.: Rehabilitation of patients with ischaemic heart disease (Present status of the question, and actual problems). *Cor Vasa, 16, 2:*81-90, 1974.
10. Winifred, M.B.: Supervised circuit training after myocardial infarction. *Physiology, 58:*340-343, 1972.
11. Carson, P., Neophytou, M., Tucker, H., and Simpson, T.: Exercise programme after myocardial infarction. *Br Med J, 27:*213-216, 1973.
12. Bjernulf, A., Boberg, J., and Froberg, S.: Physical training after myocardial infarction: Metabolic effects during short and prolonged exercise before and after physical training in male patients after myocardial infarction. *Scand J Clin Lab Invest, 33:*173-185, 1974.
13. Datey, K.K., and Dalvi, C.P.: Training programme for patients of myocardial infarction. *Singapore Med J, 14, 3:*376-378, 1973.
14. Katayama, F.: Physical training program. *Singapore Med J, 14, 3:*376-378, 1973.
15. Feifar, Z.: Problems and challenges in rehabilitation of patients with acute myocardial infarction. *Schweiz Med Wochenschr, 103:*35-40, 1973.
16. Kellerman, J.J.: Cardiac rehabilitation: A view. *Giorn It Card, 3:*617-624, 1973.
17. Datey, K.K., and Dalvl, C.P.: Training programme for patients of myocardial infarction. *Indian Heart J, 25:*144-149, 1973.
18. Nye, E.R., and Poulsen, W.T.: An activity programme for coronary patients: A review of morbidity, mortality and adherence after five years. *New Engl J Med, 79:*1010-1013, 1974.

19. Kirchheiner, B., and Pedersen-Bjergaard, O.P.: The effect of physical training after myocardial infarction. *Scand J Rehab Med, 5:*105-110, 1973.
20. Samios, R., and Watson, S.: Cardiac rehabilitation at the Royal Prince Alfred Hospital, Sydney, Australia. *Physiotherapy, 63, 4:*125-129, 1976.
21. Ressel, J., Jandova, R., Stolz, I., and Widimsky, J.: Effects of physical training on central haemodynamics and working capacity in myocardial infarction. *Cor Vasa, 17, 4:*241-253, 1975.

Chapter 14

SUMMARY

I N THIS BOOK, we have attempted to update, review, and discuss the issue of exercise and coronary heart disease. We have dealt with the historical aspects of exercise and have discussed in a practical and fundamental manner exercise physiology in normals and in patients with coronary heart disease. The American habit of sedentary living has been appraised as a likely coronary risk factor, and the efforts of exercise on this and the major coronary risk factors have been reviewed.

Exercise stress testing is discussed, as are the guidelines to exercise training with special emphasis on the exercise prescription—for both large groups of patients and in the private preventive cardiology clinic setting.

Post-myocardial-infarction rehabilitation in the hospital has been discussed, followed by a section on the potential disadvantages, dangers, and complications of exercise in normals and in patients with coronary heart disease. Outpatient exercise activities for postinfarction patients at Georgia Baptist Medical Center have been reviewed and updated, followed by a directory of current exercise programs in the United States today. Lastly, more data has been presented on cardiac rehabilitation in other countries.

Cardiac rehabilitation has many faces, ranging from the motivation of an executive to reduce coronary risk factors to the return of a professional baseball player to active status following a myocardial infarction (Fig. 14-1). As an important part of the rehabilitation process, exercise is inexpensive, enjoyable to most, and so far appears safe for the coronary-prone individual and for the postcoronary patient if done properly. The latter necessitates thorough preliminary evaluation and medical

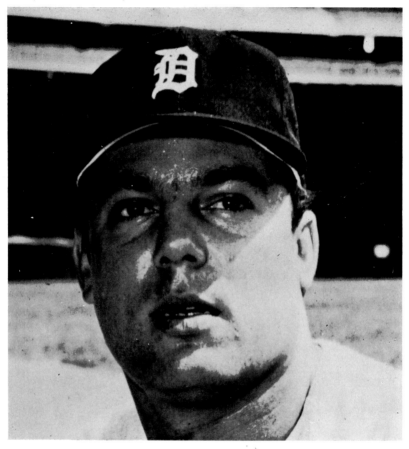

Figure 14-1. Major league baseball player who returned to stardom following a myocardial infarction. Photo courtesy of Ed Thilenius, TV-5, Atlanta, Georgia, and the Detroit Tiger baseball club.

supervision. If the only beneficial effect of exercise in the coronary patient was an *alleviation of fear, anxiety and sense of impending doom,* that alone would validate the time and cost of research in this area to date.

As this book goes to press, we continue to see more fervent interest in exercise exhibited by the American public. This is apparent in the allegedly normal population, in the coronary-prone population, and in postinfarction and postrevascularization patients. We cannot emphasize enough the importance of careful monitoring of the type, intensity, and duration of exercise for each of these groups. It seems that people, including patients, often behave in the "all-or-none" manner, and this can be self-defeating in a long-term plan of exercise. Moderation, regularity, and perseverance are "musts" in exercise programming. Adherence to these principles is mandatory if one hopes to continue the present downward trend in cardiovascular mortality and morbidity as we revert from a "sedentary, coronary-prone existence" to living habits that emphasize lifelong fitness and health enhancement.

SUBJECT INDEX

A

Achilles tendonitis, 221
Active assistive exercises, 152, 154
Active bed exercises, 152, 154
Active intervention program, 36
Active physiotherapy, 158
Activity/exercise/recreation program, 153
Acute heart overload, 15
Acute infectious disease, 123
Acute myocardial infarction, 19, 123, 158, 290 (*see also* Myocardial infarction)
Adipose triglycerides, 50
Adrenocortical activity, 15
Aerobic work capacity, 14
Age factor, 28
Air Force personnel, 82
Aircrewmen, 91
Alcohol abuse, 38
Alcohol consumption, 221
Alternate bent leg raising, 188
Alternate straight leg raising, 189
Altitude of residence, 35-36
Ambulation, 150
Ambulatory electrocardiographic monitoring, 242-243
Amputees, 113
Ancillary noninvasive techniques, 103-107
Aneurysm development, 143
Angina pectoris, 13, 21-22, 38, 61, 72, 76, 88-89, 91, 96-98, 100, 107, 123, 168-170, 226, 228
Anginal pain, 74
Animal experimental data, 28-32
  coronary arterial system, 28-31
  mitochondrial morphology, 31
  myocardial performance and efficiency, 31
  practical application of, 31-32
  size of heart muscle fibers, 28
  summary of studies, 31-32
Anterior myocardial infarction, 234
Anterior wall myocardial infarctions, 102

Antianginal medications, 228
Antiarrhythmic drugs, 242
Antiarrhythmic treatment, 232
Anticoagulant therapy, 158-159
Antismoking clinic, 298
Aortic outflow obstruction, 123
Aortocoronary saphenous vein bypass grafting, 103
Aortocoronary saphenous vein graft operations, 113
Aortocoronary vein bypass, 250
Apex-cardiography, 106
Arizona cardiac exercise programs, 251
Arm and shoulder loosening, 155, 176-177
Arm ergometer test, 113
Arm exercises, 21-22
Armchair treatment, 145
Army recruits, 53-54
Arrhythmia-prone person, 107
Arrhythmias, 75-76, 112, 215-216, 230, 242
Arterial baroreceptors, 16
Arteriovenous oxygen (A-VO₂) difference, 19
Arthritis, 123
Athlete's heart, warnings against, 27
Athletes, 34-35, 52
ATPase activity, 15
Atrial arrhythmias, 108
Australia cardiac rehabilitation, 316

B

Bad Krozingen, Germany, cardiac rehabilitation center, 308-309
Badminton, 201
Baseline resting electrocardiogram, 228
Basketball, 169, 200, 202, 210
Bayes' law, 92-93
Bed rest period, 14
Bed rest treatment, 145
Behavior patterns, 47, 58-59, 63

322

Belgium cardiac rehabilitation, 314
Bell Telephone Company employees, 91
Bench stepping, 135
Bench testing, 228-229
Beneficial effects of exercise, 31-32, 61, 320
Beta blocking agents, 228
Bicycle boom, 27
Bicycle ergometry, 72, 83-84, 95, 99, 145, 160-162, 169, 290, 300
Bicycle riding, 48, 135, 201
Bigeminy, 108, 242-243
Bipolar chest leads, 84
Bipolar lead system, 97
Black patients, 34
Blood clotting, 63
Blood clotting time, 60
Blood coagulation disorders, 47, 60-61
Blood lipid abnormalities, 47, 49-55
Blood lipids, 63
Blood pressure, 22-23, 55, 63
  control of, 227
  fall in, 145
Blood studies, 229
Blood sugar, 63
Blood uric acid, 63
Blood uric acid elevation, 47, 61-62
Blunt wounds, 222
Body fat, 171
Body weight, viii
Body weight control, 227
Boston Marathon, 27
Bowling, 200-201, 208
British cardiac rehabilitation, 314
Bruce method of treadmill testing, 77-78, 88, 108
Buddy system, 124
Bundle branch block, 108-112
Bus drivers, 33
Bypass surgery, 20, 124

C

Calf blood flow measure, 158
Calf vein thrombosis, 158
California cardiac exercise programs, 251-259
Calisthenics, 52, 225-226, 242, 297
Caloric expenditure, 11-12
Caloric intake, 58
Canada cardiac rehabilitation, 314

Capillary development, 29
Capillary/fiber ratios, 29
Capillary numbers, 29
Carbohydrate intolerance, 47, 57
Cardiac arrest, 150, 225
Cardiac capacity, 13
Cardiac catheterization, 143, 170
Cardiac complications of exercise, 215-221
Cardiac exercise programs in United States, 250-288 (*see also* specific states)
  map, 288
Cardiac glycogen metabolism, 16
Cardiac hypertrophy, 28
Cardiac output, 14
Cardiac patients, 56, 58-59
Cardiac rehabilitation in other countries, 289-318 (*see also* specific location)
Cardiac rehabilitation team, 150, 152
Cardiac rhythm disturbances, exercise testing for evaluation and detection of, 107-113
Cardiac status, 17
Cardiopulmonary endurance exercise schedule for untrained person, 134
Cardiopulmonary fitness classification, 137
Cardiopulmonary response to exercise, 17
Cardiopulmonary resuscitation equipment and trained personnel, 230
Cardiorespiratory fitness, 137
Cardiorespiratory function, 20
Cardiovascular hemodynamics, 18
Cardioversion, 76
Case histories, 135-141, 212-213
Cerebral vascular accidents, 216
Chest and leg raising, 194
Chest discomfort, 75, 77, 221, 230
Chest pain, 89-90, 107, 124, 216-217, 219
Chest x-rays, 158
Chewing gum with nicotine, 298
Chinese pedicabmen, 55, 58
Cholesterol levels, 36-38, 48-53, 63, 170, 297-299
  exercise-related lowering of, 50-51
  limited dietary intake of, vii
Chronic lung disease, 62
Chronic obstructive pulmonary disease, 62
Cigarette advertising ban, 36

Cigarette smoking, 38, 47, 49, 56-57, 63, 170, 221, 236 (*see also* Smoking)
  cessation of, 227
  control of, viii
  health hazard of, vii
Cineangiography, 97
Circulatory dynamics of exercise, 13-17
Clerks, 33
Clinical coronary heart disease, 88, 91
Clinical index of coronary artery disease, 128-133
Clofibrate, 298
Coital activities, evaluation of, 243-245
Collateral circulation, 29
Collateralization, 30
College athletes, 34-35, 52
College men, 60
College women, 51
Colorado cardiac exercise programs, 260
Competitive team games, 168
Complete heart block, 110
Compression fracture of lumbar spine, 222
Conduction disturbances, 107-113
Congenital heart disease, 123
Congestive heart failure, 123, 159
Connecticut cardiac exercise programs, 260
Conviction for drunkenness, 299
Coronary arterial system, 28-31
Coronary arteriography, 95-98, 170
Coronary artery bypass surgery, 20
Coronary artery disease, 18
Coronary atherosclerotic heart disease, 21, 97 (*see also* specific topics)
  autopsy study results, vii
  decline in mortality from, vii
  historical aspects of, 3-10
  incidence of, vii
Coronary care units, vii
Coronary collateral circulation, 29
Coronary lumen, 29
Coronary risk factors, viii, 299 (*see also* specific factors)
  booklet used in clinical practice, 131-133
  correlations with physical fitness levels, 62-63
  detection, 127-142
  effect of exercise on, 47-71

  exercise prescription, 134-141
  list of, 47
  methods of quantitating, 128-133
  modification, 233
  sedentary living, 27-46
Coumadin, 158
Couplets, 242-243
Current cardiac exercise programs in United States, 250-288 (*see also* specific states)
  map, 288
Cyanotic congenital heart disease, 123
Cycling, 135, 168, 226
Czechoslovakia cardiac rehabilitation, 316

D

Dairy farming, 36
Dangers of exercise, 215-224
  cardiac complications, 215-221
  noncardiac complications, 215, 221-223
Darts, 201
Death rate (*see* Mortality rate)
Declining vascular mortality, vii
  factors in, vii
Decreased pulmonary ventilation, 145
Deep vein thrombosis, 159
Delaware cardiac exercise programs, 261
Denmark cardiac rehabilitation, 316
Diabetes mellitus, 34, 123, 221, 228
Diabetic patients, 57
Diagnostic criteria, 100-102
Diastolic blood pressure, 18, 55-56, 63
Diet, 47-48, 58-59, 63
Dietary alterations, vii, 55
Dietary education programs, 36
Dietary fat intake, viii
Dietary interventions, 238-241
Dietary modifications, 227, 233
Digitalis, 101
Digitalis intoxication, 108
Digitalis therapy, 76
Discharge after myocardial infarction, early versus late, 144, 146-149
Dissecting aortic aneurysms, 123
District of Columbia cardiac exercise programs, 260
Dizziness, 75, 230
Dog mitochondria, 14-15
Double leg raising and lowering, 190
Drug therapy, 161, 298

Duration of exercise, 50-51, 62
Dynamic types of exercise, 11, 23
Dyspnea, 74-75, 299
Dysrhythmias, 150, 228
  screening for, 203

E

Ecchymoses, 221
Echocardiography, 107
Educational conferences, 233
Efficient types of exercise, 11
Elastic stockings, 158-159
Electrical instability, 245-246
Electrocardiographic abnormalities, 38, 47, 59-60, 63, 75
Electrocardiographic changes, 72, 170
Ellestad method of treadmill testing, 79-81
Emory University regimen, 150, 152-153
Enthusiasm for exercise, 27-28
Enzyme changes, 170
Epidemiology studies in man, 32-43
Episode hyperlactemia, 61
Eremitage Castle footrace, 27
Ergometer stress testing (*see* Bicycle ergometry)
Eskimos, 57
Exercise (*see also* specific topics)
  effect on coronary risk factors, 47-71
  goals, 11
  historical aspects, 3-10
  popularity, 3
  role of, viii
Exercise card for walk-jog, calisthenic and group activities, 175
Exercise dance routines, 244
Exercise-induced cardiac enlargement, 28
Exercise physiology, 11-26
Exercise prescription, 134-141, 233
Exercise programs, vii
Exercise stress testing, 20, 72-121
  bicycle ergometer, 72, 83-84
  cardiac rhythm disturbances, evaluation and detection of, 107-113
  diagnostic criteria, 100-102
  historical aspects, 72-73
  indications for use of, 114-115
  lead systems, 84-85
  Master 2-step, 72-74
  methods, 73-84

  predictive value of, 87-93
  prevalence of, 87-93
  prognostic value of, 94
  reasons for, 73
  recent advances in, 103-107
  risks of, 103
  sensitivity of, 93-100
  specificity of, 93-100
  target heart rates, 85-87
  treadmill, 72-83 (*see also* Treadmill testing)
Exercise test evaluation, 220
Exercise tolerance, 18
Exercise training
  contraindications to, 123
  guidelines to, 122-126
Exertional arrests, 226
External stress, 11

F

Faintness, 230
False negative, 93
False positive, 93, 95
False positive rate, 92-93
Familial tendencies, 221
Family history, 170
Fasting blood sugar, 63
Fatigue, 11, 74, 79, 217
  lessening of, 59
Fatty degeneration of heart, 3
Fibrinolysis, 60-61
Finland, 37, 289-297
Florida cardiac exercise programs, 261-262
Footrace, 27
Forced expiratory volume, 63
Framingham study, 37
Frank-Starling curve, 59
Frank-Starling mechanism, 16, 143
Free exercises, 51
Frequency of exercise, 51, 53-54

G

Gardening, 11
Georgia Baptist Hospital, 150-153, 159, 172-173, 175
  treadmill testing, 74-77
Georgia Baptist Medical Center, 245
Georgia cardiac exercise programs, 262-263

Glucose ingestion, 113
Glucose intolerance, 57
Glucose tolerance, 57
Glucose tolerance test, 63
Glycogen super-recompensation in heart, 16
Goals of exercise, 11
Golf, 202
Goteborg, Sweden, cardiac rehabilitation, 297-299
Goteborg, Sweden, study, 38, 112
Gout, 61, 221
Graded exercise, 17
Greece, 37
Group activities, 200-209
    removal from, 211
Group conferences, 151, 159-160
Gymnasium exercise program, 228-231

H

Handgrip exercise, 21
Hawaii cardiac exercise programs, 263
Health Insurance Plan (of New York) members, 34
Heart attack capital of world, 36
Heart/body ratios, 28
Heart diseased persons, exercise physiology in, 18-21
Heart failure, 228
Heart-monitoring instrument, 199-201
Heart muscle fibers, size of, 28
Heart rate, 12-13, 18, 22-23, 31, 145-146, 230, 232
Helsinki, Finland, cardiac rehabilitation, 289-297
Hemodynamic adjustment, 18
Hemodynamic assessment, 143
Hemodynamic benefits of training, 14
Hemodynamic changes, 49
Hemodynamic consequences, 23
Hemorrhage, 103
Heparin, 158
Hepatic blood flow, 19
Hepatic disorders, 123
Heredity, 47, 58-59, 63
High blood pressure, viii
High density lipoprotein (HDL) levels, 52-53
High risk population group, 78-79
    detection of, 218

High school athletes, 61
Hiking, 168
Historical aspects, 3-10
History of patient, 221, 228
Hohenried, Germany, cardiac rehabilitation center, 299-308
Home care, 144
Home exercise regimen, 161-163
    beginning two months post-coronary-incident, 172-173
    first three months post-coronary-incident, 172
Home walking program, 172
Horseback riding, 8
Hospitalization, 144
Household domestic chores, 11
Hypercholesterolemia, 38, 49-50, 298
Hyperlipemia, 61
Hyperlipidemias, 49
Hyperlipoproteinemia, 54, 98, 298
Hyperplasia, 28
Hypertension, 34, 38, 47-49, 55-56, 170, 221, 297-298
Hypertension registry, 36
Hypertensive persons, 56
Hypertrophy of myocardial cells and fibers, 28
Hypotension, 144
Hypoxemia, 15
Hypoxic air, 17

I

I-labeled Hippuran injection technique, 158
Idiopathic congestive cardiomyopathy, 21
Illinois cardiac exercise programs, 263-265
Immobilization, hazards of, 145
Impaired exercise tolerance, 145
Improved cardiac surgical techniques, vii
India cardiac rehabilitation, 315-316
Indiana cardiac exercise programs, 264-265
Indifference to exercise, 27-28
Individual patient and family conferences, 151, 159
Inferior infarction, 234
Inpatient activity regimen, 150, 153
Inpatient cardiac rehabilitation, results of, 163-165

Inspired air, measurement of, 8
Instant electrocardiograph rhythm strips, 230-234
Insulin requirements, 57
Insurance underwriters, 89
Intensity of exercise, 51, 53, 61
Intensive physical training, 14
Intermediate coronary care (ICC) unit, value of, 150
Intracellular edema, 15
Ischemic electrocardiographic changes, 16
Ischemic heart disease, 38, 75-78, 91
Isometric effect, 11
Isometric exercises, 21-23
Israel cardiac rehabilitation, 315
Italy, 37
Italy cardiac rehabilitation, 316

J

J-junctional changes, 100-101
Japan, 37
Jogger's heel, 221
Jogging, 11, 24, 32, 43, 135, 173, 209, 215-219, 223 (*see also* Walk-jog activities)
Jogging craze, 27

K

Kansas cardiac exercise programs, 265-266
Kentucky cardiac exercise programs, 266
Knee pushups, 195
Knee raising, 155, 180-181
The Kur, 310-311

L

Laceration, 222
Lactic acid, 31
Large coronary arteries, size of, 30
Lateral bending, 156, 182-183
Lawn bowling, 300
Lead systems in exercise testing, 84-85, 97
Leading threats to health and life in middle-aged man, 133
Lecithin cholestryl acyl transferase (LCAT), 53
Left ventricular aneurysm formation, 102
Left ventricular ejection time (LVET), 103-105

Left ventricular function, 18-20
Left ventricular hypertrophy, 59, 63, 101, 113
Left ventricular rupture, 19
Leg crossover, 192
Leg exercises, 21-22, 159 (*see also* specific types)
Leg raising, 188-190, 193-194
Leg rotation, 156
Leisure time activities, 38-39
Life expectancy of American men, vii
Life style changes, vii
Lipid abnormality, 298
Lipid profile, 229
Lipoprotein electrophoresis techniques, 49
London transport employees, 33
Longevity studies, 41, 43
Longshoremen, 37
Low density lipoprotein, 53
Low physical activity, 297-298
Lumberjacks, 36, 55
Lung scans, 158

M

Macromolecular synthesis, 15
Manual labor, 48
Marathon races and running, 4, 6, 32, 39, 59, 219
March fracture, 221
Marine corps recruits, 62
Marine corps trainees, 52
Maryland cardiac exercise programs, 266-267
Mass-participation sports, 27
Massachusetts cardiac exercise programs, 267
Master 2-step stress testing, 72-74, 79, 87-98
    costs compared with treadmill test costs, 83
Maximal heart rate (MHR) levels, 24
Maximal oxygen intake, 13-14, 17, 62
Maximum exercise tolerance, 31
Mayo Clinic experience, 170, 173-213
Mean peak heart rate, 79
Medications, 221
MET unit system, 134-135
    classification of activity by, 137
Metabolic alkalosis, 15

Metabolic disease, 123
Michigan cardiac exercise programs, 267-268
Microcirculation of cardiac muscle, 29
Middle-aged persons, 53-54, 133, 169
Mild strength-building activities, 168
Minidose subcutaneous heparin, 158
Minigolf, 300
Minnesota cardiac exercise programs, 268-269
Minnesota Multiphasic Personality Inventory (MMPI), 59
Missouri cardiac exercise programs, 269
Mitochondrial morphology, 31
Mitochondrial repair, 15
Mobilization, 144-145
    early versus late, 145-149, 159
Modified Balke-Ware treadmill test, 81
Morbidity rate, 103
Mortality rate, 33-34, 90, 103, 169, 171, 215, 225
Mowing grass, 11
Multiple discriminant analysis, 129
Mural thrombus formation, 143
Muscle blood flow, 19
Muscular exercise, 8
Muscular soreness, 221
Muscular strains, 222
Musculoskeletal injury, 222
Musculoskeletal problems, 123
Musculoskeletal strain, 11
Myocardial blood supply, improvement in, 20
Myocardial dysfunction, 20
Myocardial hypertrophy, 41
Myocardial infarction, 18, 29, 33-35, 38, 59, 79, 81, 87-89, 91, 98, 100, 169-170, 215-217, 296-297
Myocardial metabolism, 15
Myocardial mitochondria, 31
Myocardial oxygen consumption, 12-13
Myocardial performance and efficiency, 31
Myocardial perfusion scanning, 107
Myocardial revascularization, 221, 244-246
Myocardial rupture, 143
Myocardial stress perfusion scintigraphy, 107
Myocardial substrate uptake, 17

Myrtle Beach heart target rates, 85-86

N
National Exercise and Heart Disease Project (NEHDP) guidelines, 85-86
National Exercise and Heart Disease Project (NEHDP), 246-247
National Exercise Project treadmill test, 82-83
Near-syncope, 75
Negative studies, 51-52
Netherlands, 37
Neuropsychiatric disorders, 123
Nevada cardiac exercise programs, 274-275
New Jersey cardiac exercise programs, 269-270
New Mexico cardiac exercise programs, 270-271
New York cardiac exercise programs, 271-274
New Zealand cardiac rehabilitation, 316
Nicotinic acid, 298
Nitrates, 228
Noncardiac complications of exercise, 215, 221-223
Normal persons, exercise physiology in, 12-18
Normal postural vasomotor reflexes, loss of, 145
Normotensive persons, 56
North Carolina cardiac exercise programs, 275

O
Oarsmen, 35
Obesity (see Overweight)
Obstructive lung disease, 228
Ohio cardiac exercise programs, 275-277
Oklahoma cardiac exercise programs, 277
Oregon cardiac exercise programs, 277-278
Osteoarthritis, exacerbations of, 221
Outpatient exercise therapy, 168-214
Outpatient gym exercise program, 225-249
    data from, 234-238
Overexercise, 32, 218
Overweight, 17, 47, 57-58, 61, 63
Oxygen consumption, 20

Oxygen consumption improvement, 237
Oxygen consumption studies, 242, 244
Oxygen production, measurement of, 8

P

Pacemakers, 112-113, 123
Palpitations, 108, 230
Paradoxical cardiac pulsation, 296
Paroxysmal atrial tachycardia, 75, 79
Pathology studies, 39-42
Penetrating wounds, 222
Penile frostbite, 223
Pennsylvania cardiac exercise programs, 278-284
Peripheral vascular insufficiency, 113
Periodic exercise testing, 13
Personality patterns, 47, 58-59, 63
Petechiae, 221
Pharmacologist, 150
Phonocardiography, 106
Physical activity, significance of, 48
Physical inactivity, 38, 42, 47, 58, 63
Physical therapist, 150
Physical therapy, 159
Physical working capacity, 171, 290-293
Physically active occupations, 4, 8
Physician-supervised exercise regimen (beginning two months post-coronary-incident), 173-213
Physiological adaptation to exercise, 20
Pigs' hearts, 32
Ping pong, 201
Platelet aggregation, 16
Pool exercises, 200, 202-207 (*see also* Swimming)
Postcoronary rehabilitation studies, 41-43
Postinfarction rehabilitation (hospital phase), 143-167
Post-myocardial-infarction patients, 20-21
Posttraining bradycardia, 19
Postural hypotension, 75
Potassium content in heart cells, 15
Potassium levels, 15-16
Predictive value of exercise stress testing, 87-93
Predilection to coronary disease, 14
Predischarge and follow-up phase, 151, 159-160
Preejection period (PEP), 103-105
Premature myocardial infarctions, 48

Premature ventricular beats, 59-60, 75-76, 79, 108, 110-112, 242
Premature ventricular contractions, 63
Prerandomization exercise period (PREP), 246-247
Preventive cardiology, 127-142
  complete evaluation for, 127-128
  objectives of, 127
Preventive Cardiology Clinic, 127-142
Preventive therapy, 158
Previous exercise history, 221
Prinzmetal's angina, 113
Probability Tables of Deaths in the Next Ten Years from Specific Causes, 133
Proctoscopic examination, 133
Prognostic value of exercise stress testing, 94
Progressive exercise training, 13
Proper perspective, viii
Prospective studies, 36-39, 42
Prothrombin time, 60
Pseudogout, aggravation of, 222
Psychological testing, 159
Pulmonary blood flow, 17
Pulmonary blood volume, 17
Pulmonary dynamic changes, 17
Pulmonary emboli, 159
Pulmonary function, 229
Pulmonary function abnormalities, 47, 62-63
Pulmonary hypertension, 123
Pulmonary status, 17
Pulse rate
  measurement of, 8
  self determination of, 135
Punching bag, 169
Purpose of book, viii
Pushups, 195, 197

R

Radioactive potassium injections, 107
Radiotelemetry monitoring, 209
Railroad clerks, 33
Railroad men, 33-34
Railroad sectionmen, 33
Railroad switchmen, 55
Railroad workers, 58
Raking leaves, 11
Rapid muscle wasting, 145
Rat hearts, 15

Rate-pressure product, 19
Reach and touch, 157, 198
Recumbent position for cardiac patient, 143
Referral sheet, 150-151
Rehabilitation studies, 41-43
Reinfarction, 226
Relative risk, 92-93
Religious counseling, 159
Renal disorders, 123
Rescue units, vii
Respiratory rate, measurements of, 8
Respiratory stroke volume, measurement of, 8
Resuscitation equipment, 174, 201
Retrospective studies, 32-36, 42
Reverse pushups, 197
Rhythmic endurance exercises, 168
Risks of exercise stress testing, 103
Rocking situps, 191
Rope skipping, 135
Rowing, 8, 168
Rubidium-81, 107
Running, 52, 168, 216, 219, 226, 300
Russian cardiac rehabilitation, 314

S

San Francisco longshoremen, 37
Saturated fats
    dietary levels of, 48
    intake of, 297
    limited dietary intake of, vii
Screening of patients, importance of, 218
Seattle Heart Watch Project, 89
Sedentary bus drivers, 33
Sedentary living, 27-46
Sedentary occupations, 8, 38
Sedentary subjects, 14-15
Sensitivity of exercise stress testing, 93-100
Serum cholesterol (*see* Cholesterol)
Serum triglycerides (*see* Triglycerides)
Serum uric acid levels, 61-62
Seven Countries Study, 37-38, 48, 55, 58, 89-90
Sexual activity, 59, 159-160
Sexual tension, 59
Sheffield target heart rates, 85-86
Side leg raises, 154, 193

Silent complete occlusions of major coronary vessel, 39
Silent coronary heart disease, 169
Singapore cardiac rehabilitation, 315
Sitting position for cardiac patient, 143
Skeletal muscle oxygen deficiency, 17
Ski race, 27
Skiing, 50, 52
Sleep patterns, 59
Sleeping ability, improvement in, 59
Small jumps, 186-187
Smoking, 297-299 (*see also* Cigarette smoking)
    prohibition of, 36
    reduction in, vii
Soft tissue injury, 222
Spangler-Fox method of treadmill testing, 78-80
Specificity of exercise stress testing, 93-100
Spirometry, 229
Sportsmen, 56
Sprained fingers, 221-222
Sprinting, 11
Squirrel cage treadmill, 7
S-T segment changes, 79-81, 102, 229
S-T segment depression, 73, 75-76, 78-79, 81, 85, 87, 89-91, 97, 100-102, 113, 168, 231
    screening for, 203, 209
S-T segment responses, 96-98
Stationary bicycle exercises, 51
Step tests, 5
Stepping wheel, 7
Stepwise regression analysis, 291, 293
Stool guaiac sampling, 133
Stress electrocardiograms, 107
Stress relationships, 59
Stress scans, 107
Stress testing (*see* Exercise stress testing)
Strict bed rest period, 143
Stroke volume, 14, 18-19, 31, 145-146
Subcutaneous fat loss, 58
Subendocardial infarction, 234
Sudden death, 9, 91, 112, 215, 219-220
Sudden vigorous exercise, 16
Superprecipitation of actomyosin, 15
Supine exercise, 145
Supraventricular arrhythmias, 75
Supraventricular rhythm disorders, 123

Supraventricular tachyarrhythmias, 108
Supraventricular tachycardia, 76
Sweden cardiac rehabilitation, 315
Swimming, 8, 11, 15, 50, 52, 135, 168-169, 173, 200, 218, 244, 300
Swiss cardiac rehabilitation, 315
Symptom-linked peak oxygen uptake, recording of, 202-203
Syncope, 75
Systemic arterial hypertension, 123
Systolic blood pressure, 12-13, 18, 38, 55-56, 63, 75, 299
Systolic time intervals, recording of, 103-105

T

T-wave abnormalities, 76
T-wave changes, 59-60
Tachyarrhythmia, 76
Tachycardia, 15, 75
Tagged on fibrinogen scanning technique, 158
Target heart rates, 85-87
Tennessee cardiac exercise programs, 284-285
Tennis, resurgence of, 27
Tension time index, 18
Testing the individual, 5
Texas cardiac exercise programs, 285
Thallium-201, 107
Thromboembolic vascular disease, 16
Thrombophlebitis, 123
Thrombosis formation, 159
Thrombosis prevention, 61
Thyroid disorders, 123
Tobacco consumption, health hazards of, vii (*see also* Cigarette smoking; Smoking)
Toe touching, 178-179
Tolerance for a workload, 161
Total energy expenditure, 55
Toxemias of pregnancy, 123
Track exercises, 201, 209
Transient ventricular tachycardia, 79
Treading the wheel, 7
Treadmill exercises, 8, 13, 29, 60
Treadmill studies, 16, 32
Treadmill testing, 5, 20, 29, 72-84, 88, 91, 96-99, 146, 172, 202, 228-229

Bruce method, 77-78
costs compared with step test costs, 83
Ellestad method, 79-81
Georgia Baptist Hospital, 74-77
modified Balke-Ware method, 81
National Exercise Project, 82-83
Spangler-Fox method, 78-79
USAFSAM, 82
Treadmills, 7-8
Trigeminy, 108
Triglycerides, 38, 49-50, 53-55, 63, 171
elevation of, 298
True negative, 93
True positive, 93
Trunk twisting, 157, 196
Twelve-lead systems, 84
Two- to three-vessel coronary disease, 100-101

U

Uncompensated congestive failure, 169
Uncomplicated patient defined, 148-149
United States, 37
Urate excretion, 61
Uric acid levels, 61
USAFSAM treadmill test, 82
Utah cardiac exercise programs, 285

V

Valvular disease, 169
Vasa cross-country ski race, 27
Vector lead systems, 84
Venous occlusion plethysmography, 158
Venous thrombosis, 158
Ventilation, 62
Ventricular aneurysm, 19, 123
Ventricular ectopic beats, 112
Ventricular ectopy, 60, 231, 242, 245
Ventricular fibrillation, 81, 103, 152, 220, 232, 245-246
Ventricular rhythm disorders, 123
Ventricular tachycardia, 209, 231
Vibrating table exercises, 51
Virginia cardiac exercise programs, 285-286
Vital capacity, 63
Vital capacity changes, 62
Volleyball, 168-169, 200, 202, 209, 217, 222, 242, 244

W

Walk-jog activities, 199-200, 209-211, 220, 225, 231, 242 (*see also* Jogging; Walking)
Walk tests, 5
Walking, 4, 135, 297
 brisk, 11
Wall-tennis, 201, 208
Warfarin, 159
Warm-up period in exercise, 16-17, 124
Washington cardiac exercise programs, 286
Weekend activity, 38-39
Weight-independent changes due to exercise, 50

Weight lifting, 52, 168
Weight loss, 58, 171
West Germany cardiac rehabilitation
 diagnostic center, 312-313
 private facility, 312-313
 sophisticated Kur, 312-313
 status, 309-314
Wisconsin cardiac exercise programs, 286-287
Women, 51, 101
Work classification scheme, 11, 13
Work load, 62

Y

Yugoslavia, 37

NAME INDEX

A

Abelmann, W. H., 145, 165
Abraham, A. S., 148, 166
Adam, C., 46
Adams, C. W., 9
Adams, John Quincy, 27
Adams, W. C., 20, 26
Addison, 3
Adgey, A. A. J., 166
Albrink, M. J., 68
Aldinger, E. E., 44
Aleen, C., 116
Alexander, E. R., 67
Alexander, J. K., 9
Allen, W., 115
Alvaro, A. B., 121
Anderson, L. F., 68
Aravanis, C., 67
Arcos, J. C., 44, 218, 224
Argus, M. F., 224
Armstrong, Neil, 27
Armstrong, R., 25, 68, 248
Aronov, D. M., 317
Aronow, W. S., 91, 94, 106, 117, 119-121
Astrand, P. O., 72, 83, 115-116
Astrup, T., 60, 70
Atkins, J. M., 25
Attar, O. A., 121
Auchincloss, J. H., 20-21, 26

B

Baekeland, F., 69
Bahl, O. P., 119
Bailey, I. K., 120
Balasubramanian, V., 70
Balke, B., 24, 84, 116, 203
Banister, E. W., 31, 43
Barach, A. L., 62, 71
Barbarin, P., 66
Barnard, R. J., 16, 25
Bass, N. M., 166
Beard, E. F., 89, 94, 117

Belknap, E. L., 66
Bellet, S., 91, 94, 117
Benade, A. V. S., 116
Benchimol, A., 106, 120
Bergman, H., 25, 67
Bergstrom, K., 20, 26
Berkson, D., 50, 65
Berkson, D. M., 64, 67
Bernauer, E. M., 26
Beuresy, J., 119
Beyer, J., viii
Bhan, A., 25
Biern, R. O., 117
Billings, F. T., 65
Bjernulf, A., 26, 317
Blackburn, H., 45, 118-119, 165, 220, 224
Blackburn, H. W., 60, 67, 69, 89, 94, 117, 166
Blackman, J. R., 67, 115
Bloch, Antoine, 147-148, 166, 315
Block, W. D., 64
Blomqvist, G., 25, 65, 165
Bloor, C. M., 28, 43-44
Blotner, H., 57, 68
Boberg, J., 317
Bogard, D. L., 67
Bohannon, R. L., 116
Boileau, R. A., 69
Bonchek, L. I., 119
Borer, J. S., 98, 118
Bosco, J. S., 70
Bowerman, W., 68, 216, 221, 224
Bowman, J. L., 26
Boyer, John L., 56, 68, 172, 214, 248
Brakman, P., 60, 70
Braunwald, E., 24
Brensike, J. F., 118
Brest, A. N., 116
Brody, A. J., 87, 94, 117
Brown, D. L., 165
Browse, N. L., 158, 166
Brozek, J., 45

Bruce, E. H., 171, 203, 214, 225, 248
Bruce, R. A., 67, 77-78, 84, 89, 94, 116-117, 171, 203, 214, 225, 248
Bruhn, J. G., 69
Brumbach, W. B., 52, 66
Brunner, E., 43-44
Bryson, A. L., 119
Bulkley, B. H., 46
Burch, G. E., 224
Burke, G. E., 117
Burt, J. J., 30, 44, 60, 69
Buskirk, E. R., 69
Buzina, R., 70
Bygdemon, S., 21-22, 26

C

Cady, L. D., 66
Cake, D., 120
Calvy, G. L., 62, 66
Campbell, D. E., 50, 65
Cantwell, J. D., 27, 64, 104-105, 110, 120, 164, 167, 173, 221, 224, 235, 237, 243, 248-249, 315
Carson, P., 314, 317
Carson, P. H. M., 166
Cary, Bruno, 136
Cassidy, J., 120
Castelli, W. P., 67, 69
Celander, D. R., 70
Chahine, R. A., 102, 119
Chailley-Bert, 50, 65
Chaniotis, L., 213
Chapman, C. B., 9, 24
Chaturvedi, N. C., 166
Chave, S. P. W., 46
Cheitlin, M. D., 119-120
Chiang, B. N., 55, 67, 69
Choquette, G., 213
Chung, A., 25
Cicero, 3, 9
Clancy, R. E., 64
Clausen, J. P., 18, 26, 56, 65, 70, 214
Cobb, F. R., 29, 44
Coe, W. S., 165
Cohen, H., 54, 67
Cohen, H. L., 224
Cohen, P. F., 73-74, 96, 99, 102, 115
Cohn, K., 118, 120
Cohn, P. F., 119, 129, 131
Cohne, M. V., 119

Colvard, M. D., 69
Conner, W. T., 166
Cooksey, J. D., 119
Cooper, J. A., 150, 166
Cooper, K. H., 71, 81, 116
Cooper, M. N., 117
Corrigan, T., 167
Crawford, 39
Cubitt, William, 7
Cullen, K. G., 69
Cumber, W., 69
Cumming, G. R., 85, 101, 116, 118
Cunningham, D. A., 317
Cureton, T. K., 68
Currens, J. H., 9, 46
Cvorkov, N., 43

D

Dalderup, L. M., 65
Dalvl, C. P., 317
Daniel, B. J., 51, 53, 65
Danlievicious, Z., 70
Datey, K. K., 317
Davia, J. E., 119
Davids, D. J., 45
Davidson, P. C., 57, 68
Davies, C. T. M., 17, 25
Dawber, T. R., 64, 70
Dayton, S., 219, 224
Debacker, G. D., 314, 317
de Castro, C. M., 119
Demany, 99
DeMar, Clarence, 32, 39-40, 46
De Marion, A. N., 166
DeMots, H., 102, 119
Depew, Chauncey, 3
Deporter, A. M., 317
Derick, C. L., 68
De Sanctis, R., 166
Detry, J. M. R., 19, 26, 103, 119
Dimond, E. G., 106, 120
Doan, A. E., 67, 115
Dodge, H. T., 119
Dolder, M. A., 64
Doll, E., 17, 25
Donoso, S., viii
Doyle, J. T., 64, 67, 88, 94, 117
Dufresne, C., 118
Dunbar, S. A., 25

E

Easton, J., 3, 9
Eckstein, Richard W., 29-30, 44
Edgill, M., 70
Egeberg, O., 70
Ellestad, M. H., 79-80, 84, 115, 118
Elmfeldt, D., 214, 248, 317
Enos, W. F., viii
Epstein, F. H., 69
Epstein, S. E., 70, 85, 116, 118
Erikson, U., 26
Evans, A., 166

F

Fabre-Chevalier, 65
Falls, H. B., 11-12, 24
Fareeduddin, K., 145, 165
Farhi, A., 65
Fariss, B. L., 44
Feifar, Z., 317
Feigenbaum, H., 120
Feil, H., 72, 115
Feleki, V., 44
Ferguson, J. H., 70
Ferguson, R. J., 213
Firstbrook, J. B., 67
Fisch, C., 101, 118
Fisher, L. D., 248
Fitzgibbon, 99
Fletcher, G. F., 24, 115, 164, 167, 224, 235, 237, 243, 248-249
Floyd, W. L., 120
Fortuin, N. J., 97, 118
Foss, M. L., 64
Fox, S. M., III, 9, 32, 44, 56, 68, 82-83, 116, 136, 215, 224
Frank, C. W., 42, 45
Franks, B. Don, 66
Frederick, R., 214, 248
Frederick, R. C., 224
Fredrickson, D. S., 64
Frence, G. N., 24
Frick, M. H., 14, 18, 24-25, 57, 68, 213, 248
Friedan, J., 150, 166
Friedman, E. H., 69, 160, 167
Friedman, M., 59, 64
Friesinger, G. C., 97, 118
Froberg, S., 317
Froelicher, V. F., 32, 43-44

Froelicher, V. F., Jr., 82, 84-85, 91, 93, 101, 116-117
Frye, R. L., 248
Fullerton, H. W., 60, 70

G

Garcia, E., 117, 119
Garrard, C. L., Jr., 119
Garrett, H. L., 65
Garrison, G. E., 120
Gastineau, C. F., 68
Gershengorn, K. M., 120
Gertler, M. M., 66
Gey, G. O., 117
Gilbert, C. A., 26
Gilbert, C. G., 104-105, 120
Gilbert, R., 26
Gima, A. S., 45
Godfrey, S., 25
Goldbarg, A. W., 116
Goldberg, C., 67
Goldhammer, S., 72, 115
Golding, L. A., 50, 65
Goldschlager, N., 100-101, 118, 120
Gollnick, P. D., 49, 64
Gooch, A. S., 108, 120
Goode, R. C., 67
Gordon, B., 68
Gordon, T., 67, 69
Gorlin, R., 118-119
Gorman, P., 249
Goss, F. A., 65
Gottheiner, V., 42, 46, 168, 213, 248
Greenleaf, J. E., 70
Gregoratos, G., 64
Griffith, L. S. C., 120
Grimby, G., 25, 248
Grossman, J., 166
Guest, M. M., 70
Gulbrandsen, C. L., 66
Gustufson, A., 298, 317

H

Haissly, J-C., 166
Hakkila, J., 43
Halhuber, M. J., 301, 317
Hames, C. G., 16, 25, 42, 45, 64
Hamilton, M., 166
Hanafee, W. N., 213
Handley, A. J., 158, 167

Harpur, J. E., 166
Harris, C. N., 119, 121
Harris, W. E., 61, 68, 216, 221, 224
Harris, W. S., 119
Haskell, William L., 116, 215, 220, 224,
    226, 248, 250
Heady, J. A., 44, 46, 69
Hellerstein, H. K., 42, 46, 58-59, 65, 69,
    82, 84, 116, 160, 165, 167-169, 203,
    213-214, 248
Herman, M. V., 119
Hershkowitz, M., 224
Hirsch, E. Z., 69
Hodge, M. F., 67
Hofer, V., 115
Hoffman, A. A., 54, 65
Holloszy, J. O., 31, 44, 52-53, 66, 68
Holmes, R. H., viii
Holroyd, A. M., 166
Hood, W. B., Jr., 44
Horman, M. J., 115
Hornstein, T. R., 115-116
Horstman, D. H., 69
Horwitz, L. D., 16, 25
Hosmer, D., 116
Houk, P., 25, 67
Howard, G. E., 70
Hughes, J. L., 166
Huhti, E., 166
Hultgren, 99
Hunder, G. G., 224
Hurych, J., 17, 25
Hutchins, G. M., 40, 46
Hutter, A. M., 147, 166

I

Iatridis, S. G., 70
Ibsen, H., 167
Ishimori, T., 119
Ismail, A. H., 59, 69

J

Jackson, R., 30, 44
James, Curtis, 34
Jandova, R., 318
Jefferson, Thomas, 3, 27
Jelliffe, R. W., 117
Jenzer, H. R., 26
Jessop, W. J., 64

Jeyasingh, K., 166
Johnson, T. F., 50, 65
Johnston, B. L., 164, 167
Jones, K. W., 64
Jones, W. B., 118
Jorgensen, C. R., 117

K

Kagan, A., 44, 66
Kakkar, V. V., 167
Kang, B. S., 55, 67
Kannel, William B., 37, 42, 45, 64, 69
Kansal, S., 119
Kaplan, M. A., 121
Kaplinsky, E., 30, 44
Karava, R., 68
Karvonen, M. J., 50, 55, 65, 67
Karvonen, M. W., 66
Kasch, F. W., 56, 68
Kassebaum, 99
Katayama, F., 317
Katila, M., 25, 57, 68, 248
Kattus, A. A., 89, 94, 117, 121
Kattus, A. A., Jr., 170, 213
Kavanagh, T., 121, 314, 317
Kaye, R. L., 70
Keiser, N., 116
Keller, J. B., 67
Kellerman, J. J., 315, 317
Kemp, H. G., 118
Kennedy, C. C., 170, 213, 226, 248
Kentala, E., 57, 68, 170-171, 213, 289, 292,
    297, 317
Keul, J., 17, 25
Keys, A., 42, 44-45, 64, 67, 69-70, 117, 131
Khanna, P. K., 70
Kinch, S. H., 88, 117
Kirchheiner, B., 318
Kjoller, E., 167
Klein, G. J., 120
Klein, H., 66
Klepetar, E., 44
Knoebel, S. B., 118
Kobernick, S. D., 49, 64
Konttinen, A., 24, 51, 53, 66, 67
Korge, P., 15, 25
Kostuk, W. J., 120
Krzywanek, H. J., 67
Kuller, L., 219, 224
Kusumi, F., 116

L

Laird, J., 166
Lampman, R. M., 54, 67
Lamus, J. G., 118
Lancaster, M. C., 116
Larse, N. O. A., 65, 70, 214
Larsen, O. Andree, 44, 68, 70
Lategola, M. T., 68-69
Laughlin, M. E., 45
Leaf, Alexander, 41, 43, 46
Lees, R. S., 64
Lefcoe, N. M., 71
Leon, A. S., 28, 43-44
Levine, S. A., 57, 68, 145, 165
Levy, R. I., 64
Lewis, S., 66
Lewis, W. J., 96, 99, 118
Libignette, P., 65
Lichty, J. A., 45
Likar, I., 116-117
Likoff, W., 69, 99
Lind, A. R., 26
Lindberg, H. A., 64, 67
Lindsay, M. I., Jr., 248
Lindsey, M. I., 213
Linhart, J. W., 101, 118-119
Lintgen, A. B., 119, 220, 224
Logan, James, 9
Lohrbauer, L. A., 26
Longmire, W. P., Jr., 213
Lown, B., 19, 26, 145, 165
Lynch, J. D., 118

M

Maca, R. D., 25
MacAlpin, R., 25
MacAlpin, R. N., 121
MacDonald, G. A., 60, 70
MacMahon, B., 45
Makin, G. S., 166
Malder, J-P., 166
Malmborg, R. D., 68, 70
Malmborg, R. O., 44
Mankin, H. T., 248
Mann, G. V., 50, 56-57, 61, 64-65
Marks, H. H., 90, 94, 117
Martin, C. M., 96, 99, 118, 120
Martin, N. D., 120
Martin, R. L., 71
Mason, D. T., 16, 69

Mason, J. K., viii
Mason, R. E., 84-85, 99, 116-117
Masso, R., 25
Master, A. M., 72, 115
Mather, H. G., 165
Mattingly, T. W., 87, 94, 117
Maurer, B., 167
Mayer, Jean, 58, 68
Mayes, F. B., 166
McCallister, B. D., 118, 248
McCarthy, B., 44
McConahay, D. R., 95-96, 99, 104, 118, 120
McCoy, J., 68
McDonough, J. R., 45, 64
McFadden, R. B., 68, 224
McHenry, M. M., 26
McHenry, P. L., 96, 99, 101, 118
McNeer, J. F., 148, 166
McPherson, B. D., 69
McRitchie, R. J., 16, 25
Mead, W. F., 220, 224
Mellerowicz, H., 56, 68
Mengeot, P., 119
Metivier, J. G., 51, 66
Metzner, H. L., 67
Meyknecht, E. A., 65
Miall, W. E., 55, 67
Miller, S. W., 115
Miner, M. M., 46
Mirkin, G., 52, 66
Mitchell, H. J., 13, 24
Mitchell, J., 26
Mitchell, J. H., 25, 65, 165
Mohiuddin, S. M., 118
Monroe, R. G., 12, 24
Monson, R. R., 45
Montoye, H. J., 55, 61, 64, 67, 70
Morgan, C. M., 248
Morris, J. N., 38-39, 42, 44, 46, 55, 67, 69
Morris, Jerry, 33
Morse, D., 120
Mortimer, E. A., Jr., 45
Morton, W. E., 45
Most, A. S., 97, 99, 115, 118
Mouratoff, G. J., 68
Moyer, J. G., 69
Moyer, J. H., 116
Mufson, M. A., 66
Murray, H., 65

Murray, J. A., 113, 121
Myasnikov, A. L., 49, 64
Myron, B. R., 119

N
Nasrallah, A., 119
Naughton, John P., 18, 25, 41, 56, 58-59, 68-69, 82, 104-105, 116, 119, 248-249
Nelson, W. R., 58, 65, 68
Neophytou, M., 317
Niawayama, G., 64
Nichols, G. J., 117
Nierman, J., 66
Nikkila, E. A., 53, 67
Noguera, I., 116
Nutter, P. O., 26
Nye, E. R., 316-317

O
Oberman, A., 44, 121
Ogirimah, A. M., 314, 317
Oilinki, O., 166
Oks, M., 25
Oldham, P. D., 55, 67
Oliver, M. F., 64
Olson, H. W., 52, 66
Opie, L. H., 219, 224
Oppenheimer, E. T., 72, 115
Orgain, E. S., 120
Orma, S., 67
Oscai, L. B., 53, 67
Ostadal, B., 43-44
Ostrander, L. D., 69
Ostrander, L. D., Jr., 64

P
Paffenbarger, R. S., 37, 42, 45
Page, Irvine, 127
Paige, Satchel, 27-28
Paivio, A. U., 46, 213, 248
Paivo, A., 69
Pandit, V., 317
Parisi, A. F., 119
Parker, B. M., 119
Parker, D. P., 119, 121
Parmley, L. F., 9, 224
Pasyk, S., 43
Paterson, N. A. M., 71
Patterson, J. A., 67
Pattison, D. C., 44

Pearlman, D., 44
Pearson, N. G., 165
Pedersen-Bjergoord, O. P., 318
Penpargkul, S., 25, 44
Perlman, L. V., 69
Peterson, D. R., 67, 115
Peterson, K., 120
Petty, T. L., 62, 71
Phillips, L., 51, 65, 118
Pickard, H. A., 46, 68, 70, 213, 248
Pillow, C., 117
Pohndorf, R. H., 51, 66
Polednak, A. P., 35, 42, 45
Pollock, M. L., 51, 53, 65, 71, 84, 116
Pomeroy, W. C., 34, 42, 45
Pouget, J. M., 104-105, 119
Poulsen, W. T., 317
Poupa, O., 29, 43-44
Proudfit, W. L., 121
Prout, C., 35, 42, 45
Punsar, S., 68
Pyfer, H. R., 224
Pyorala, K., 60, 68

R
Raab, W., 67
Raffle, P. A., 44
Raffle, P. A. B., 46, 69
Raizner, A. E., 119
Rakusan, K., 43-44
Rantaharun, P. M., 67
Read, K. L. Q., 165
Rechnitzer, P. A., 42, 46, 62, 68, 70, 169, 213, 248, 317
Rechnitzer, R., 44
Redwood, D. R., 70, 85, 116, 118
Reeves, T. J., 116, 118
Ressel, J., 316, 318
Reynell, P. C., 150, 166
Rhoads, G. G., 66
Rich, A., 64
Riley, C. P., 121
Rios, J., 249
Robb, G. P., 90, 94, 117
Robinson, B. F., 13, 24
Rochelle, R., 66
Rochelle, R. H., 50, 65
Rochmis, P., 119, 220, 224
Rodahl, K., 115-116
Roitman, D., 97, 99, 116, 118-119

Roman, L. R., 117
Romanova, D., 66
Ronleau, J., 120
Roosson, S., 25
Rosch, J., 119
Rose, Geoffrey, 67, 145, 147, 149-150, 165
Rose, K. D., 16, 25
Rosenbaum, F. F., 66
Rosengarten, D. S., 166
Rosenman, R. H., 64
Rosing, D. R., 70
Roskamm, H., 310-311, 313
Rotman, M., 69
Rousseau, M., 26
Rousseau, M. F., 119
Rubin, I. L., 166
Ruby, R. L., 44
Rulli, Vincenzo, 316
Ruskin, J., 69

S

Salcedo, D., viii
Salel, 132
Saltin, B., 25, 145, 165
Samios, R., 316, 318
Sammon, J., 118
Sanne, H., 214, 248
Santinga, J. T., 67
Sarajas, H. S., 24
Sarnoff, S. J., 12, 24
Satinsky, J. D., 118
Schechter, E., 119
Schelbert, H., 120
Scherf, D., 72, 115
Scheuer, J., 15, 25, 44
Schnohr, P., 35, 42, 45
Schoenfeld, C. D., 119
Scott, E. M., 68
Segel, L. D., 16, 25
Seltzer, F., 90, 117
Selzer, A., 118
Seth, H. N., 70
Sever, Y., 166
Shaffer, R. D., 64
Shames, D. M., 120
Shanbour, K., 25, 68, 248
Shane, S. R., 68
Shaper, A. G., 64
Shapiro, S., 45
Shaw, L. W., 249

Sheffield, L. T., 23, 85, 116, 118-119, 121
Shepard, R. V., 116
Shephard, R. H., 317
Shephard, R. J., 64, 67, 219, 224
Shillingford, J., 167
Shine, K. I., 166
Shkhvatsabaya, L. K., 317
Sidel, V. W., 166
Siegel, I. M., 224
Siegel, M. L., 72, 115
Siegel, W., 21, 25-26, 50, 54, 65, 121
Siltanen, Heikki, 36
Simpson, M. T., 16, 25
Simpson, T., 317
Singer, E., 112, 120
Sketch, M. H., 101, 118
Skinner, J. S., 9, 44, 52, 56, 66, 68
Smith, E., 115
Smith, Edward, 7-10, 73
Smith, R. E., 118
Smith, W. G., 69
Sohal, R. S., 44, 224
Song, S. J., 67
Spangler, R. D., 78, 115
Spann, J. F., Jr., 69
Spiekerman, R. E., 213, 248
Spindler, J., 167
Sproule, B. J., 24
Stamler, J., 42, 64, 67
Stanek, J., 25
Steele, Richard, 3
Stevenson, J. A. F., 30, 44
Stocksmeier, V. U., 301, 317
Stokes, 3
Stolz, I., 318
Straus, R., 64
Strauss, H. W., 120
Strauss, M., 9
Stuart, R. J., Jr., 118
Stubb, S. C., 45, 64
Stvinick, E. H., 120
Styperek, J., 160, 167
Suh, C. S., 67
Sun, S. C., 44, 224
Swan, H. J. C., 166
Swenson, E. W., 52, 66

T

Takkunen, J., 146, 166
Taylor, H. L., 42, 44-45, 55, 67, 69, 117

Taylor, Henry, 33
Taylor, J., 249
Tepperman, J., 30, 44
Thilenius, Ed, 320
Thomas, M. M., 117
Thompson, A. J., 117
Thompson, A. J., Jr., 116
Thompson, P. L., 19, 26
Thorburn, I. O., 69
Tibblin, G., 38, 45, 248, 299, 317
Timaeus, 3
Tomanek, R. J., 29, 43-44
Toto, G., 66
Trachtman, L. E., 59, 69
Trap-Jensen, J., 26, 65, 70, 214
Trombold, J. C., 224
Trulson, M. F., 64
Tsuji, J., 120
Tucker, H., 317
Tucker, H. H., 146, 166
Turnoff, H. B., 119

U

Ursick, J. A., 25
Uyeyama, R. R., 120

V

Vandenbrouche, G., 26
Van Fossan, D. D., 24
Varewijck, E., 317
Varnauskas, E., 18, 25, 67
Vatner, S. F., 25, 224
Vedin, J. A., 112, 120
Viel, B., viii
Vismara, L. A., 150, 166
Vokonas, P. S., 115, 119
Voogd, N. de, 65

W

Wagner, G. S., 166
Wahren, J., 21-22, 26
Walker, W. J., viii, 64
Wallace, A. G., 166
Walsh, M. J., 166
Wan, M. C., 115

Wan, M. K. C., 80, 115
Ware, K., 116
Warnock, N. H., 60, 70
Watson, S., 316, 318
Watt, E. W., 50, 64, 248
Wedel, H., 248
Weinblatt, E., 45
Weinstein, M., 166
Weissler, A. M., 103, 119
Welch, G. F., Jr., 24
Wells, J. G., 13, 24
Wenger, N. K., 144, 165-166
Wenger, Nanette, 250
Werko, L., 42, 45, 317
White, Paul Dudley, 4-5, 9, 34, 42, 45-46,
    72
Whitsett, T. L., 104-105, 119
Widimsky, J., 318
Wiley, J., 248
Wilhelmsen, Lars, 45, 120, 214, 226-227,
    248, 297, 299, 317
Wilhelmsson, C. E., 120
Willems, P., 317
Wilson, W. J., 96, 118
Winifred, M. B., 317
Wolfeth, C. C., 87, 116
Wollenberger, A., 14, 25
Wolthius, R., 116-117
Wood, J. H., 70
Wood, P. C., 87, 116
Wood, P. D., 52, 66
Worden, R. E., 117
Wray, R., 158, 167
Wyatt, H. L., 20, 26

Y

Yuhasz, M. S., 68-70, 317

Z

Zaret, B. L., 107, 120
Zauner, C. W., 52, 66
Zelis, R. F., 69
Zuehlewski, A. C., 64
Zukel, 42